P9-CFT-134

Evidence-Based NURSING

The Research–Practice Connection

Sarah Jo Brown, PhD, RN

Consultant
Practice–Research Integrations
Norwich, Vermont

JONES & BARTLETT
LEARNING

World Headquarters
Jones & Bartlett Learning
5 Wall Street
Burlington, MA 01803
978-443-5000
info@jblearning.com
www.jblearning.com

Jones & Bartlett Learning books and products are available through most bookstores and online booksellers. To contact Jones & Bartlett Learning directly, call 800-832-0034, fax 978-443-8000, or visit our website, www.jblearning.com.

Substantial discounts on bulk quantities of Jones & Bartlett Learning publications are available to corporations, professional associations, and other qualified organizations. For details and specific discount information, contact the special sales department at Jones & Bartlett Learning via the above contact information or send an email to specialsales@jblearning.com.

Copyright © 2014 by Jones & Bartlett Learning, LLC, an Ascend Learning Company

All rights reserved. No part of the material protected by this copyright may be reproduced or utilized in any form, electronic or mechanical, including photocopying, recording, or by any information storage and retrieval system, without written permission from the copyright owner.

Evidence-Based Nursing: The Research–Practice Connection, Third Edition is an independent publication and has not been authorized, sponsored, or otherwise approved by the owners of the trademarks or service marks referenced in this product.

Some images in this book feature models. These models do not necessarily endorse, represent, or participate in the activities represented in the images.

The author, editor, and publisher have made every effort to provide accurate information. However, they are not responsible for errors, omissions, or for any outcomes related to the use of the contents of this book and take no responsibility for the use of the products and procedures described. Treatments and side effects described in this book may not be applicable to all people; likewise, some people may require a dose or experience a side effect that is not described herein. Drugs and medical devices are discussed that may have limited availability controlled by the Food and Drug Administration (FDA) for use only in a research study or clinical trial. Research, clinical practice, and government regulations often change the accepted standard in this field. When consideration is being given to use of any drug in the clinical setting, the health care provider or reader is responsible for determining FDA status of the drug, reading the package insert, and reviewing prescribing information for the most up-to-date recommendations on dose, precautions, and contraindications, and determining the appropriate usage for the product. This is especially important in the case of drugs that are new or seldom used.

Production Credits
Executive Publisher: Kevin Sullivan
Acquisitions Editor: Amanda Harvey
Editorial Assistant: Sara Bempkins
Associate Production Editor: Sara Fowles
Marketing Communications Manager: Katie Hennessy
V.P., Manufacturing and Inventory Control: Therese Connell
Composition: Paw Print Media
Cover Design: Theresa Day
Cover Image: © Ensuper/ShutterStock, Inc.
Printing and Binding: Edwards Brothers Malloy
Cover Printing: Edwards Brothers Malloy

To order this product, use ISBN: 978-1-4496-9749-5

Library of Congress Cataloging-in-Publication Data
Brown, Sarah Jo.
Evidence-based nursing : the research-practice connection / Sarah Jo Brown.
-- 3rd ed.
p. ; cm.
Includes bibliographical references and index.
ISBN 978-1-4496-9099-1 (pbk.)
I. Title.
[DNLM: 1. Evidence-Based Nursing. 2. Nursing Research. WY 100.7]
610.73--dc23
2012025528

6048

Printed in the United States of America
17 16 15 14 13 10 9 8 7 6 5 4 3

Contents

	Lead-In	xi
	Contributor	xiv
PART I	**NURSING RESEARCH**	**1**
Chapter 1	**The Research–Practice Connection**	**5**
	Research to Practice	5
	Evidence	6
	Evidence-Based Clinical Protocols	6
	Evidence-Based Care	7
	Short History of Evidence-Based Nursing Practice	11
	Your Path to Evidence-Based Practice	12
	References	14
Chapter 2	**Research Evidence**	**15**
	Types of Research Evidence	15
	Findings from an Original Study	16
	Conclusions of a Systematic Review	20
	Recommendations of an Evidence-Based Clinical Practice Guideline	22
	Going Forward	24
	References	24

Chapter 3	**Reading Research Articles**	**25**
	Starting Point	26
	Format of Study Reports	27
	Reading Approach	34
	Wading In	35
	References	36
Chapter 4	**Qualitative Research**	**37**
	Data Collection and Analysis	38
	Qualitative Description	41
	Uniqueness of Qualitative Studies	42
	Exemplar	43
	Profile and Commentary	61
	References	65
Chapter 5	**Descriptive Research**	**67**
	Natural Conditions	67
	Study Variables	68
	Target Population and Sampling	75
	Results	83
	Exemplar	84
	Profile & Commentary	103
	References	110
Chapter 6	**Correlation Research**	**111**
	Relationship	111
	Measuring Relationship	112
	Correlational Design	122
	Exemplar	123
	Profile & Commentary	136
	References	143

Chapter 7 **Experimental Research** **145**

Chapter Layout 145

Section 1: Understanding Experimental Methods 146
Key Features of Experimental Studies 146
Limitations of Randomized Experiments 157
Quasi-Experimental Designs 157
Exemplar 159
Profile & Commentary: Introduction and Methods 173

Section 2: Understanding Study Results 176
Was One Intervention More Effective Than the Others? 176
Exemplar 188
Profile & Commentary: Results and Discussion 188
References 192

Chapter 8 **Cohort Research** **193**

Cohort Studies 193
Case-Control Studies 195
Wrap-Up 197
Exemplar 197
Profile & Commentary 206
Discussion 212
References 212

Chapter 9 **Systematic Reviews** **213**

Types of Systematic Reviews 214
The IRR Production Process 216
Use of IRRs 224
Exemplar 224
Profile & Commentary 248
References 250

Chapter 10 Evidence-Based Clinical Practice Guidelines 251
Forerunners to Clinical Protocols 251
EbCPG Production Process 253
Formats 259
Comorbidity 261
Exemplar 261
Profile & Commentary 274
Wrap-Up 276
References 276

PART II EVIDENCE-BASED PRACTICE 279
The Evidence-Based Practice Impact Model 281
References 283

Chapter 11 Asking Clinical Questions 285
Triggers 285
Questions Not Answerable by Research Evidence 287
Forming a Useful Project Question 288
References 292

Chapter 12 Searching for Research Evidence 293
Ellen F. Hall
Searching for EbCPGs and SRs 293
Sources of EbCPGs and SRs 294
Searching Databases 298
A Final Word and a Few Tips 308
References 309

Chapter 13 Appraising Research Evidence 311
Appraisal Systems 312
Appraisal in General 312
Synopsis 313

Credibility 313
Clinical Significance 315
Applicability 316
Practical Considerations 318
Reference 319

Chapter 14 Appraising Recommendations of Clinical Practice Guidelines 321
AGREE and GRADE 322
An Appraisal Guide for Use by the Nurse with a BSN 322
Your Turn 326
References 327

Chapter 15 Appraising Conclusions of Integrative Research Reviews 329
Synopsis 330
Credibility 330
Clinical Significance 331
Applicability 332
Your Turn 332
References 333

Chapter 16 Appraising Findings of Original Studies 335
Broad Credibility Issues 336
Appraisal of the Findings of a Qualitative Study 338
Appraisal of the Findings of a Quantitative Study 339
Clinical Significance 342
Applicability 342
Your Turn 343
Across-Studies Analysis 343
Wrap-Up 346
References 347

Chapter 17 Evidence-Based Practice 349

Professional Action 349
Evidence-Based Care Design 350
Prespecification: Evidence-Based Care Protocols 352
Point-of-Care Design: Individualized Care 353
Goal: Quality Care 354
EBP Projects 360
Organizational Integration of EBP 366
Research–Practice Lag 368
Recap 369
References 370

Chapter 18 Evidence-Based Practice Participation Scenarios 375

Join a Project Team 375
Make a Poster 376
Present an Idea or Concern 377
Contribute to a Patient Care Conference 379
Build Your EBP Knowledge and Skills 380
References 381

Chapter 19 Research-Informed Practice 383

RIP Opportunities 385
The Information Intersection 386
Point-of-Care Formats Resources 387
Clinical Decision Support 391
My Ending—Your Beginning 392
References 393

Appendix A Appraisal Guide: Recommendations of a Clinical Practice Guideline 395

Appendix B Completed Appraisal: Recommendations of a Clinical Practice Guideline 399

Appendix C Appraisal Guide: Conclusions of an Integrative Research Review 405

Appendix D Completed Appraisal: Conclusions of an Integrative Research Review 409

Appendix E Appraisal Guide: Findings of a Qualitative Study 415

Appendix F Appraisal Guide: Findings of a Quantitative Study 419

Appendix G Completed Appraisal: Findings of a Quantitative Study 423

Appendix H Completed Findings Table 429

Appendix I List of Evidence-Based, Point-of-Care, Summary Resources 433

Glossary 435

Index 447

Lead-In

"Evidence is stronger than argument."
—*from* The Celebrity
by Winston Churchill, 1897

In our modern world, opinions abound. However, when much is at stake, it is essential to get beyond opinion to reliable knowledge and information. That is the case with the health care given to patients. And that is why all the healthcare professions are committed to evidence-based practice.

Evidence-based practice involves seeking out and incorporating into care the most reliable sources of evidence available—and knowledge produced by research is one of those. Scientific knowledge is reliable because it is (1) methodically developed and (2) open to review by all interested parties.

A body of scientific knowledge about a particular issue is built over many years. One study examines *this* aspect of an issue; another study examines *that* aspect. Some studies are conducted because the researcher wants to better understand an aspect of existing knowledge that was not fully explored by earlier studies. Other studies are conducted to challenge the findings of an earlier study. In a sense, all studies build on the findings of earlier studies in some way. Gradually, like a jigsaw puzzle, the picture gets put together.

The fact that reports of studies are published in professional journals or reported at professional meetings makes science self-correcting. Open reporting allows colleagues to consider and challenge the claims of a study. In the years to come, they then conduct studies under similar or slightly different circumstances to verify, refute, fine tune, or add to the knowledge claim of the earlier study. This continuous tweaking and adding to earlier knowledge claims leads us to say that science is accretive, meaning that it grows over time like . . . the picture of a jigsaw puzzle.

In nursing, we have an ever-increasing body of research-derived knowledge to use in designing care for populations of patients and for individual patients. Nursing departments and agencies use research-derived knowledge when developing clinical protocols and standards of care. At the point of care, individuals seek out research-derived knowledge to guide them when they are confronted with situations in which routine knowledge is insufficient.

Importantly, scientifically based care has the highest likelihood of producing optimal patient outcomes. To contribute to and give scientifically based care, the 21st-century nurse must be able to read research reports and decide whether and how to use research evidence in clinical decision making and care planning. This book is offered to assist nursing students in acquiring the knowledge required to engage in evidence-based practice, which includes basic knowledge about research methods and knowledge about how to incorporate credible research evidence into practice.

Features of Note

- *Companion website:* I call your attention to the companion website for this book, which is available at ***go.jblearning.com/brown3e***. Formatted by chapter, the site offers interactive study guides, supplementary papers, references for additional reading, and links to interesting information.
- *Easy-to-read text.* Students, some of whom admitted to dreading their research course, have told me that they found this text easy to read and understand—even interesting. I hope you will find it so.
- *Incorporation of statistical tests:* You will note that there is not a chapter about statistics; instead specific statistical tests and interpretation of their results are incorporated into the chapters about the different types of research. This enables statistical tests and results to be explained in the research context in which they most often are used. The index indicates the page(s) on which each statistic is discussed.

- *Changing gender references:* As with all texts that include examples with unknown persons, there is the old she-he/her-him conundrum. There are various ways to deal with it, but I have chosen to sometimes refer to the nurse as *she* accompanied by the possessive *her* when needed. Other times I refer to the nurse as *he* accompanied by the possessive *his* when needed.

This Edition

Because certain areas of the field of evidence-based practice (EBP) are changing rapidly, this edition followed the previous more quickly than a new edition might have in another field. In particular, there is new information in the following areas:

- Evidence-based practice as a component of the safety and quality movement.
- Research examining implementation of evidence-based changes in practice; i.e., translational research.
- Standards for producing clinical practice guidelines and systematic reviews.
- Evidence formatted for point-of-care reference.

To reflect these trends, changes and additions have been made throughout this edition and on the website.

Sarah Jo Brown, PhD, RN

Contributor

Chapter 12: Searching for Research Evidence

Ellen F. Hall, MALS, AHIP
Library Director Emerita and Professor
Norwich University
Northfield, Vermont

PART I

Nursing Research

1 The Research–Practice Connection

2 Research Evidence

3 Reading Research Articles

4 Qualitative Research

5 Descriptive Research

6 Correlation Research

7 Experimental Research

8 Cohort Research

9 Systematic Reviews

10 Evidence-Based Clinical Practice Guidelines

The level of knowledge required to understand research reports published in clinical journals is somewhat akin to being a savvy computer user. To be a competent computer user, you do not have to understand binary arithmetic, circuitry, program architecture, or how central processing units work. You just need to know some basic computer language and be familiar with the features of the hardware and software programs you use.

Similarly, as a professional nurse in clinical care, you do not need to know all the different ways of obtaining samples, how to choose an appropriate research design, or how to decide on the best statistical test. But you do need to know the basics of how various types of research are conducted and what results mean. You also need to know how good data are obtained and how incorrect conclusions are avoided.

The goal of the first part of the book is to introduce you to research methods and different kinds of research evidence. To accomplish this, seven research articles have been reprinted in full. I chose this learning strategy because I have found that explaining research methods by pointing them out in an actual study is more vivid than explanations without an example at hand.

Importantly, a grasp of the basics of research methodology lays the groundwork for evidence-based practice. For readers who like to know where their learning will take them, an overview of the book's learning progression is graphically displayed in **Figure PI-1**. The main learning goals are in the diamonds on the left side. More specific learning issues associated with each goal are shown to the right.

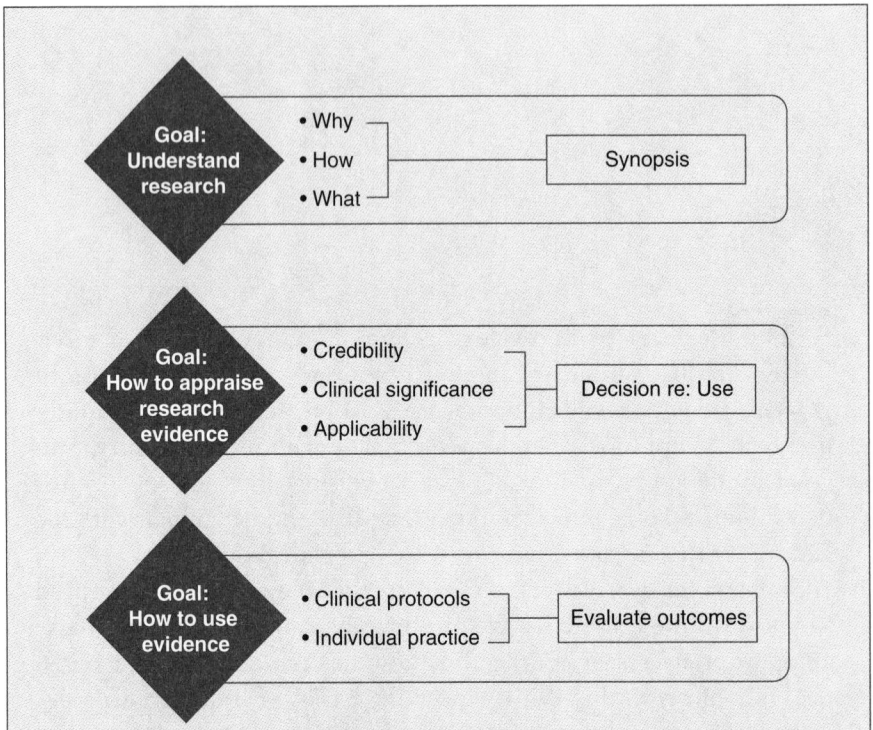

Figure PI-1 Overview of the Book's Learning Progression

CHAPTER ONE

The Research–Practice Connection

Effective nursing practice requires knowledge, information, judgment, skills, caring, and art. This book is about the knowledge component—more specifically, about knowledge used to make decisions regarding the care patients should receive. An important part of the knowledge used in making decisions about care is produced by research. Ideally, all key decisions about how patients are cared for should be based on research evidence (Institute of Medicine, 2001). Although this is not a completely attainable goal, large bodies of healthcare research provide considerable guidance for the design of nursing care.

Research to Practice

The findings of a research study are raw materials, like petroleum and iron ore that must undergo transformations to become everyday products such as gasoline and steel. Similarly, research findings undergo several transformations before they become the basis for clinical protocols that guide clinicians' decisions and actions. The path from researchers conducting studies to clinicians giving care based on what has been learned from research is a long one with many transformations—which you will learn about in detail in later chapters.

Evidence

To produce effective and useful clinical protocols, research evidence must be used in combination with other sources of information. Thus, when developing nursing protocols, project teams actually use several different sources of evidence, including the following:

- Research findings
- Agency quality monitoring data
- Data from national databases
- Expert opinion
- Scientific principles

There is wide agreement among healthcare providers that research evidence is the most trustworthy source of evidence and that clinical protocols should be based on it to the extent possible. However, when research evidence is not available or does not sufficiently address the clinical issue, the other forms of evidence come into play. In recognition of the fact that multiple sources of knowledge and information are used to develop clinical protocols, they are commonly called *evidence-based* protocols—as opposed to calling them research-based protocols. Thus, from here forward I will use the descriptor *evidence-based* to describe protocols and practice that rest to a large degree on research evidence.

Having said this, the focus of the book is on research evidence. The fact that this book focuses on research evidence is not meant to devalue the other forms of evidence; rather, a focus on research evidence allows a close consideration of this very important source of information for clinical practice.

Evidence-Based Clinical Protocols

Clinical protocols are standards of care in that they define care that should be given to patients who are part of a defined population. (A population is a group of patients who have the same health condition, problem, or treatment. A population can be defined broadly, for example, persons having surgery; or narrowly, as elderly persons having hip replacement surgery.) Some clinical protocols set forth a comprehensive plan of care for the specified population, for example, perioperative and postoperative care of elderly persons having hip surgery, whereas others address just one aspect of care such as body temperature maintenance in the elderly having hip surgery. Still others are even narrower and could be called a clinical procedure, for example, blood salvage and transfusion during hip surgery. Generally, multidisciplinary groups produce protocols that address many aspects of care, whereas nursing staffs produce protocols that address clinical issues that nurses manage.

Clinical protocols can be set forth in various formats: plans of care, standard order sets, clinical pathways, care algorithms, decision trees, care bundles —all are guides for clinicians regarding specific actions that should be taken on behalf of patients in the specified population. An appropriate committee or authority in the agency, nursing department, or clinical service line endorses each clinical protocol.

In short, clinical protocols are tools for achieving consistent, high-level care; they set forth clear standards of care for a defined patient population by specifying the care actions that should be performed.

Evidence-Based Care

When research findings are used to develop a protocol and the protocol is followed in daily practice, everyone involved (patients, healthcare professionals, the agency, third-party payers, and accrediting agencies) can be confident that patients in that population are receiving nursing care that is based on the best available scientific evidence.

The protocol approach to care design and delivery is in contrast to each nurse deciding what care she or he will give to patients—an approach to caregiving that often results in considerable variability in care because of omissions and differing opinions regarding the best method of care. Evidence-based protocols are increasingly being used as standards of care and being integrated into computerized clinical information systems.

Using Clinical Protocols

In any care agency, there is not a care protocol for every patient population and every care situation. Agencies develop protocols to promote effective clinical management and to reduce variability in the care of their high-volume and high-risk patient groups. If a protocol exists, it should be followed unless there is a good reason for not following it. Generally, following scientifically based protocols is in the best interest of patients because doing so increases the likelihood that patients will achieve good outcomes. This is the case because the recommended actions have been scientifically studied, and people with expertise in the field have considered their application.

Protocols Are Not Recipes Protocols should be adhered to when they exist, but they should not be blindly followed. Nurses are patient advocates and as such look out for patients' welfare; this requires that nurses be constantly aware of patients' responses to protocols. If a nurse observes that a protocol is not producing good results with a patient, she should discuss this with a nurse leader and decide if a different approach to care should be used. A protocol may be evidence based and it may work well for most patients, but it may not be right for every patient.

Consider this scenario: Suppose you are providing care to a patient who had a cervical fusion and recognize that he does not seem as comfortable as he should be even though the pain protocol is being followed. This recognition should cause you to ask yourself questions such as, "Why isn't he getting good pain relief? Should we be doing something different?" The advisable course of action would be to talk with a nurse leader so as to get better pain relief for the patient.

If, however, you notice the same problem with two or three similar patients, you would have cause to wonder if some aspect of the protocol is not effective. You would then look into when the protocol was written and on what evidence it was based. If further investigation reveals recent research literature indicating that a different positioning approach is helpful or a different medication dosing schedule is more effective for this population, you should bring this information to the attention of your nurse manager or the quality improvement council for your unit.

Even when a protocol is being carried out and is effective for most patients, there are still many aspects of care that nurses do at their discretion. Some of these discretionary acts are nursing art—that is, personal style, whereas others are actions taken to fulfill a protocol's recommendations. For example, a protocol regarding fall prevention required assessing newly admitted elderly patients for orthostatic hypotension. However, the protocol did not spell out exactly how to do this assessment. The staff nurse asked an advanced practice nurse, who told her about a research article comparing four procedures for evaluating positional/orthostatic blood pressure changes (Guss, Abdelnur, & Hemingway, 2008). The article reported that arm positions while supine and upright affect the blood pressure values obtained; therefore arm position should be held constant from measurement to measurement. Thus, the gap in the protocol's recommendation could be filled by a research-informed decision made by the individual nurse. The take-away message is that care protocols are not detailed recipes for care; rather, they are guides to care that should be followed in conjunction with patient preference, attentive observation, clinical judgment, and additional research information.

Protocols ≠ Recipes

As a Student

At this point in your career, as a student nurse with placements in several hospitals, clinics, and agencies, you will find that some clinical settings have care protocols that clearly are based on research evidence, whereas others have care protocols, but their rationale is not clear. You might wonder: Do the required actions represent the opinions of nurses on a practice committee? Were they based on an article someone read in a professional journal? Did the chief doctor on that service stipulate how things should be done? Did the salesperson for a piece of medical equipment recommend the care actions? As a person who will enact the protocol, you have a right to information about its basis, and for that reason clinical protocols are more frequently being written in ways that provide a description of the amount of research support for the recommended actions and/or references of supporting research articles.

As a Staff Nurse

After you start to work as a professional nurse, you may be asked to participate in a project to develop or update a care protocol or procedure. Often, your agency will be adapting an evidence-based guideline that was issued by a professional association, leading healthcare system, or government organization. Other times, an evidence-based guideline will not be available, but a research summary relative to the clinical issue has been published, and its conclusions will be used in developing the protocol. To contribute to a protocol project, you will need to know how to read and understand research articles published in professional nursing journals and on trustworthy healthcare Internet sites.

Let us assume that you are working in a well-baby clinic and are asked to be a member of a work group revising the protocol for preventing and managing diaper dermatitis in infants. You may be asked to read, appraise, and report to the group about an evidence-based clinical guideline produced by a nursing specialty association. To fulfill this assignment, you should be able to formulate a reasonably informed opinion as to the extent to which the guideline recommendations are evidence based and were produced in a sound manner. If the recommendations are deemed credible, then the work group will rely heavily on them while developing their protocol.

Another scenario could be that you read in the specialty journal for your area of practice a research report about an effective way of managing fever in young children. You note that the recommended sequence of actions is different from that used in the clinic where you work. You look in a nursing database and find a research summary article about the issue that brings together the findings from six studies. It offers conclusions about the temperature level at which antipyretic drugs should be given that are different from the standard of care in your clinic. You and your colleagues now have an opportunity to improve the care you give by designing care that is based on nursing research.

GUIDELINE: A set of recommendations for the care of a patient population that is issued by a professional association, leading healthcare center, or government organization. Guidelines are not agency specific.

PROTOCOL: A set of care actions for a patient population that has been endorsed by the hospital, agency, clinic, or healthcare facility. Protocols are agency specific.

Regardless of whether you come to question the effectiveness of the care being provided through clinical observation, by reading a research article in your professional journal, or by learning of a possibly better way at a conference, the next step is to act on your insight. Talk with your nurse manager, nurse leader, or a member of your unit's quality council. From this discussion, you will learn how the protocol came to be as it is and stimulate dialogue regarding its effectiveness.

Short History of Evidence-Based Nursing Practice

The nursing profession—*discipline* to use the more academic term—has been conducting scientific research since the 1920s, when case studies were first published, and calls for research about nursing practice were first issued in the *American Journal of Nursing*. Now, nursing research is being conducted in countries around the world, and reports of clinical research studies are published in research journals and clinical journals in many languages. In many countries, nursing research is funded by the government, and over 30 countries have doctoral programs in nursing. The growing cadre of nurses with doctoral degrees has propelled both the quantity and quality of clinical nursing research being conducted. In the United States, the National Institute of Nursing Research (www.ninr.nih.gov), a component of the National Institutes of Health, is a major source of funding for nursing research. Many other countries have similar organizations.

In the mid-1970s, visionary nurse leaders realized that even though clinical research was producing new knowledge indicating which nursing methods were effective and which were not, practicing nurses were not aware of the research. As a result, several projects were started to increase the utilization of research-supported actions by practicing nurses. These projects gathered together the research that had been conducted on issues such as preoperative teaching, constipation in nursing home residents, management of urinary drainage systems, and preventing decubitus ulcers. Studies were critiqued, evidence-based guidelines were developed, and considerable attention was paid to how the guidelines were introduced into nursing departments (Horsley, Crane, & Bingle, 1978; Krueger, Nelson, & Wolanin, 1978). These projects stimulated interest in the use of nursing research in practice throughout the United States; at the same time, nurses in other countries were also coming to the same recognition. By the 1980s and 1990s, many research utilization projects using diverse approaches to making nurses aware of research findings were under way.

During this time, interest in using research findings in practice was also proceeding in medicine. In the United Kingdom, the Cochrane Collaboration at Oxford University was formed in 1992 to conduct rigorous research summaries with the goal of making it easier for clinicians to learn what various studies found regarding the effectiveness of particular healthcare interventions. At the McMaster Medical School in Montreal, Canada, a faculty group started the evidence-based practice movement. This movement brought to the forefront the responsibility of the individual clinicians to seek out the best evidence available when making clinical decisions in everyday practice. The evidence-based practice (EBP) movement in medicine flowed over into nursing and reenergized the use of research by nurses.

Three other things were happening in the late 1990s and early 2000s:

- Considerably more clinical nursing research was being conducted.
- The EBP movement was proceeding in a somewhat multidisciplinary way.
- National governments in the United States, United Kingdom, Canada, and many other countries funded efforts to promote the translation of research into practice.

Today, high-quality evidence-based clinical practice guidelines and research summaries are being produced by healthcare organizations around the world, and nursing staffs are increasingly developing agency clinical protocols based on those guidelines and summaries. Also, individual clinicians are increasingly seeking out the best available evidence to use as a guide for the care they provide to patients.

The most recent development is a new area of research called implementation research or translational research. These studies examine how to implement evidence-based changes in practice so the changes become part of routine care and bring about good patient outcomes. That's all I will say about this new area of study for now—more in Chapter 17.

Your Path to Evidence-Based Practice

This book and your classroom experiences should help you acquire a solid base of research knowledge to launch you into becoming a 21st-century professional nurse. I want to emphasize that the point of this book and of the course you are taking is not to make you into a nurse researcher, but rather to help you be an informed consumer of nursing research.

Clearly, there is a lot for you to learn. As you read this book, you will learn how to do the following:

- Get comfortable reading research articles
- Locate evidence-based guidelines and research summaries
- Develop basic skills in judging whether a clinical practice guideline or research summary was soundly produced
- Decide if the research evidence available is strong enough to use as a basis for nursing care
- Participate in the development and implementation of evidence-based protocols in the agency, unit, or clinic in which you work

The research articles you will be reading in Part I were published in clinical journals, not research journals. They were written for clinicians; thus they emphasize the clinical implications of the findings, not the fine points of research methodology. In Part I your goal in reading the reports is to grasp *why* the study was done, *how* it was done, and *what* was found.

Because the book is a primer, only the most widely used and important types of research are presented. Also, the information provided is selective, which means that it is not a comprehensive reference source regarding research methodology. It does not delve deeply into methodological issues; it does not explain all research designs, methods, and statistics. However, it does provide an introduction to methodological issues that must be appreciated to understand most nursing research reports.

In Part II you will learn about using research evidence in nursing practice. You will revisit the studies you read in Part I, learn to critically appraise their soundness, and consider their applicability to a particular setting You will also learn about how to use research evidence in your own individual clinical practice. I call individual use of research evidence *research-informed practice*. Most often, individual practice is *informed* by research, not solidly *based* on it.

Evidence-based practice is designed by clinical project teams.
Research-informed practice is engaged in by individual clinicians.

Assumptions About You, the Learner

The exploration of evidence-based nursing in this book assumes that you (1) have had an introduction to statistics; (2) have some experience in clinical settings; and (3) are committed to excellence in your professional practice. Becoming a nurse who contributes to evidence-based quality improvement on your unit or in your agency requires that you be an active learner by developing the following professional habits:

- Questioning what you see in practice
- Seeking additional knowledge when care protocols seem less than effective
- Reading research articles in clinical journals
- Thinking about the application of new knowledge to your practice

- Participating in evidence-based quality improvement projects on your unit or in your agency
- Adopting evidence-based protocols when they are introduced into your work setting

Other Learning Resources

In reading this book, and indeed in your later reading of research articles, you may want to have a statistics book handy to look up statistical terms and tests you have forgotten or never learned. Your statistics text need not be new. Earlier editions are often available very inexpensively—and statistics do not change much from edition to edition. Do make sure you use a basic book, not an advanced one written for researchers. If in doubt, ask your instructor for a suggestion.

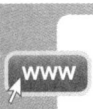

For a full suite of learning activities and resources, use the access code located in the front of your book to visit this exclusive website: http://go.jblearning.com/brown3e. If you do not have an access code, you can obtain one at the site.

References

Guss, D. A., Abdelnur, D., & Hemingway, T. J. (2008). The impact of arm position on the measurement of orthostatic blood pressure. *Journal of Emergency Medicine, 34*(4), 377–382.

Horsley, J. A., Crane, J., & Bingle, J. (1978). Research utilization as an organizational process. *Journal of Nursing Administration, 8*, 4–6.

Institute of Medicine. (2001). *Crossing the quality chasm: A new health system for the 21st century.* Washington, DC: National Academy of Sciences. Retrieved from http://www.nap.edu/html/quality_chasm/reportbrief.pdf

International Network for Doctoral Education in Nursing (2012). Directory of International Doctoral Programs. Retrieved from: http://nursing.jhu.edu/academics/programs/doctoral/phd/inden/programs.html

Krueger, J. C., Nelson, A. H., & Wolanin, M. O. (1978). *Nursing research: Development, collaboration, and utilization.* Germantown, MD: Aspen.

CHAPTER TWO

Research Evidence

In Chapter 1, reference was made to research evidence, but it was not explained in full. That needs to be done. As a student new to the science of nursing, when mention is made of research evidence, you will naturally think of the findings of a scientific study. However, as you proceed through this course, you will come to see that research evidence can take several forms, namely:

- Findings from a single, original study
- Conclusions from a summary of several (or many) original studies
- Research-based recommendations of a clinical practice guideline

Types of Research Evidence

Building Knowledge

A finding of a single original study is the most basic form of research evidence. Most studies produce several findings, but each finding should be considered as a separate piece of evidence because one finding may be well supported by the study whereas another finding may be on shaky ground. Although a finding from an original study is the basic building block of scientific knowledge, knowledge is really more like a structure made up of many different kinds of blocks (see **Figure 2-1**).

Findings from many soundly conducted studies are necessary to build a reliable body of clinical knowledge regarding an issue. Insistence on confirmation of a finding from more than one study ensures that a knowledge

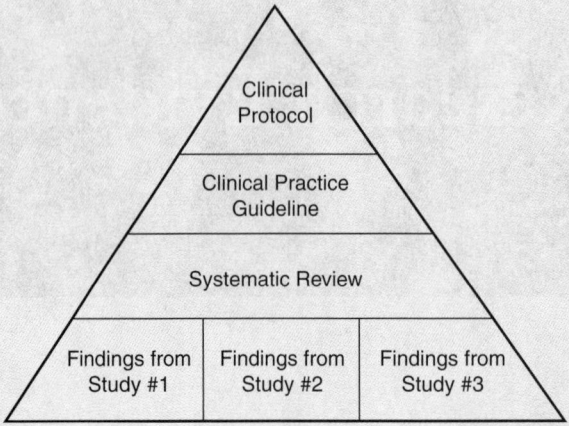

Figure 2-1 Building Knowledge for Clinical Practice

claim (or assertion) is not just a fluke unique to the patients, setting, or research methods of one study. If a finding is confirmed in several different studies, clinicians have confidence in that knowledge because it held up across diverse settings, research methods, patient participants, and clinician participants.

There are several recognized ways of combining findings from two or more studies; as a group these methods are called systematic reviews. Conclusions from systematic reviews may then be translated into evidence-based recommendations by expert panels. A group of e-b recommendations is called an evidence-based clinical practice guideline. Although evidence-based recommendations are not technically research evidence, if they were directly derived from research findings and summaries, they are considered so for practical purposes. In this chapter, each of these forms of research evidence is introduced briefly in turn. Later in the book, each is considered in depth.

Findings from an Original Study

Most people think of a research study as involving (1) a large number of subjects who are (2) randomly assigned to be in one of several intervention groups; (3) research environments that are tightly controlled; and (4) data that are meticulously obtained and then analyzed using statistics to produce results. In fact, research using these methods is common and valuable; however, it is only one type of scientific study—there are many other kinds. The most common way of thinking about research methods is to categorize them as qualitative and quantitative.

Qualitative Research

Qualitative research methods collect data in the form of what people say, observations of events, and written material. The data are not quantified by scales or number values; rather verbal descriptions that convey the meanings in the data are constructed. The goal of qualitative research is understanding—not counting, averaging, or quantifying in any way.

Qualitative research is used to study what it is like to have a certain health problem or healthcare experience such as being a physically disabled parent or recovery after a major head injury. Qualitative research methods are also used to study social settings, social interaction, and social processes. The following are examples of situations a nurse researcher might study using qualitative methods:

1. The interpersonal support dynamics at a social center for persons with chronic mental illness (a subculture setting)
2. How intensive care unit (ICU) staff members interact with family members of unconscious patients (social interaction)
3. How a family who has entered a family weight loss program makes changes in eating and physical activity over time (social process)

These kinds of social situations are typically tangles of issues, forces, perceptions, values, expectations, and aims. They can be understood and sorted out best by a researcher embedding herself in the situation and using methods of inquiry that will get at participants' perceptions, feelings, daily thoughts, beliefs, expectations, and behavior patterns. Data collection methods such as in-depth conversations, diary keeping, extensive interviewing, extended observation, and focus groups are used to acquire insights regarding these subjective realities. The data are analyzed in ways that preserve the life meanings of the stories and comments the participants offer. Qualitative research is described in more depth in Chapter 4.

Quantitative Research

Quantitative research methods are also used to examine how the world works. However, numerical measurement is used to explore and confirm the level at which the phenomena are present and the nature of relationships among them. I realize I introduced a new word in that last sentence, so a bit of a diversion is needed because the word is used in research articles. The word *phenomena* (the plural word) is used throughout the research world as a catchall phrase to describe the realities that exist in a field of study. The phenomena of interest in nursing can be grouped into five categories (adapted from Kim, 2000). The categories and examples of phenomena within each are:

1. The client as a person (motivation, anxiety, hope, exercise level, and adherence to treatments)
2. The client's environment (social support, financial resources, and peer group values)
3. Nursing practice (risk assessment for skin breakdown, patient teaching, and wound care)
4. The nurse–patient relationship and communication (person-centered talk, participative decision making)
5. The healthcare system (access to health care, quality of care, cost)

In brief, nursing phenomena are personal, social, physical, and system realities that exist or occur within the realm with which nursing is concerned. When phenomena are examined in a quantitative research study, they are called the research variables.

Getting back to types of research, exploring the nature of phenomena can be done using qualitative research methods. However, the workings of many phenomena can be explored more extensively when the phenomenon is measured quantitatively. For instance, body temperature could be described using the qualitative words *cool, warm*, and *hot*, but using the quantitative standard of thermometer degrees is a more precise way of conveying and tracking body temperature.

Moreover, quantifying phenomena allows exploration of how a change in one relates to a change in another, as when the relationship between body temperature and white blood count is analyzed using a correlation statistic. Quantitative methods are also used to test how well a nursing intervention works compared to another intervention. In intervention studies, the outcomes expected to be produced by the intervention are carefully measured in each patient participant and a determination is made regarding how many participants in each intervention group attained the outcomes of interest.

Study Purpose and Study Method

The researcher's decision to use either a qualitative method or a quantitative method is determined by the nature of the question. As just described, qualitative methods yield better understanding for some types of research questions, whereas quantitative methods provide better answers to other questions. Together, qualitative and quantitative methods serve a range of purposes:

- Understand a health, illness, or healthcare experience (e.g., How do 18–20-year-old, black women view mammography?)
- Develop a theory about responses to an illness condition (e.g., a theory about determinants of exercise in urban-dwelling adolescents)
- Describe a health-related situation (e.g., mother–infant interaction)
- Measure the strength of relationships between several health-related phenomena (e.g., hours worked outside the home and mother fatigue)
- Test a hypothesis about the effectiveness of an intervention (e.g., A smoking cessation program delivered to small groups of sixth graders by a school nurse will result in a lower level of smokers in 3 years than will an interactive computer program delivered and evaluated in the same time frame.)

Generally, each of these purposes requires a different research strategy and approach, although researchers sometimes use qualitative and quantitative methods in combination with one another. Using mixed methods may produce a more complete portrayal of an issue than can one method alone. For instance, researchers used mixed methods to identify health concerns in an African American community; they conducted focus groups and analyzed the results of a community health survey. They concluded that "Although quantitative approaches yield concrete evidence of community needs, qualitative approaches provide a context for how these issues can be addressed" (Weathers et al., 2011, p. 2087).

Qualitative research methods are generally inductive, meaning researchers produce findings by working from particular observations to groupings of observations, to general statements. Qualitative researchers have strategies and plans before they enter the settings in which they will make observations and inquiries, but they are also flexible to revise their investigative approach and to follow leads that arise.

In contrast, quantitative researchers tend to have specific research questions and choose a research design that will produce answers to those questions. A research design is a framework or general guide regarding how to structure studies conducted to answer a certain type of research question. The four quantitative research designs used most often in nursing research are:

1. Descriptive designs
2. Correlation designs
3. Experimental designs
4. Quasi-experimental designs (Burns & Grove, 2009)

You will be learning about each of these.

Researchers choose the design that will provide the best approach to their research question or purpose and that is feasible given the resources available. Using the design features as a template, they develop a detailed study plan that spells out specifically how their study will be conducted. A study plan includes the following:

- The theoretical framework that will be used (if any)
- Sites and settings that will be involved
- How the sample will be obtained
- Ethical protections that will be put in place
- Information that will be provided to participants
- Design of the interventions (if any)
- Measuring instruments that will be used
- The sequence of study activities
- Data collection procedures
- How unwanted influences will be controlled
- How data analysis will be performed

In summary, the two major categories of research methods used in clinical nursing studies are qualitative and quantitative. Both methodological approaches are needed to develop the full range of knowledge needed by clinical nurses.

Conclusions of a Systematic Review

Systematic reviews are an important and useful form of research evidence. A systematic review is a research summary that produces conclusions by bringing together and integrating the findings from all available original studies. The integration of findings from several or many studies can be done using tables and logical reasoning and/or with statistics. The cumulative findings are formulated as new knowledge claims, which are unifications of the separate findings of the original studies. The methods for accomplishing the unification are widely agreed upon and serve to reduce bias resulting from the process used to summarize the findings.

Systematic reviews, when well done, bring to light trends and nuances regarding the clinical issue that are not evident in the findings of individual studies. I suggest that now you take a look at an abstract of a systematic review. I suggest this because reading and using the conclusions of systematic reviews is one of the destinations on your learning path, and looking at one will give you a sense of this important learning destination.

1. Go to the CINAHL database in your library's website or go online to PubMed (http://www.ncbi.nlm.nih.gov/pubmed). PubMed is a free, online database of healthcare articles.
2. Type the following text in the search box: "facilitated tucking Obeidat, 2009" and click on the *Search* button. (Facilitated tucking involves holding or swaddling an infant so his arms and legs are slightly flexed and close to his body.)
3. That should bring up the citation and abstract for a systematic review of five studies about facilitated tucking of preterm infants during invasive procedure to modulate their responses to pain; the review was conducted by Obeidat, Kahalaf, Callister, & Froelicher and published in 2009.
4. Note that the abstract provides information about how many articles were included in the review, the outcomes that were examined, and the main conclusion of the review. Remember: You are reading a very short synopsis of the review, not the entire report.

From this quick look at the abstract of a systematic review, you should get a sense of the groundwork that has been done by the persons who did this review. In the process of doing the review, they did the following:

- Searched for articles
- Sifted through them for relevant studies
- Extracted information from each study report
- Brought the findings together in a coherent way

Clearly, this saves clinical nurses a great deal of time when they are looking for the research evidence about an issue in care. You will delve more deeply into systematic reviews in later chapters.

Recommendations of an Evidence-Based Clinical Practice Guideline

The third form of research evidence is the recommendations of an evidence-based clinical practice guideline. A clinical practice guideline consists of a set of recommendations, and when the recommendations are based on research evidence, the whole guideline is referred to as an evidence-based clinical practice guideline. These guidelines are most often developed by organizations with the resources (money, expertise, time) required to produce them. Again, I suggest taking a look at one, as follows:

1. Go to the website of the Registered Nurses' Association of Ontario (RNAO; http://www.rnao.org).
2. Click the *Best Practice Guidelines* tab; enter "dyspnea" into the search box and click *Search*. The search result will include the guideline *Nursing Care of Dyspnea: The 6th Vital Sign in Individuals With Chronic Obstructive Pulmonary Disease*.
3. Double click to open the page for the guideline
4. Under Downloadable Files you will see *COPD Summary*. Open that by double clicking and you will see a list of recommendations.

The developers of this guideline looked at the research evidence regarding nursing assessment and management of stable, unstable, and acute dyspnea associated with COPD. Based on the evidence, they derived the recommendations listed. (I suggest that you look at the Practice Recommendations [1–5] and ignore the Education and Organization and Policy Recommendations that follow.)

The strength of the evidence supporting each recommendation is indicated in the right column and definitions of those levels are provided at the end of the table; do not get caught up in that right now, although you should know that level Ia is very strong research evidence whereas level IV evidence was obtained from expert opinion evidence (i.e., no research exists, so consensus of an expert panel was the best available evidence). The evidence levels that support the recommendations are mostly either Ia or IV, indicating that considerable research evidence is available for some issues but none for others.

Remember that you are looking at part of a much larger report. The other document, the complete 166-page guideline (viewable by clicking on *Free Download*), presents more specific guidance and detailed review of the evidence that led to each recommendation. It also informs the reader how the search for evidence was conducted and how the 2010 update of the original 2005 guideline was done.

RESEARCH EVIDENCE

- **Findings from original studies**
- **Conclusions of systematic reviews**
- **Recommendations of evidence-based clinical practice guidelines**

As you can see, evidence-based clinical practice guidelines are much more ready to go for clinical application than systematic reviews and definitely more ready to go than tracking down the original research articles and working forward from there. For time-pressed protocol development teams, evidence-based clinical practice guidelines and systematic reviews are the short roads to evidence-based protocols (see **Figure 2-2**).

If starting the development of a care protocol by retrieving individual research articles is like baking a cake from scratch, and systematic reviews

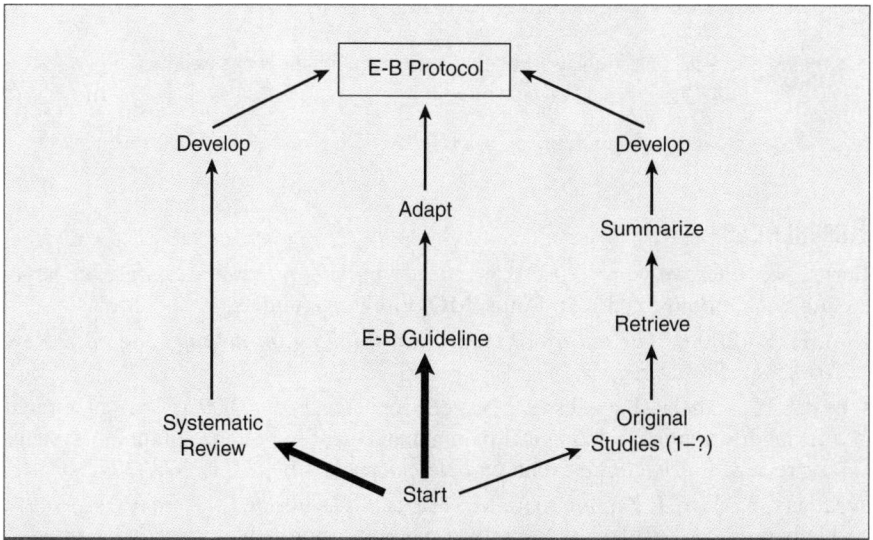

Figure 2-2 Roads to E-B Protocols

are like using a cake mix, then starting with an evidence-based clinical practice guideline is like buying a cake at the bakery and adding a personalized topping or presentation.

Going Forward

In the next chapter, you will begin to learn how to read research reports of individual studies. Then in Chapters 4 through 8, you will be guided through reading of exemplary articles reporting five different types of research (one qualitative study and four types of quantitative studies). After that, you will read a systematic review and learn how one type of systematic review is conducted, and then you will read an evidence-based clinical practice guideline and learn how they are produced.

Note that this order is the reverse of the order in which care design project teams search for research evidence—they first look for evidence-based guidelines and systematic reviews. If they exist and are well done, the team can build on them rather than reinventing the wheel. The order of presentation in this book is reversed because proceeding from original studies to systematic reviews to evidence-based clinical practice guidelines is a more natural learning order.

For a full suite learning activities and resources, visit the book's website: http://go.jblearning.com/brown3e.

References

Burns, N., & Grove, S. K. (2009). *Practice of nursing research: Conduct, critique, and utilization* (6th ed.). St. Louis, MO: Elsevier Saunders.

Kim, H. S. (2000). *The nature of theoretical thinking in nursing* (2nd ed.). New York, NY: Springer.

Obeidat, H., Kahalaf, I., Callister, L. C., & Froelicher, E. S. (2009). Use of facilitated tucking for nonpharmacological pain management in preterm infants: A systematic review. *Journal of Perinatal and Neonatal Nursing, 23*(4), 372–377.

Weathers, B., Barg, F. K., Bowman, M., Briggs, V., Delmoor, E., Kumanyika, S., . . . Halbert, C. H. (2011). Using a mixed-methods approach to identify health concerns in an African American community. *American Journal of Public Health, 101*(11), 2087–2092.

CHAPTER THREE

Reading Research Articles

Although some kinds of reading are intended to be a passive experience, reading professional articles, especially research reports, should be anything but passive. One way to be an active reader is to annotate or mark your copy of the article: underline, circle phrases, highlight, or jot comments in the margin—whatever helps you keep track of important information and connect the various parts of the study. Some people prefer to make notes in a file on their laptop—fine, whatever works for you.

I annotate right on my paper copy of articles. I write something like "n = 54" in the margin so I can quickly locate the sample size. I underline important definitions, outcomes, or findings. I circle abbreviations that will be used in the report and the parts of a table that are most important to me or unexpected. I put question marks where a statement does not fit with what was said earlier or does not make sense. Of course, it is possible to overannotate and in so doing produce clutter. However, if you annotate selectively, you will be able to find important information easily when you return to the article at a later time.

In this chapter, I make suggestions about how to read reports of individual studies. At this point in your learning, the goals in reading a research article about a study are to identify: (1) why the study was done, (2) how it was conducted, and (3) what was found. After you are comfortable reading research articles, you will add the goals of: (4) determining whether the study was soundly conducted , and (5) relevant to the care of patients to whom your agency or unit provides care (see text box).

GOALS IN READING A RESEARCH REPORT

1. **Determine the purpose of the study**
2. **Understand how the study was done**
3. **Understand what was found**
4. **Appraise the credibility of the findings**
5. **Determine if the findings are relevant to the care of your patients**

The emphasis in this chapter and in all of Part I of the book is on goals 1, 2, and 3 in the text box, although goals 4 and 5 may pop into your thinking as you read. For instance, you will undoubtedly note whether the patient groups that were studied are similar to a patient you have taken care of. You may make a mental note about this for now; however, serious consideration of the applicability of the study to a particular patient group is on hold until later in the book.

In reading this chapter, you may see a few terms that are unfamiliar to you. For now, just look them up in the glossary to get a sense of what they mean. Most of them are explained in full as you proceed through the first part of the text.

Starting Point

Is this a report of an original research study? This seems like it should be an easy question to answer, but at times it is not. Some articles read like research articles, but they are in fact other kinds of reports. When you see tables with numbers and percentages, you may think you are reading a research study, but the article may just be providing numerical data to describe a clinical program. Such data is anecdotal and naturally occurring with no control over its quality or the conditions under which it was collected. As you will learn, it takes more than numerical data to call an evaluation report "research."

Most often, the author of a research article will refer to the study early in the report, but sometimes you have to read quite far into an article to determine that it has the essential elements of a study. The essential elements of a research study include the following:

- A specified research question, **hypothesis**, or purpose
- Specified, systematic methods of data collection and analysis

- Results of data analysis
- Findings (interpreted results)
- Conclusions

If all these elements are present, then the likelihood that you are reading a research study report is very high. Remember, however, that there are many types of research methods and designs, and the essential elements of each type look quite different. Most quantitative studies address specific research questions or hypotheses, whereas qualitative studies may have a broad aim or purpose. Quantitative studies report results with tables, graphs, and statistics, whereas the findings of qualitative studies consist of extended quotes, narratives, descriptions, or themes. Qualitative studies often have small sample sizes (e.g., N = 6); some quantitative studies use a very large number of participants (e.g., N = 3,200). In short, research articles are diverse but should include at a minimum a clear purpose statement, a description of methods used to collect and analyze data, results and/or findings, and conclusions.

Format of Study Reports

Research reports of original studies are organized in a very logical way, and the formats used are similar from one journal to another. This standardization can help you as a reader because you will learn where to expect, and later locate, various kinds of information about the study. The following is a brief orientation to the format of research reports.

Title and Abstract

The title tells the reader what the study examined and often the patient group of interest. These are your first clues as to whether the report is likely to be of interest to you. However, titles can be misleading because a phrase or term used in the title may be different from the one used in your practice setting.

Abstracts almost always precede the main body of the article. An abstract provides a brief summary of the study—typically 300 words or less. Note the section headings used in the abstract because they are useful in beginning to organize your thinking about the study. The abstract distills the main points of the study, and after reading it you should know whether the study is of interest.

Let us assume that you have decided to read the whole study. Rather than read straight through the first time, you might want to read the introduction and then jump to the discussion section. The discussion summarizes the important findings and places them in the context of findings from earlier studies. Having read the introduction and the discussion, you should have a sense for the context of the study—and be ready to read the article from start to finish in its entirety.

Introduction

In the introduction of a research report, the researcher presents his view of the current state of knowledge regarding the issue or problem being investigated; this includes what is known and what the gaps in knowledge are. Study purposes are often set forth in the introduction section. Mark them in some way because they are important and you will want to refer to them.

Theoretical Frameworks In the introduction section of a research report, there may be a discussion of a theory that has been used to organize thinking about the issue and that serves as a conceptual context for the study. A theory is made up of assumptions, concepts, definitions, and/or propositions that provide a cohesive, although often tentative, explanation of how a phenomenon in the physical, psychological, or social world works. Propositions are suggested linkages among the concepts of the theory that have not yet been proven.

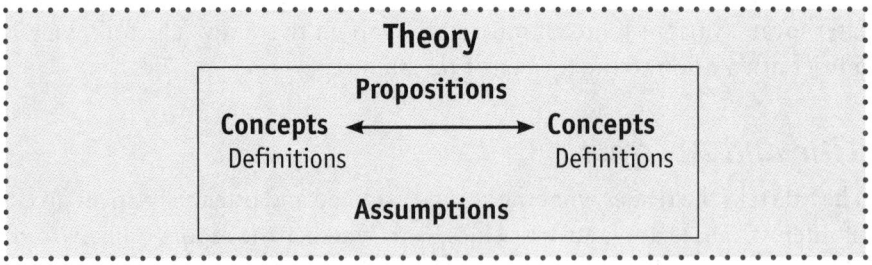

To make the preceding paragraph a bit more rooted in the real world, consider the following illustration. The *theory of community empowerment* was developed to provide direction for improving health in communities (Persily & Hildebrandt, 2008). Consider two propositions from this theory:

1. Involving lay workers in a community health promotion program extends access to health promotion opportunities.
2. Access to health promotion information leads to adoption of healthy behaviors.

Lay workers, access, health promotion opportunities, and *adoption of healthy behaviors* are concepts of the theory.

A researcher conducting a study about improving the health of elders living in their own homes might use the *theory of community empowerment* as a source of ideas for the study. By translating the two theoretical propositions into more concrete terms, the following two study hypotheses are formed:

1. Trained volunteers who collect healthy living questions from elders once a month at the weekly senior lunch and deliver answers the following week will increase access to health promotion information.
2. Health promotion information of personal interest will produce changes in health-related behaviors.

The questions submitted are given to a nurse practitioner who answers them via video recording shown at the next week's lunch. Adoption of new health behavior outcomes will then be measured at 3-month intervals for 1 year. Thus, the theory has served the research by bringing into a trial program a component that otherwise might not have been included and by providing a knowledge context for the findings. At the same time, the study acts as a test of the theory because the study has translated the abstractions of the theory into concrete realities that can be examined. If the study hypotheses are supported, the theory is supported because the hypotheses represent the theory.

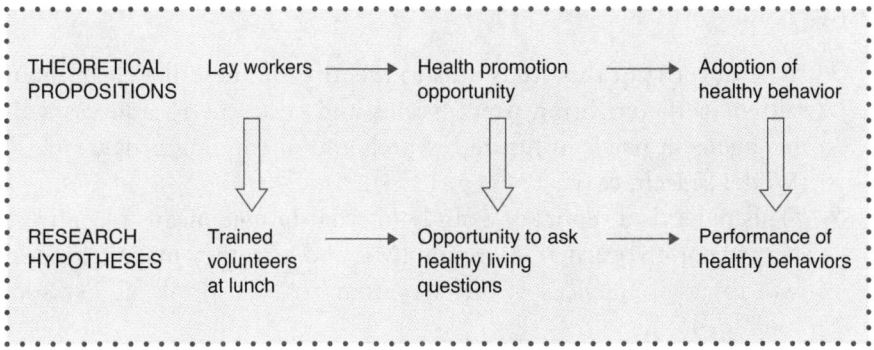

Not all study reports stipulate a theoretical framework; many researchers, particularly those testing physiological hypotheses, do not locate their studies within a theoretical framework; instead, they locate their study in a review of what is known from previously conducted research and what is still not known with certainty.

Clearly, much more could be said about the relationship between theory and research; however, doing so would be a diversion from the topic of this chapter, which is how research articles are formatted.

Study Purposes A reason for doing a study may be stated as a purpose statement, aims, objectives, research questions, or as hypotheses that will be tested by the study. Purpose words and phrases you will encounter in nursing study reports include:

- Acquire insights about . . .
- Understand
- Explore
- Examine
- Describe
- Compare
- Examine the relationship/association between
- Predict
- Test the hypothesis that . . .

In the early stages of studying an issue, research is directed at acquiring understanding of the various aspects of the issue—the problems people with the condition are experiencing, forces at work, and what the condition or experience means to individuals. Generally, these early studies use qualitative research methods. The following are study purposes from qualitative studies:

- "The purpose of this study was to identify and describe clean intermittent catheterization users' issues and concerns to address self-management needs in future research and/or training programmes" (Wilde, Brasch, & Yi, 2011, p. 1254).
- "This paper is a report of a study of what fatigue means to patients with recent myocardial infarction (MI) and how they manage to deal with the consequences of this symptom" (Alsén, Brink, & Persson, 2008, p. 459).

Note how both purposes set forth issues that will be examined, but they do not get highly specific about what they are looking for because they want the study participants to highlight the important aspects of their situation and experiences.

After the condition or situation is well understood at the experiential or social process level, subsequent studies may determine the frequency with which it occurs in different populations or measure the degree to which aspects of the condition or situation are present. Later, when several studies have been done and the situation is fairly well mapped, researchers will propose and quantitatively test associations between aspects of the situation or effectiveness of interventions directed at it. The following examples illustrate several ways of stating quantitative research purposes:

- "The specific research question [of this study] was 'What patient characteristics, clinical conditions, nursing unit characteristics, medical pharmacy, and nursing interventions are associated with falls during hospitalization of older adults?" (Titler, Shever, Kanak, Picone, & Qin, 2011, p. 129).
- "The purpose of this study was to compare the time needed to reach a specified temperature and the efficiency of two warming methods—warm cotton blankets and a radiant warmer—for hypothermia patients in a postanesthetic care unit (PACU) after spinal surgery" (Yang et al., 2012, p. 2).
- "The hypothesis is that the outcomes from nurse-led clinics will not be inferior to those obtained by the rheumatologist-led clinics, but at a lower cost and greater patient satisfaction" (Ndosi et al., 2011, p. 996).
- In a study of the association between depression and health-risk behaviors in high school students, two competing explanations became the hypotheses that were tested in the study: (1) Early depressive symptoms predict increases in risk behaviors over time; and (2) Early participation in health-risk behaviors predicts increases in depressive symptoms over time (Hooshmand, Willoughby, & Good, 2012).

These study purpose statements illustrate the variety of ways used to set forth quantitative study aims.

Methods

In the methods section, the author describes how the study was conducted, including information about the following:

1. The overall arrangements and logistics of the study
2. The setting or settings in which the study was conducted
3. The institutional review board (IRB) that gave ethical approval to the study
4. How the sample was obtained

5. The number of people in the sample
6. How data were collected
7. Any measurement instruments that were used (i.e., scales, questionnaires, physiologic measurements)
8. How the data was analyzed

Each of these steps will be discussed in detail specific to different research designs in later chapters. Briefly here, I will just say that the information about the sample should be sufficient to inform the reader about the likelihood that the sample is a good representation of the target population or provide enough profile information about the sample to let readers decide to whom the results would likely apply.

The information about how the data were obtained includes a statement about the organization that gave ethical approval to the study, procedures used to collect data, and descriptions of the measurement instruments used. For now, you should come away from reading the methods section of the reports with an understanding of the characteristics of the people who were included in the study, the sequence of steps in the study, and the data collected.

Results/Findings

In the results/findings section, the results of the data analysis are reported. Results are the outcomes of the analyses. In quantitative studies, results are shown in tables, graphs, percentages, frequencies, and statistics. There should be results related to each of the research questions, hypotheses, or aims. To illustrate, consider the following hypothetical statement that might be found in the Results section of a quantitative study: "The *t*-test comparing the functional status scores of those in intervention group A and intervention group B indicated a significant difference (mean A = 8.4; mean B = 6.1; $p = .038$)." This is a result statement; it reports the results of the statistical analysis.

The interpretation of a result is called a finding. A finding for the result statement just given would be stated something like, "The group who received nursing intervention A had a significantly higher functional level than did the group who received intervention B." Note how the findings statement interprets the statistical result but does not claim anything more than the statistical result indicated. Findings statements are usually found in the conclusions or discussion section of quantitative study reports.

To illustrate further, consider the results and findings of a hypothetical quantitative study comparing the effects of a new method for osteoporosis prevention education to standard education. A t-test was used to compare the scores of the two groups on an osteoporosis prevention questionnaire; the result of that test was $t = 1.99$, $p = .025$. This result indicates that the statistical calculation comparing the scores of the two groups resulted in a t-value of 1.99, which is statistically significant at the $p = .025$ level (I will explain p-values in a later chapter). The finding was this: The new educational method on average produced higher osteoporosis knowledge levels than standard education did, and there is a very low chance that this claim is wrong.

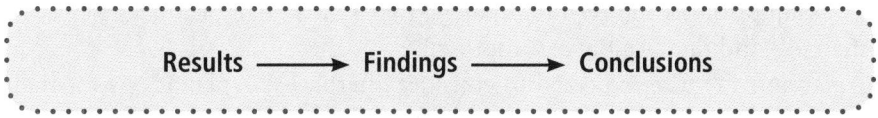

In qualitative research reports, data (observations, quotes) and findings (e.g., themes) are often intermingled. Generally, qualitative study reports do not have a Results section; rather, they have a findings section in which themes, narrative descriptions, or theoretical statements are presented along with examples of data that led to them. A later chapter provides more explanation of the analytical processes used by qualitative researchers.

When you first begin reading research articles, you may have a tendency to skip over the tables and figures. This is not advisable because the real meat of the results is often in them. Most authors highlight or summarize in the text what is in the tables, but others assume the reader will get the information from the tables, thus they do not restate that information. In examining tables and figures, it is important to carefully read their titles so you know exactly what you are looking at. Also, within tables, the column and row labels are critical to understanding the data provided. Reading tables is a bit like dancing with a new partner—with a bit of practice, you will quickly get good at it.

Discussion or Conclusions

In the discussion section, the researcher ties together several aspects of the study and offers possible applications of the findings. The researcher will usually open this section by stating the most important findings and placing them in the context of what other studies on the topic or question have found. In discussing the findings, many researchers describe what they think are the clinical implications of the findings. Here, they are allowed some latitude in saying what they think the findings mean. In the osteoporosis education for high school students example just given, the researcher might say, "The findings indicate that a short educational session is effective in increasing high school students' knowledge regarding osteoporosis prevention." This conclusion statement is close to the findings. On the other hand, if the researcher said, "Short educational sessions are an effective way of increasing osteoporosis prevention behaviors in high school students," the findings statement would be beyond the results. Because the study only measured the outcome of knowledge, not behaviors, the author is adding an assumption to the results, namely, that knowledge produces behavior change—and that is a big assumption.

Authors are also expected to consider alternative explanations for their findings. This would include noting how research methods may have influenced the results, such as "The sample size may have been too small to detect a difference in the treatment groups" or "The fact that a high proportion of patients in the intervention group didn't return for follow-up may have made the outcomes of the intervention group look better than they would have been if post-data had been available from everyone in that group." At the end of this section, the authors usually comment on what they view as the limitations of the study and the implications of the findings for future research.

References

The reference list should include complete information for all citations made in the text. You might find it useful to circle in the text and in the reference list any articles that you want to obtain and read for greater understanding or because they studied a population of interest to you, for example, elderly persons living independently in the inner city. Perusal of the reference list also reveals other current work on the issue, who has done research on the issue, and which journals have published research articles about the issue.

Reading Approach

When you first read research reports, they may seem difficult to read. It is really like any new undertaking—at first it is confusing. However, the fog lifts rather quickly, the whole picture comes into focus, and the relationships between the parts become clear. For now, you should set three simple goals for yourself. You should come away from your reading of a research report knowing:

WHY? HOW? WHAT?

- **Why was the study done—to what purpose?**
  Found in Introduction and its subsections: background, literature review, theoretical framework, purpose, and hypotheses
- **How was the study done?**
  Found in Methods and its subsections: design, setting, sample, data collection, measuring instruments, data analysis
- **What was found?**
  Found in Results, Discussion, Conclusions.

Importantly, even seasoned readers of research reports find it necessary to read a research report at least twice. The first time you may only get a general sense of why the study was done, how it was done, and what was found. During the second reading, the why, how, and what should become clear to you.

During the second read, you also may begin to notice issues that make you wonder, such as the following:

- Why did the researchers exclude persons with heart disease?
- Did they take into account patients' balance when evaluating capacity for self-care?
- Did the fact that a study was going on put the nurse participants on best behavior?

These are important observations and questions; they will become important later when you are also required to appraise the credibility of study findings. For now, your aim is to get a grasp of the *why*, *how*, and *what* of the study.

Wading In

Having considered how research reports are organized and having noted some difference between the formats of qualitative and quantitative study reports, it is now time to delve into reading one of them. Your instructor may have you choose one or assign one for everyone in the class to read.

The research reports reprinted in full in subsequent chapters are considered exemplars in that they are typical or representative of a particular type of healthcare research. Most of the exemplar studies were also very well conducted, but they were not chosen because they are perfect models—all studies have warts. Rather, they were chosen because they used a research design that is widely used in healthcare research. I hope you will figuratively wade around in these studies enough to acquire a thorough understanding of them.

http://go.jblearning.com/brown3e

References

Alsén, P., Brink, E., & Persson, L. O. (2008). Living with incomprehensible fatigue after recent myocardial infarction. *Journal of Advanced Nursing, 64*(5), 459–468.

Hooshmand, S., Willoughby, T., & Good, M. (2012). Does the direction of effects in the association between depressive symptoms and health-risk behaviors differ by behavior? A longitudinal study across the high school years. *Journal of Adolescent Health, 50*(2), 140–147.

Ndosi, M., Lewis, M., Hale, C., Quinn, H., Ryan, S., Emery, P., . . . Hill, J. (2011). A randomized controlled study of outcome and cost effectiveness for RA patients attending nurse-led rheumatology clinics: Study protocol of an ongoing nationwide multi-centre study. *International Journal of Nursing Studies, 48*(8), 995–1011.

Persily, C. A., & Hildebrandt, E. (2008). The theory of community empowerment. In M. J. Smith & P. R. Liehr (Eds.), *Middle range theory for nursing* (2nd ed., pp. 131–144). New York, NY: Springer.

Titler, M. G., Shever, L. L., Kanak, M. F., Picone, D. M., & Qin, R. (2011). Factors associated with falls during hospitalization in an older adult population. *Research and Theory for Nursing Practice: An International Journal, 25*(2), 127–134.

Wilde, M. H., Brasch, J., & Yi, Z. (2011). A qualitative descriptive study of self-management issues in people with long-term intermittent urinary catheters. *Journal of Advanced Nursing, 67*(6), 1254–1263.

Yang, H-L., Lee, H-F., Chu, T-L., Su, Y-Y., Ho, L-H., & Fan, J-Y. (2012). The comparison of two recovery room warming methods for hypothermia patient who had undergone spinal surgery. *Journal of Nursing Scholarship, 44*(1), 2–10.

CHAPTER FOUR

Qualitative Research

Research methods that delve deeply into experiences, social processes, and subcultures are referred to as qualitative research. As a group, qualitative research methods:

- Recognize that every individual is situated in an unfolding life context—that is, a set of circumstances, values, and influences
- Respect the meanings each individual assigns to what happens to and around him or her
- Recognize that cultures and subcultures are diverse and have considerable effect on individuals

Qualitative researchers feel strongly that a person's experiences, perceptions, and social interactions are not reducible to numbers and categories—they are much too complex and situated in the context of a person's life. They believe that the researcher attempting to understand experiences, perception, and social interaction must enter into a person's lifeworld and let the participant's words and accounts lead the researcher to understandings that would remain hidden without deep and open-minded exploration (Munhall, 2007). Thus, qualitative researchers go into their exploration with as few assumptions as possible.

Data Collection and Analysis

The data collection techniques used to understand subjective realities include:

- Nonintrusive, often prolonged, observation
- Conversational interviews
  - ✓ Open-ended questions
  - ✓ Careful listening
  - ✓ Follow-up questions
  - ✓ Helping persons to be reflective about their experiences
  - ✓ Requesting elaboration
- Validation (when making an interpretation of observations or what was said, they ask the informant if the interpretation is accurate)

Often, detailed notes are kept or interviews are recorded and subsequently transcribed. The researcher spends considerable time going back and forth through the notes to identify important connections. As the researcher gains greater insight into the issue, the questions asked of subsequent study participants may change (Swanson, 2001). The researcher works inductively—that is, moving from details to a slightly more general encompassing phrase or concept and finally to a set of themes or patterns that portrays important aspects of the experience, social process, or culture.

The term *qualitative research* actually refers to methodological traditions and methods with diverse aims, data collection techniques, and analysis techniques. The methodological traditions were developed in disciplines such as sociology and anthropology—and nursing has adopted them (see **Table 4–1**).

The phenomenological research tradition is useful in gaining insight into human experiences, whereas the grounded theory tradition enables researchers to understand the fundamental social processes involved in healthcare situations, say, the workings of emergency care transports or how families make the decision for a child to have an organ transplant. The ethnographic research tradition creates descriptions of healthcare subcultures, such as chronic renal dialysis units or Alzheimer's disease support groups—from the insider perspective. Two other qualitative research traditions are discourse analysis and historical analysis. Discourse analysis is used to analyze the dynamics and structure of conversations, such as patient–provider dialogue. Historical research examines past events and trends, usually through records, documents, articles, and personal diaries from the past.

TABLE 4–1 Qualitative Research Traditions

Tradition	Common Aim in Nursing Studies	Data Collection Techniques	Data Analysis Techniques
Phenomenologic research	Understanding and description of the lived experience of persons with a particular health condition or situation	1. Select persons who are living or have lived the experience. 2. Set aside preconceived ideas. 3. Engage in dialogue with each participant. 4. Explore the person's lifeworld. 5. Assist person to be reflective about his or her experiences and what they mean to him or her. 6. Stay in the setting until no new insights are emerging and all issues are understood.	1. Transcribe interviews. 2. Look for segments in the account. 3. Identify significant phrases. 4. Group phrases with common thoughts into themes. 5. Confirm themes with the participants.
Ethnographic research	A rich portrayal of the norms, values, language, roles, and social rules of a health or healthcare culture or subculture	1. Immerse self in the culture/setting, typically for long periods of time. 2. Observe social interactions. 3. Seek out and informally question good informants. 4. Analyze documents. 5. Take detailed notes.	1. Identification of social rules and understandings. 2. Analysis of social networks. 3. Confirmation of interpretations. 4. Produce a coherent account of the culture. 5. Check out description with key informants.

(continued)

TABLE 4–1 Qualitative Research Traditions (continued)

Tradition	Common Aim in Nursing Studies	Data Collection Techniques	Data Analysis Techniques
Grounded theory research	A theory (i.e., a tentative, coherent explanation) about how a social process works, particularly social interaction	1. Gain access to the social setting. 2. Observe social interactions. 3. Conduct informal interviews. 4. Keep field notes. 5. Identify useful written materials. 6. Stay in the setting until no new insights are emerging and all issues are well understood.	1. Intermix data collection and analysis. 2. Name what is happening in the data with codes. 3. Analyze the use of language. 4. Proceed from concrete codes to theoretical ones. 5. Constantly compare new data with previously acquired data. 6. Generate core concepts and hypotheses and check them out with participants.

Each of these traditions requires techniques for collecting and analyzing data appropriate to its purposes. After looking across the rows of Table 4–1, which will give you a sense for each tradition, look down the columns and note how the purposes and methods of these traditions differ.

Qualitative Description

Not all questions in nursing and health care can be investigated in a clinically useful way using the methods of one of the traditions just described. As a result, another method that draws on features from the traditional approaches has evolved. This somewhat eclectic approach is called **qualitative description** (Neergaard, Olesen, Andersen, & Sondegaard, 2009; Sandelowski, 2010). The goal of qualitative description is to produce a straightforward description of participants' experiences in words as similar to what the participants said as possible. Most often, but not always, the participants are patients. Commonly used methods of qualitative description include, but are not limited to the following:

1. Sampling for diversity
2. Data collection by interviews of individuals or focus groups
3. Data analysis by qualitative content analysis
4. Generation of themes or patterns that capture what has been said

Even quantitative data collection and analysis techniques can be incorporated into a study using the qualitative description method.

Understanding how **qualitative content analysis** is done is key to understanding this qualitative research method. If you think about it, you will realize that qualitative data collection produces an abundance of data—pages and pages of transcripts of interviews and dialogue or of written material. To extract meaning from all this raw data, researchers identify sections of data that convey an idea and assign it a word or phrase code that conveys its essence. The code should be data derived, i.e., generated from the data itself (Sandelowski, 2010). In assigning a code to a section of transcribed narrative or a section of a diary, the researcher is always aware that she is making an interpretation and therefore must be careful that the code does not change the original meaning of what was said.

Content analysis is not a linear, constantly forward-moving process. Rather, it is dynamic and reflexive. If none of the previously used codes captures the meaning of a section of text, the researcher will create a new code. The new code may or may not lead the researcher to revise the coding of already coded text.

A list of codes can be informative, but it may be more useful if coding is taken a step further. That step involves identifying similarities in the codes; it may be possible to group similar codes without losing the meaning of the first round of codes. This broader grouping may be a category, a chronological order, or a theme. Again, the researcher is on guard not to lose the meaning of the original data and codes. For example, in a study using grounded theory methods to understand the experiences of mother of infants who cry persistently, "Level one codes such as "staying at home," "feeling judged as a parent," and "protecting image of perfect infant" became the level two code "isolation" (Megel, Wilson, Bravo, McMahon, & Towne, 2011, p. 146). The term isolation referred to the mothers' decisions "to stay at home to protect themselves and the baby from unwanted advice and criticism" (p. 148).

Original quote → Code
Several similar codes → Theme

Importantly, even though qualitative description is somewhat eclectic in the methods used, researchers who use it remain committed to rigor of method by using methodological principles widely recognized by other qualitative researchers. In summary, qualitative description is a very pragmatic approach to doing qualitative research. It is characterized by using a combination of methods that will produce a useful description of the experience, perceptions, or events of interest. Any interpretation produced should not be far removed in meaning from the data provided by the study participants.

Uniqueness of Qualitative Studies

Some findings from qualitative research are useful in their own right, whereas others produce hypotheses that require further study using quantitative methods. Certainly, in-depth descriptions of patients' experiences of illness and health care are directly useful to nurses in understanding what their patients are experiencing and in communicating helpfully with them. They may also be useful in developing nursing assessment guides and teaching plans.

Other findings from qualitative research are hypotheses about associations and causal relationships at work in the situation of interest. These hypotheses require further study using quantitative methods—to acquire knowledge regarding the degree to which the identified associations are true across different segments of the population or to test possible causal relationships identified by the qualitative study.

At first, qualitative research methods may seem unscientific to you. Although it is true that they are very different from what most people view as scientific, the reality is that these methods have been developed to acquire insights into subjective experiences and social processes—complex human realities that cannot be broken apart, manipulated, and examined the way physical realities can be. The rich and nuanced understandings of human experiences and social interaction produced by qualitative methods cannot be achieved using methods that reduce human characteristics to numbers and the context of human lives to the status of variables.

Qualitative studies are sometimes criticized for having small sample sizes or for not being objective. These criticisms are based on a lack of understanding of what qualitative studies aim to produce and how their methods produce unique and valuable forms of knowledge for the clinical professions. Both qualitative and quantitative research methods have a place in the scientific toolbox of the clinical professions. Just as a house cannot be built with only one type of tool, e.g., saws, so it is that producing the full range of knowledge required for clinical practice requires the use of both qualitative and quantitative research methods.

Exemplar

Reading Tips

I want to call your attention to the structure of this chapter because the same structure will be used in the rest of the chapters in Part I of the book. Each chapter is made up of three sections:

1. Introductory information about the featured research method in an opening section such as you have just read about qualitative methods
2. A reprinted exemplar article of an actual study using the featured method
3. A profile and commentary on the exemplar article

The Jacobson et al. (2008) article uses qualitative description methods. After reading the Methods section in the text, read the box titled *More on Methods and Analysis* before proceeding to read the Results section. The Profile & Commentary that follow the article reprint will refer quite a bit to the information provided in that box.

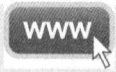

Patients' Perspectives on Total Knee Replacement

Ann F. Jacobson, Rodney P. Myerscough, Kirsten DeLambo, Eileen Fleming, Amy M. Huddleston, Natalie Bright, and Joseph D. Varley (2008).

American Journal of Nursing 108(5), 54–63.

Abstract

Objective: Because patients' perspectives on total knee replacement (TKR) surgery have rarely been the topic of research, this study sought to describe their pre- and postoperative experiences.

Methods: Using a qualitative descriptive design, researchers collected data from a convenience sample of 27 patients who were about to undergo or had recently undergone TKR. Preoperative data were obtained in focus group sessions (n = 17); postoperative data were obtained in individual interviews (n = 10). All data-collection sessions were tape-recorded and transcribed, and transcripts were analyzed. The researchers isolated themes by identifying recurrent words and phrases and then sorted the data into thematic categories.

Results: Four main themes emerged. First, many participants delayed surgery for months to years, despite increasing pain and limitation. Second, once participants decided to proceed with surgery, they entered a period of waiting and worrying about what would happen during and after surgery. Third, both pre- and postoperative participants struggled with the need for independence, as well as with learning to accept the new knee. And fourth, patients experienced postoperative pain associated with surgery and rehabilitation, yet reported having hope that they'd regain function.

Conclusions: These findings suggest that patients need to be better educated and supported before and after TKR surgery. More research is needed to shed light on how patients' experiences influence their decisions about the surgery and its outcomes.

Key Words

total knee replacement, total knee arthroplasty, patient response to surgery, pain, functional ability, patient education

* * *

Total knee replacement (TKR) is one of the most common orthopedic operations in the United States,[1,2] but few researchers have examined patients' experience of the procedure. The operation, performed to improve function and relieve pain in people with osteoarthritis or rheumatoid arthritis, involves resurfacing damaged bone and cartilage and replacing them with plastic or metal parts.[2] Yet numerous studies of total joint replacement (of the hip or knee) indicate that eligible patients delay or decline the procedure for reasons that aren't well understood.[3,4] One recent literature review reported that a significant proportion of people who were eligible for joint replacement were unwilling to consider surgery.[4] It concluded that patients' expectations of outcomes are significantly influenced by factors such as sex, race, ethnicity, and socioeconomic status and that patient education materials "may not address the concerns of many individuals." (For more on total knee replacement, see *Facts About Total Knee Replacement Surgery*.)

One orthopedic surgeon who has written on this topic, Peter Bonutti, put it this way: "Maybe we don't understand what our patients care about."[5] He cited two studies' findings that one-third of patients who'd had TKR were dissatisfied with it, and he identified the need to consider the procedure from the patient's, rather than the surgeon's, point of view. The difference in perspective was highlighted in another study of 108 patients who underwent 126 TKRs: patients' subjective and physicians' objective assessments of outcomes correlated poorly.[6] The researchers concluded that "surgeons are more satisfied than patients."

In 2003 the National Institutes of Health held the Consensus Development Conference on Total Knee Replacement, calling in particular for research into patients' decisions about surgery and the factors that affect outcomes.[7] Members of the expert panel also suggested that the use of qualitative rather than quantitative methods might reveal a fuller range of experiences. And a British review examining qualitative research concluded that it "has particular strengths in uncovering evidence that is discrepant with researchers' or practitioners' prior assumptions" and revealing "significant but unanticipated factors."[8]

Facts About Total Knee Replacement Surgery

- The first hinged knee prosthesis, made of ivory, was inserted in 1891 by German surgeon Themistocles Gluck to replace a tubercular joint.[1]
- According to the Agency for Healthcare Research and Quality's Healthcare Cost and Utilization Project (HCUP) (http://hcupnet.ahrq.gov), the number of total knee replacements (TKRs) performed in the United States almost doubled between 1995 (293,086) and 2005 (549,867).
- The proportion of patients ages 40 to 49 years and 50 to 59 years having TKRs increased by 95% and almost 54%, respectively, from 1990 through 2000.[2]
- Significantly fewer eligible black patients elect to have TKR than do eligible white patients.[3,4]
- According to the HCUP, acute care discharge disposition for TKR in 2005 was 41% to another institution such as a rehabilitation center or nursing home, 32% to home health care, and 26% to home.
- Indications for TKR include "radiographic evidence of joint damage, moderate to severe persistent pain not adequately relieved by an extended course of nonsurgical management, and clinically significant functional limitation resulting in diminished quality of life."[3]
- Advances in implant composition and placement techniques have increased the popularity of TKR surgery. The longevity of the implant depends on individual factors such as the amount and type of postsurgical activity and the patient's weight, age, and sex.[5-8]

References

1. Shetty AA, et al. The evolution of total knee arthroplasty. Part II: the hinged knee replacement and the semi-constrained knee replacement. *Curr Orthop* 2003;17(5):403-7.
2. Jain NB, et al. Trends in epidemiology of knee arthroplasty in the United States, 1990-2000. *Arthritis Rheum* 2005;52(12):3928-33.
3. NIH Consensus Development Conference on Total Knee Replacement. NIH Consensus Statement on total knee replacement. *NIH Consens State Sci Statements* 2003;20(1):1-34. http://consensus.nih.gov/2003/2003TotalKneeReplacement117main.htm.
4. Weng HH, Fitzgerald J. Current issues in joint replacement surgery. *Curr Opin Rheumatol* 2006;18(2):163-9.
5. Beadling L. TKA can be an option for the young active patient. *Orthop Today* 2003;23(10):43.

6. Dennis DA. Trends in total knee arthroplasty. *Orthopedics* 2006;29(9):S13-S16.
7. Jenabzadeh AR, Haddad FS. Novel strategies in joint replacement. *Br J Hosp Med Lond* 2006;67(6):294-8.
8. Vazquez-Vela Johnson G, et al. Patient demographics as a predictor of the ten-year survival rate in primary total knee replacement. *J Bone Joint Surg Br* 2003;85(1):52-6.

Methods

In seeking to describe patients' experiences with TKR, we used a qualitative descriptive design, collecting data from 17 preoperative and 10 postoperative patients during focus group and individual interviews, respectively. The focus group session immediately followed the hospital's joint-replacement class. Because of the limitations imposed by postoperative recovery and the variety of care sites, we collected data on patients' postoperative experiences during individual interviews. Table 1 shows the demographic characteristics of the sample. (For additional details about the methods, see *More on Methods and Analysis*.)

More on Methods and Analysis

Design. The qualitative descriptive method entails collecting data and presenting findings in everyday language, with minimal inference and interpretation by researchers, unlike other qualitative methods (such as grounded theory).[1] As Sandelowski states, this method is "especially amenable to obtaining straight and largely unadorned . . . answers to questions of special relevance to practitioners."[1]

The study was approved by the institutional review boards at the university where the first author (AFJ) worked and the hospital where the patients were scheduled for their operations, a large urban medical center with an active orthopedic surgery department. All participants were informed of the nature of the study and signed consent forms. At the end of data collection, each participant was paid $25.

Sample. Data were obtained from a convenience sample of 27 patients (see Table 1) who either were scheduled for total knee replacement (TKR) surgery within one month or had undergone the surgery within the previous two months.

Preoperative data were obtained in four focus group sessions in which a total of 17 patients participated; postoperative data were obtained in individual interviews with 10 patients. Inclusion criteria were being able to speak English, being 21 years of age or older, having had no previous total joint replacement, and either being scheduled for (preoperative sample) or having undergone (postoperative sample) a single TKR within the periods specified. Exclusion criteria were having cognitive impairment, rheumatoid arthritis of the operative joint, or significant postoperative complications (such as surgical site infection or thrombophlebitis). In addition, participants in the preoperative sample could not be in the postoperative sample, to avoid the possibility that participation in a preoperative focus group might influence postoperative views. Participants were recruited into both samples until data saturation occurred (with the additional interviews yielding only redundant information).

Instrument. All data collection sessions were tape-recorded and transcribed, with the transcripts serving as the units of analysis.

Preoperative focus groups. Four different focus groups with patients scheduled to undergo their first TKR within one month were held. The focus groups were moderated by one of the authors (RPM), a clinical psychologist with extensive experience in facilitating group discussion. One or two other research team members, RNs with research experience (AFJ and EF), served as assistant moderators, organizing participant recruitment and consent, keeping track of time, observing and recording nonverbal cues, and making other field notes.

Focus group participants were recruited from among people attending a class on total joint replacement, which was held in a conference room of the hospital where they would have the surgery. The nurse leading the class (not a research team member) mentioned the study at the end of class and invited attendees scheduled for a single TKR to remain if they wanted more information. Those who were interested met with one of us (AFJ), who explained the study. Participants signed a consent form and remained for the focus group session, at which participants and moderators were seated around a conference table. The session started with the moderator explaining basic concepts and expectations (for example, that there are no right or wrong answers in descriptive research and that it's hoped that everyone will participate).

The moderator then facilitated the discussion. First, to discourage "group think" (a phenomenon marked by a failure to express views that differ from the perceived group consensus), participants were asked to write down their three main concerns for later discussion. Next, the moderator prompted discussion by asking questions that progressed from the general (such as "As you've been thinking about the surgery, what's been on your mind the most?") to the more specific (such as "What are some of your concerns?"). (The complete list of Questions for Focus Group and Interview Sessions is available at http ://links.lww.com/A422.) Follow-up questions were based on the participants' responses and were asked as they arose during the sessions. Each focus group session lasted about one hour, after which the moderators held a debriefing session to review responses and note emerging themes.

Postoperative interviews. Potential participants—patients who had undergone TKR in the previous two months—were identified by the orthopedic unit's patient care coordinator, an RN, who notified them of the study and obtained their permission to be contacted by the research team. Those who were interested in participating signed a consent form and scheduled a date for the interview with the research team member (NB), an RN graduate assistant with perioperative experience. Interviews took place on the post-acute rehabilitation unit or the patient's home. The researcher interviewed the patient using open-ended questions. Interviews ranged from about 15 minutes to about 60 minutes in length.

Data analysis. Transcripts from the focus group, debriefing, and interview sessions were first read through. Next, each transcript was read and analyzed using principles of qualitative content analysis, an approach that's "oriented toward summarizing the informational contents of [the] data" with minimal inference and interpretation.[1] Using the study's stated purpose as a guide, the researchers selected relevant sections of the transcripts, defined themes by identifying recurrent words and phrases, sorted the data into the thematic categories, and drew conclusions. Two members of the research team (AFJ and KD) analyzed the data independently and met periodically to compare findings and resolve category coding discrepancies ("check coding"). Codes were repeatedly revised as similarities and differences were noted across categories, until the final categories were considered robust and complete with agreement between coders.

Reference

1. Sandelowski M. Whatever happened to qualitative description? *Res Nurs Health* 2000;23(4):334-40.

Table 1 Participant Characteristics (N = 27)

Mean age, in years (SD)	66.5 (12.8)	65.6 (11.9)	66.03 (12.1)
Range in years of age	45–83	49–83	45–83
Race, n (%)			
African American	1 (7.7)	2 (14.3)	3 (11.1)
White	12 (92.3)	12 (85.7)	24 (89.9)
Marital status, n (%)			
Married	8 (61.5)	7 (50)	15 (55.6)
Widowed	3 (23.1)	2 (14.3)	5 (18.5)
Divorced	1 (7.7)	1 (7.1)	2 (7.4)
Single	1 (7.7)	4 (28.6)	5 (18.5)

SD = standard deviation
Note: Percentages in the middle columns are percentages of the column totals (n) rather than the total cohort (N). Demographic data are not categorized by pre- and postoperative samples because the study did not investigate the differences between these groups; rather, it sought to fully describe patients' experiences.

Results

We identified four overarching themes in patients' experiences of TKR, which we named "putting up and putting off," "waiting and worrying," "letting go and letting in," and "hurting and hoping." Our purpose was to describe overall experience; we did not compare and contrast the data from the pre- and postoperative samples.

Putting up and putting off characterized the period before the decision to have surgery was made. It typically lasted for years and involved "putting up" with knee pain and resulting limitations and "putting off" TKR by modifying activities, using adaptive equipment, and undergoing less drastic treatments.

Putting up: pain limits what you can do. Participants described a gradual increase in knee pain, which they usually characterized as constant and aggravated by walking and other movements. Sometimes the joint gave out unexpectedly when they were walking or climbing stairs. They frequently described the knee as "bone on bone" with "no cartilage." Some reported that the knee was bending to the side or "bowing out."

One participant said, "Pain limits what you can do," a sentiment echoed by many. Another said,

> I'm tired of it. . . . I am a very active person. My favorite comment is 'I can't.' I can't take the trash to the street. I can't cut the grass. . . . I am a car salesman. I feel like a flat tire, and in my business you can't have a flat tire. [Emphasis added]

Knee pain limited participants' ability to perform many daily activities, including dressing, cooking, cleaning their homes, shopping, using stairs, dancing, and playing golf. Many activities required careful planning, such as bringing crutches or a wheelchair, premedicating with analgesics, and planning routes.

> If I went to the store, I had to know exactly what I could get and just hold onto the shopping cart. . . . [Eventually] I could only go to the stores that had [electric shopping carts]. I really couldn't even walk. . . . [The physician] even encouraged me to get handicapped parking, which I did.

Outings often resulted in fatigue and prolonged or exacerbated pain. Some participants described crying because of the pain and becoming depressed and isolated. As the condition worsened, participants began to limit their activities to those that required little walking or could be accomplished with frequent rest breaks or the use of mobility aids. Some relied on others for transportation; some obtained handicapped parking permits. One participant took her cell phone everywhere, even inside her own home, so that she could "call someone in case I get stuck." Others described modifying the way they approached tasks—for example, placing pillows under the knees when kneeling, sitting or lying down instead of kneeling, and crawling instead of walking.

For some, knee pain and functional limitations changed how they viewed themselves or how they believed others viewed them. They considered themselves active people who had been forced into inactivity. They saw their knee problems as constricting, and even controlling, their lives.

Putting off: getting to the point. Most participants delayed surgery for as long as possible, and for many, that was years after the option was first presented.

> It was something I knew I had to do, but you just keep hoping that it will get better. . . . You get to the point where finally you figure, "I got to do something."

Some said that they'd put off surgery because they'd hoped that medical science would eventually offer a less drastic alternative or because they wanted to first try to strengthen their knees. Most participants said they wished they hadn't delayed surgery for as long as they had and would advise others not to wait so long. But that view was not universally shared. One postoperative participant "wanted to make sure that . . . there wasn't any doubt, that [surgery] was my only recourse."

During this period, participants often received treatments such as cortisone or hylan G-F 20 (Synvisc) injections. These gave transient relief to some; others said the treatments either weren't effective or worsened their condition. Participants referred to these treatments as "Band-Aids," "just temporary," or "a prelude to having [TKR] done."

Waiting and worrying. Once participants decided to proceed with TKR, they entered a period of waiting and worrying about what would happen during and after surgery.

Waiting: let's get it over with. As participants prepared for TKR, they became anxious to put the surgery behind them: "I put this off for years. I can't wait to get it over with." They described the waiting period as one filled with apprehension; one spoke of "anxiety that is cursing my life."

Many participants prepared by maintaining or increasing their activity level, believing that would aid recovery: "The better shape you are in, the better you get through surgery." Some worked to get "everything in as much order as [they] possibly can" to prepare for a postoperative period of limited functioning.

Worrying: 'something can go wrong.' Participants reported having concerns about anesthesia, surgery, and complications. Many viewed anesthesia as particularly risky. Participants were given the choice of a spinal or a general anesthetic. Most chose general, even if they felt it was riskier and would prolong recovery; they didn't want to be aware of any aspect of surgery.

> I had general anesthesia, it was my choice. . . . [I'm] a nurse; I didn't want to wake up in the middle and hear things. . . I've been scrubbed in for orthopedic surgeries so I kinda know the sounds and noises, and I didn't want to wake up and hear the jigsaw or anything.

Some expressed a generalized fear about surgery:

"Any time you have surgery, anything can happen." Specific fears involved the risk of complications, such as a blood clot, infection, or death. Some had had complications with prior procedures or knew someone who had, which led to their current fear. But some said they had no concerns. Many said they tried to maintain a positive attitude, believing a negative one would worsen their outcome.

> I sure don't want to be negative going into it. . . . I mean, it's either go [in] up, or go in down and out. And if you go in down and out, there's . . . a worst-case scenario, that you will have complications.

One factor contributing to worry was having too little information about the operation: "I have no idea how long it will take. . . . Everything is ambiguous. . . . Please tell me what you are going to do." Most wished they'd received more information from their surgeons preoperatively and had better understood what to expect during recovery. One postoperative participant said that understanding the "backward-and-forward" nature of recovery beforehand would have made it "less scary and less traumatic than afterwards thinking, 'Why, what's wrong?'" (For more, see *Questions Participants Had About Surgery*.)

Some participants reported feeling well prepared for surgery and recovery. Those who'd received detailed and graphic information from their physicians appreciated it: "He was very explicit about what . . . the surgery would entail. [The surgeon] was great. . . . He let me hold the [replacement] joint in my hand."

Questions Participants Had About Surgery

- When can I take a shower?
- How can I get up and down stairs?
- Will they give me a temporary wheelchair card for my car?
- How much pain will I have?
- When can I drive?
- What will the incision look like?

Letting go and letting in. Pre- and postoperatively, participants struggled with the need for independence and with allowing others to help, comfort, and support them. "Letting in" also involved learning to accept the knee implant as part of their bodies.

Letting go: accepting a loss of control. Participants described themselves as independent people who found it difficult to rely on others: "I had to accept the loss of control." Many said they'd needed increasing assistance in performing activities of daily living preoperatively. Participants worried about being dependent on others, usually family members, while recovering.

> When you're used to being the caregiver, that's hard, having somebody take care of you. . . . The first night I came home from the hospital . . . I went to the bathroom and I made a mess and I couldn't clean it up. . . . That night [my partner] was fine, he didn't mind cleaning up my mess or doing all that but I asked him to just leave the room and just let the music play and shut out the lights. I put the pillow over my head and I cried.

Sometimes, participants resisted relinquishing control and exercised their independence, ignoring the advice of clinicians or family members. One participant planned to sip ginger ale after surgery during the period when fluids weren't allowed, believing that it would relieve postoperative nausea. Some planned to get out of bed on their own right after surgery: "I can't be tied down." One planned to bring his pajamas to the hospital, saying he couldn't sleep in anything else. A participant with diabetes planned to adhere to his usual diet after surgery, rather than the one prescribed.

Religion helped some participants; one spoke of God: "He will take care of this." Others articulated a philosophical acceptance: "Life is a road and you have to go down it, and this is something that I have to do."

We observed that letting go was accompanied by letting in—receiving encouragement from others, establishing trust with clinicians, and accepting the new knee.

Letting in: accepting encouragement. Many participants knew others who'd undergone TKR and found their accounts of successful outcomes encouraging: "It is wonderful . . . just thinking that I am going to come out the same way." Some of these acquaintances had spoken about wishing they'd had the procedure years earlier and being happy with the results; they told our participants that after TKR they'd "feel brand-new." But reports of negative outcomes (such as continuing pain or poor knee function) left participants feeling frustrated or fearful, and many said they tried to avoid hearing such stories: "I don't want any negativity around me right now. I want the positive stuff."

Several participants said that having more opportunities to talk with people who'd had the surgery or with providers would have increased their confidence going into surgery.

> **Don't let me just read it in a book or in a pamphlet or whatever.** [Emphasis added] That's all well and good, but I want to talk to somebody. **I want to bounce things off of them.** [Emphasis added] I want to put myself more at ease. I want to get rid of that stress.

They would also have appreciated a structured peer-support group: "[It helps] knowing that other people have the same discomforts that I have. . . . You know, misery loves company and I'm sure we can compare notes."

Letting in: trusting the team. Participants spoke favorably of physicians who took the time to explain the surgery and answer questions. They valued a direct approach: "He's the nuts-and-bolts type of doctor that I like"; "He's not into fooling around. He tells you what's happening." They related having "100% confidence" in their physicians and their recommendations. Many chose a surgeon based on the recommendations of friends and family; some had solicited opinions about surgeons from others who'd had TKR.

Participants also noted the caring and skills of nurses and other hospital workers, especially those who had helped with transferring and walking. They appreciated nurses who assessed their pain and suggested or administered analgesia. They felt cared for by nurses who "hovered over" them or helped with personal care.

Letting in: accepting the new knee. Participants referred to how "bad" their own knees were and asked questions about the new one. (For more, see *Questions Participants Had About the New Knee*.) Postoperative participants said their muscles needed to "learn" to work with the new knee, which they described as stable and strong.

> I just feel like it's part of my knee. I don't feel like there's anything metal in there, or there's anything different, and if you hold one of those joints in your hands, they're real heavy. But I don't feel it at all. . . . In fact, it feels more steady than [the other] leg, to stand on it. Many wished they had seen an actual model. One preoperative participant had, but only after asking the surgeon to show it to her. Another asked his surgeon whether the operation would be videotaped so that he could watch it later.

Questions Participants Had About the New Knee

- What is it made of?
- How long will it last?
- What if the implant wears out?
- Is it heavy?
- Can I get through airport security?
- Do they use the original kneecap?
- Can I kneel on it?
- Will I sink if I go swimming?

Hurting and hoping. During the recovery period patients were in pain, and they hoped that regaining lost function would make it worthwhile.

Hurting: pain is the thing. Pain was a prevalent theme. Preoperatively, participants anticipated postsurgical pain; as one said, "The pain is the main thing with the knee." They expressed the hope that adequate analgesia would be given; some discussed pain management preoperatively with the surgeon or anesthesiologist. One quoted her anesthesiologist's advice to take pain medications at regular intervals rather than as needed, "because if you let that pain get ahold of you, it is really hard to get rid of." Another's physician had said, "Take pain medicine when I tell you to take it and you won't hurt."

Many preoperative participants said that postoperative pain was inevitable and that they would endure it.

> I don't care how much pain medicine you give—it's still going to hurt. The pain medicine's going to wear off. And I know I'm probably going to go through . . . about two weeks of just a lot of pain. And then once that passes, the healing begins, it gets better.

All who underwent surgery reported immediate postoperative pain that was intensified by movement of the leg and by physical therapy. For some, the pain level diminished daily. Several reported being pleasantly surprised to find that they were in less pain than they'd anticipated: "I thought it would be a lot more painful than what it was. . . . I thought it would be a different type of pain." Yet others described severe, continuous pain. One explained how she would prepare someone else considering TKR for postsurgical pain.

> Even if they give you morphine, the pain's still there. . . . I think that would be one thing I would tell a patient: that we can relieve the pain afterward, but you're gonna have pain. And the pain medications will ease it a little bit, but it will never take it away completely.

Pharmacology was the primary pain management strategy—nonpharmacologic measures such as meditation, walking, transcutaneous electrical nerve stimulation, and topical application of ice were less frequently reported. Some participants' care teams advised them about pharmacologic strategies preoperatively. Some noted that nurses' postoperative strategies helped. For example, a home health care nurse advised a participant to take smaller doses of oxycodone with acetaminophen (Percocet) more often, rather than larger doses at greater intervals, with good results: "That really worked for me." Another participant said, "I feel really good in the morning because they medicate me during the night. . . . They said they should give it to me before I start to hurting real bad." But another described losing sleep because of pain and repeatedly asking for analgesia.

> I . . . just cried this morning 'cause it hurt so bad I couldn't stand it. And I couldn't get no more pills. . . . Just wish I could get a doctor in here to . . . give me something a little stronger.

Some participants worried about potential problems with analgesics (such as constipation, nightmares, becoming addicted, breakthrough pain, and reduced mental acuity), and some reported adverse effects.

Hurting: rehabilitation is work. Preoperative participants viewed the rehabilitation period as necessary to returning to normal life, saying that they knew it would involve "slow, hard work." Postoperative participants described physical therapy regimens including exercise, walking, and other measures as a necessary stage: "You have to give it time." Adaptive devices such as canes, walkers, and dressing aids (a trouser pull, for example) were used. Regular supervision was important to ensure adherence to the physical therapy program.

> My second physical therapy session in outpatient was tough. . . . They put you on your stomach and they bend your knee. . . . They try to break up the scar tissue, and push on it until you scream. . . . I know they have to do it. I know I can't do it all on my own.

Some made steady progress: "I expected to be able to get up and walk right away, and I did." One found rehabilitation to be "not as bad as what I figured it would be," as did others. But many voiced frustration over a lack of progress. How long is it gonna take? 'Cause I haven't felt like anything has changed. Everybody says it looks like it has, but I can't see that and I don't feel that.

Hoping: eyes on the prize. Participants envisioned a timeline for recovery, although the duration of the timeline varied, and some patients were more specific than others. Many predicted that they'd be independent, able to return to work, or both within three weeks. Some predicted it would take several months to a year. They emphasized the need to stay motivated during recovery: "Gotta keep your eye on the prize." They talked about pushing themselves or being pushed by providers or family members.

> Since I couldn't go outside much, [the physical therapist] told me, "Just walk." So I walk from one end of the house to the other. I try to keep walking.

Participants believed that if they didn't perform the prescribed rehabilitation exercises, their new knees would be "stiff" or painful or wouldn't bend. Some said they thought that if they didn't bend their knees as prescribed, the surgeon would "take you back to surgery and bend it for you."

> So I'm telling myself, and I'll tell somebody else, "Don't give up until you get full mobility back." Because if you don't gain it in this window of time . . . you're not gonna. You can't decide a year from now, "I'm gonna rehabilitate my knee and get more mobility." It's gone.

Many identified having a positive attitude, before and after surgery, as being necessary. One referred to this as "mind management."

Hoping: back to normal. Participants articulated specific activities they hoped to be able to perform as a result of the surgery, especially those they had been capable of doing "without having to think about it" and without pain, such as housework, gardening, and walking the dog. (For more, go to http://links.lww.com/A423) The phrase "normal human being" was often used.

> I'm going to be back out hiking and biking and doing all those things I haven't been able to do. Get down on the floor with my grandkids. I have no fear that it's not going to be good; I know it's going to be good.

Discussion

Many of our 27 participants reported delaying the surgery for months to years, despite increasing pain and limitation. Similarly, prolonged "enduring" was identified in a qualitative study of nine people in New Zealand who had had TKR surgery.[9] While our study included only people who ultimately did have the operation, their comments suggest that possible reasons for delay include the hope that the knee would get better on its own or that surgical advances would offer less drastic alternatives to total joint replacement. The latter reason echoes findings from a 1997 study of 30 people with osteoarthritis of the hip or knee, in which women were more likely than men to delay surgery because they expected that technology would improve.[10]

Once participants decided to proceed with surgery, they typically anticipated it with anxiety and felt a desire to "get it over with." Common sources of anxiety were general fears about anesthesia, surgery, and complications. Another frequent concern was their lack of information about the implant and what surgery and recovery would entail. In contrast, two quantitative surveys of patients planning to undergo total joint replacement identified more specific concerns, the most prominent of which involved postsurgical pain and mobility and the ability to care for oneself.[11,12] This discrepancy may result from the selection of items included in the quantitative surveys and the forced-choice responses they entailed. In our study, participants' responses were not so restricted.

Although we conducted the preoperative interviews after patients had met with their surgeons and attended the hospital's joint-replacement class, our findings strongly suggest that patients wanted more information. But does additional information improve outcomes? A recent review of nine studies involving a total of 782 patients about to undergo joint replacement suggests that it does not. The researchers concluded that "there is little evidence to support the use of preoperative education . . . to improve [most] postoperative outcomes," although they said that "there is evidence that preoperative education has a modest beneficial effect on preoperative anxiety."[13] Similarly, a Swedish study found that giving patients specific information about pain management before TKR lessened their anxiety.[14] Such educational programs are increasingly common, but because they don't report on the theoretical or empirical basis for their design, the mechanisms that might explain their effectiveness remain obscured, limiting their applicability.[15,16] More research is needed. Approaches tailored to a patient's age, race, and sex may be most effective.[11,12]

Many participants indicated that they would have liked to have talked with others who had had successful TKR; those who had done so reported feeling that it was helpful. Other qualitative studies of people considering total joint replacement have described similar findings.[10,17] Further investigation into the efficacy of formal peer-support interventions—which have been effective in other patient populations (such as people with cancer[18] or diabetes[19])—for people preparing to undergo TKR is warranted.

The adequacy of participants' postoperative analgesia was inconsistent. For some, acceptable pain control was obtained with strategies such as routine dosing (rather than dosing as needed) and consultation with providers. Some comments reflected acceptance of postoperative pain, which was perceived as inevitable. Because preoperative expectations of postoperative pain and doubt about one's ability to manage it can increase pain levels,[20] effective pain management strategies should be developed and shared with patients before surgery.

Limitations. The study has several limitations. Participants were recruited by convenience sampling from one healthcare institution, and their experiences may not be representative of all patients in all geographic regions. Another limitation was a lack of control over variables (such as the surgeon, the surgical technique, and the analgesic regimen) that could influence participants' experiences. And although we attempted to encourage participants to respond candidly, the fact that we identified focus group moderators and interviewers as healthcare professionals may have altered some of the responses we received.

Further Considerations

Our study revealed four themes reflecting patients' experiences of anticipating and recovering from TKR, extending the findings of several other studies in this population.

Findings from this and similar studies suggest that patients need better education and support and highlight the role of the healthcare team, particularly nurses and physicians, in providing both. Patients aren't prepared to make the decision to undergo TKR, and they don't know what to expect in the postoperative period. Anxiety and pain, which were common before and after surgery, may adversely affect outcomes. Participants emphasized the benefits of peer support and of having competent and caring surgeons, anesthesiologists, and nurses. Descriptive and interventional studies should be conducted to evaluate strategies designed to eliminate or reduce the negative aspects of TKR (such as preoperative pain and anxiety) and promote positive influences (such as peer support). More research focusing on the patient's perspective is also needed to explore how patients' experiences influence their decisions about TKR surgery and affect their outcomes.

* * *

Ann F. Jacobson is an associate professor at Kent State University (KSU) College of Nursing in Kent, OH. Rodney P. Myerscough is a clinical psychologist at Summa Health System in Akron, OH; this study was conducted at St. Thomas Hospital, a Summa site. Kirsten DeLambo was a postdoctoral fellow at the Summa Health System-KSU Center for the Treatment and Study of Traumatic Stress in Akron at the time of the study and is now a psychologist with KSU Health Services. Eileen Fleming is the nursing research coordinator and Amy M. Huddleston is a clinical psychologist at Summa Health System. Natalie Bright was a master's-degree candidate at KSU College of Nursing at the time of the study and is now an organizational learning and performance specialist at Hillcrest Hospital in Mayfield Heights, OH. Joseph D. Varley is chairman of the Department of Psychiatry at Summa Health System.

The study was funded by the Summa Health System-KSU Center for the Treatment and Study of Traumatic Stress; the KSU Research Council; and Sigma Theta Tau, Delta Xi Chapter. The authors have disclosed no other significant ties, financial or otherwise, to any company that might have an interest in the publication of this educational activity. They thank Patty Costigan, MSN, RN, and LeAnn Speering, MS, CCRP, for assistance with data collection; Claire Draucker, PhD, RN, for guidance on qualitative methods and analysis; and Elizabeth H. Winslow, PhD, RN, FAAN, for her review of a previous version of this article. Contact author: Ann F. Jacobson, ajacobso@kent.edu.

References

1. Agency for Healthcare Research and Quality. *HCUPnet, healthcare cost and utilization project* [database online]. http://hcupnet.ahrq.gov.
2. Kane RL, et al. *Total knee replacement*. Rockville, MD: Agency for Healthcare Research and Quality; 2003 Dec. AHRQ publication no. 04-E006-2. Evidence report/technology assessment, no. 86. http://www.ncbi.nlm.nih.gov/books/bv.fcgi?rid=hstat1a.chapter.16930.
3. Ballantyne PJ, et al. A patient-centered perspective on surgery avoidance for hip or knee arthritis: lessons for the future. *Arthritis Rheum* 2007;57(1):27-34.
4. Hawker GA. Who, when, and why total joint replacement surgery? The patient's perspective. *Curr Opin Rheumatol* 2006;18(5):526-30.
5. Bonutti PM. *Improving patient satisfaction through technique: minimally invasive TKA*. Clinical counterpoints: new techniques in total knee arthroplasty and pain management; 2005 Feb 24; Washington, D.C.: Medscape and the Postgraduate Institute for Medicine; 2005. http://www.medscape.com/viewarticle/502313_9.
6. Bullens PH, et al. Patient satisfaction after total knee arthroplasty: a comparison between subjective and objective outcome assessments. *J Arthroplasty* 2001;16(6):740-7.
7. NIH Consensus Development Conference on Total Knee Replacement. NIH Consensus Statement on total knee replacement. *NIH Consens State Sci Statements* 2003;20(1):1-34. http://consensus.nih.gov/2003/2003TotalKneeReplacement117main.htm.
8. Murphy E, et al. Qualitative research methods in health technology assessment: a review of the literature. *Health Technol Assess* 1998;2(16):iii-ix, 1-274.
9. Marcinkowski K, et al. Getting back to the future: a grounded theory study of the patient perspective of total knee joint arthroplasty. *Orthop Nurs* 2005;24(3):202-9.
10. Karlson EW, et al. Gender differences in patient preferences may underlie differential utilization of elective surgery. *Am J Med* 1997;102(6):524-30.
11. Macario A, et al. What questions do patients undergoing lower extremity joint replacement surgery have? *BMC Health Serv Res* 2003;3(1):11.
12. Trousdale RT, et al. Patients' concerns prior to undergoing total hip and total knee arthroplasty. *Mayo Clin Proc* 1999;74(10):978-82.
13. McDonald S, et al. Pre-operative education for hip or knee replacement. *Cochrane Database Syst Rev* 2004(1):CD003526.
14. Sjoling M, et al. The impact of preoperative information on state anxiety, postoperative pain and satisfaction with pain management. *Patient Educ Couns* 2003;51(2):169-76.
15. Prouty A, et al. Multidisciplinary patient education for total joint replacement surgery patients. *Orthop Nurs* 2006;25(4):257-61.
16. Tribbey F. Total joint replacement program. *Med-Surg Matters* 2005;14(1):9.
17. Clark JP, et al. The moving target: a qualitative study of elderly patients' decision-making regarding total joint replacement surgery. *J Bone Joint Surg Am* 2004;86-A(7):1366-74.
18. Ussher J, et al. What do cancer support groups provide which other supportive relationships do not? The experience of peer support groups for people with cancer. *Soc Sci Med* 2006;62(10):2565-76.

19. McPherson SL, et al. The benefits of peer support with diabetes. *Nurs Forum* 2004; 39(4):5-12.
20. Granot M, Ferber SG. The roles of pain catastrophizing and anxiety in the prediction of postoperative pain intensity: a prospective study. *Clin J Pain* 2005;21(5):439-45.

Profile & Commentary

STUDY PURPOSE

In the introduction, the authors set forth the reasons *why* they conducted this study, namely that patients' subjective experiences of having a total knee replacement (TKR) are not well understood. The lack of understanding is reflected in the findings of several previous studies. Several studies found patients delayed having a TKR for a long time even though they were having considerable pain and functional limitations. Also, two studies found that after surgery, a third of the patients were dissatisfied with their outcomes. Note that the reasons for doing the study are rooted in: (1) what prior studies have found; (2) what is not yet known; and (3) facts about TKR. The goal of the study was to describe patients' experiences before and after uncomplicated TKR. The restriction to patients with uncomplicated results is important as it limits the variation in the data; patients with complications undoubtedly have very different views than patients with relatively smooth postoperative recoveries.

METHODS

How the study was done is described in a short section in the body of the report and in greater detail in the box called *More on Methods and Analysis*.

Design In the text and the box we are told that the researchers used qualitative descriptive methods with the goal of conveying what patients said in everyday language.

Ethics Review The study was approved by the institutional review boards at the university where the first author worked and the hospital where the patients were seen. An institutional review board (IRB) is a group of people appointed by a university, hospital, or other healthcare organization who are charged with the responsibility of ensuring that the rights of human subjects are protected when a study is conducted under their auspices. Federal law requires that IRBs be nationally registered.

A researcher must receive IRB approval prior to beginning a study and provide reports to the IRB about the ongoing status of the research. In reviewing proposals, IRBs consider the following information:

- How participants will be protected from discomfort and harm and treated with dignity
- How informed consent (knowledgeable choice to participate or not) will be ensured
- Whether pressure or coercion to participate in the study is completely absent
- How participants in the study will be informed about the purpose of the study, the basis of subject selection, the experimental treatments, assignment to treatment groups, and risks associated with each treatment
- How privacy, confidentiality, and anonymity will be ensured

Importantly, an informed consent document must be signed and dated by the participant or the participant's legal guardian. The informed consent document must include a statement giving the researcher access to the participant's protected health information, if that is needed to conduct the study.

Some studies, by their very nature, involve minimal risk of violating human rights, whereas others are very sensitive. Studies involving infants, children, reproductive issues, imposed pain or distress, and risks are considered sensitive, and thus the procedures of the study must be spelled out in great detail. Only individuals who are 18 years of age or older and legally competent can give their own informed consent. Parents or guardians must give consent for minors. The capacity of persons with cognitive and mental limitations to give consent is considered carefully by IRBs.

Recognizing the great diversity of studies, an IRB chairperson or committee designates a study as (1) exempt from review, (2) eligible for expedited review, or (3) requiring complete review (Office of Human Subjects Research, 2005). The criteria for exempt-from-review status are spelled out in a U.S. Department of Health and Human Services policy. If the risk is minimal, an expedited review can be carried out by the IRB chairperson or by one or more experienced reviewers. A study that has greater than minimal risk must receive full review by the entire IRB. From the exemplar article, we do not know if this study underwent expedited review or full review; we do know that it was approved.

Sample A brief demographic profile of the sample participants is provided in Table 1. Of the 27 total participants, 17 participated in preoperative focus groups, and 10 participated in postoperative individual interviews. Focus group participants were excluded from postoperative interviews to avoid having the preoperative focus group discussions influence what the patients said in the postoperative interviews. Note the inclusion and exclusion criteria used to enable full participation in the focus groups and interviews and to control extraneous influences (e.g., postoperative complications). The sample size was not predetermined; rather, recruitment of new participants was closed when no new information was being contributed (i.e., data saturation). The high percentage of white participants imposes limits on the generalizability of the findings to other racial groups.

Data Collection The preoperative focus group participants were recruited during classes on joint replacement held in the hospital; the focus groups were held immediately after the classes. The moderators, who were experienced in leading group discussions, used prompts that at first encouraged participants to say what was on their minds but subsequently asked participants to talk about more specific issues. Do look at the questions used for the focus group and the interview sessions that are provided at the online site given in the article. I would say that the questions are slightly more focused than what might be used by some other qualitative researchers. The postoperative interviews were held within 2 months of having undergone the TKR; they lasted 15 to 60 minutes. Transcripts of both the focus group dialogue and the interviews were produced to facilitate analysis.

Data Analysis The researchers analyzed the data of transcripts using the principles of qualitative content analysis. They marked sections of the data relevant to understanding the patients' experiences and perceptions with word or phrase codes that conveyed the meaning of the section or comment. The codes were then grouped into themes based on similarity of the ideas expressed. Do note that the researchers took steps to control their own preconceptions during this interpretation process by having two members of the research team independently code the data and then resolve discrepancies.

Four overarching themes comprise the findings; after reading the article and referring to notes you took, you should be able to list these themes. Under the heading for each of these themes, the researchers provide general statements portraying participants' experiences. These statements expand on the abbreviated theme labels. Illustrative participants' quotes that led to the development of each theme are also provided. Notice how these quotes give life to the more abstract overall description. This is how it should be—the linkage between the themes and the quotes should ring true; the themes should not seem forced. The researchers provide these quotes to demonstrate to the reader that the themes did indeed arise out of the data and are close to it. Each reader then makes a judgment about the credibility of the themes.

Discussion

In the discussion section, the researchers link their findings to findings from other studies. This is crucial to producing a coherent and broad body of knowledge about the issue. These authors (1) link their finding to similar finding in a New Zealand study; (2) contrast their findings to two qualitative surveys of patients planning to have total joint replacement; and (3) discuss the implications of participants' views that they would have liked more information preoperatively. To further place the findings in a larger knowledge context, the limitations of the study as perceived by the researcher themselves are set forth. Finally, clinical implications and issues needing further research are offered.

http://go.jblearning.com/brown3e

References

Jacobson, A. F., Myerscough, R. P., DeLambo, K., Fleming, E., Huddleston, A. M., Bright, N., & Varley, J. D. (2008). Patients' perspectives on total knee replacement: A qualitative study sheds light on pre- and postoperative experiences. *American Journal of Nursing, 108*(5), 54–63.

Megel, M. E., Wilson, M. E., Bravo, K., McMahon, & Towne, A. (2011). Baby lost and found: Mothers' experiences of infants who cry persistently. *Journal of Pediatric Health Care 25*(3), 144- 152.

Munhall, P. (2007). The landscape of qualitative research. In P. Munhall (Ed.), *Nursing research: A qualitative perspective* (4th ed., pp. 3–36). Sudbury, MA: Jones and Bartlett.

Neergaard, M. A., Olesen, F., Andersen, R. S., & Sondergaard, J. (2009). Qualitative description—the poor cousin of health research? *BMC Medical Research Methodology, 9*, 52–57. Advance online publication. Retrieved from http://www.biomedcentral.com/1471-2288/9/52/prepub

Office of Human Subjects Research (2005). *Basic HHS policy for protection of human research subjects*. Retrieved from http://www.hhs.gov/ohrp/human subjects/guidance/45cfr46.html/

Sandelowski, M. (2010). What's in a name? Qualitative description revisited. *Research in Nursing & Health, 33*, 77–84.

Swanson, J. M. (2001). Questions in use. In J. M. Morse, J. M. Swanson, & A. J. Kuzel (Eds.), *The nature of qualitative evidence* (pp. 75–110). Thousand Oaks, CA: Sage.

CHAPTER FIVE

Descriptive Research

When building knowledge about patients' wellness behaviors, illnesses, or caregiving situations, a useful early step is learning about the elements and features that comprise them. Quantitative descriptive studies create detailed descriptions of phenomena by obtaining structured data—that is, categorical or numerical data—about them. Structured data include:

- Measurements of physiologic states that produce a number value
- Questionnaires with choice answers that can be scored
- Observations and verbal responses that are categorized and/or counted

Often, but not always, the content of the questionnaires and scales used in quantitative research is influenced by earlier qualitative research that identified important issues.

Some quantitative data are obtained directly in numerical form (e.g., white blood cell count), whereas other quantitative data are produced by converting occurrences or behaviors from their natural form to categories or numerical values (e.g., exercise behaviors described by patients are converted into defined levels of exercise by the data collector). An advantage of quantitative data is that it can be summarized to create a concise snapshot of an experience or situation.

Natural Conditions

In quantitative descriptive research (from now on just called descriptive research), data are obtained from participants under natural conditions, with no attempt to manipulate the situation in any way—no treatment or intervention is given. For this reason, descriptive studies are classified as nonexperimental or observational designs. The aim is to capture naturally occurring variations in the features of the phenomenon being studied. After the data about the features are collected from individuals, they are summarized to produce a rather detailed, composite picture of the phenomenon. The composite picture portrays the frequency with which the elements or features of the phenomenon are present and the different levels at which they are present.

A descriptive study examined the phenomenon of hospital arrival time of persons experiencing a stroke (Maze & Bakas, 2004). Among the features examined were stroke warning signs, the decision to seek hospital care, and mode of transportation to the hospital. Data were collected from 50 stroke survivors and/or their companions in face-to-face interviews using a structured interview guide. The data about warning signs were categorized by the interviewer from what the patient said, and then the cases in each category were counted. The data about time to arrival at the hospital were quantified as minutes by the interviewer based on the information provided by the patient or companion.

The findings included the following:

1. "The most common stroke warning sign resulting in the decision to seek medical care was sudden confusion and trouble speaking or understanding speech, followed [in frequency] by sudden numbness or weakness on one side of the body" (Maze & Bakas, 2004, p. 136).
2. "Only 28.9% of patients arrived at the hospital within 3 hours of the first warning sign, with the mean arrival time for the group being 330.4 minutes (5.5 hours)" (Maze & Bakas, 2004, p. 136).

Study Variables

In descriptive research, the elements, features, or characteristics of persons, experiences, situations, or things studied are referred to as variables. By definition, a variable changes or varies from person to person, thing to thing, or situation to situation. In other words, it is not constant. In fact, most characteristics of human nature and of situations vary. Examples of variables are anxiety level, blood pressure, gender, weight, pressure ulcer rate, length of breastfeeding, attitudes toward birth control, family unity, and frequency of hand washing—quite a diverse list. To expand on one of these: Not every person on the day of surgery has the same level of anxiety;

moreover, a person's level of anxiety varies over time depending on what is happening to him or her. Thus, anxiety varies across time in a person and across persons—it is a variable. Gender is an example of a variable that usually has just two variations, that is, categories (female and male), whereas ethnic identification could have several categorical variations (Asian American, black or African American, Hispanic or Latino, white or Caucasian, and so on).

Measurement of Variables

The variables are categorized, counted, or measured; i.e., a numerical value is determined. A person's overall anxiety level at any point in time can be measured using a questionnaire with a scale that the responder uses to indicate to what degree each statement is true for him or her (see **Figure 5-1**). The scores for all the statements are then summed to produce a total score.

Measurement involves determining one or all of the following:

- Whether the variable is present or absent
- At what level it is present
- The aspects of the variable that are present
- At what level the aspects are present

Aspects of anxiety could include frequency, degree of perceived threat, physiological sensations, interference with functioning, and duration of the experience. A subscore for each of these aspects and a total anxiety score could be calculated. The devices used to measure variables are called tools or **instruments**. Commonly used nursing research instruments include rating scales, questionnaires, physiological measurement, and observational scoring.

Circle the number of the phrase that describes your experience of each statement.

My worries interfere with my ability to do my job.

Strongly Disagree	Moderately Disagree	Neither Agree nor Disagree	Moderately Agree	Strongly Agree
1	2	3	4	5

Figure 5-1 Example of a Likert Scale

In the clinical professions, healthcare providers are interested in the following information about variables of interest:

- Their level (average and range) in various populations.
  Example: How much knowledge do middle-age men have regarding the symptoms of heart attack?
- How they change over time.
  Example: How does hope fluctuate across time for women diagnosed with breast cancer?
- How they affect one another.
  Example: How does general health affect the exercise level of women in their 60s and 70s?

These interests stem from the nature of clinical practice, which uses information about expected levels, manifestations, and components to diagnose the problems of individual patients and plan preventive, therapeutic, and restorative care for them.

Good Data In quantitative research, data are considered good when the measurement of variables is consistent and true. Consistent means the measurement method obtains values that are very close to actual values across time, persons, and settings. A measurement method that consistently yields values close to actual values is described in research terms as *reliable*.

A true measurement method captures the essence and attributes of what it is intended to measure. In other words, it really zeroes in on the variable of interest and captures it in its totality. When a measurement method captures to a high degree the totality of a variable of interest, researchers say the measure is valid. As you will learn, there are ways of testing a measurement method's reliability and validity, and the results of these tests are often provided in research reports.

Reliability Measurement is not as objective as one might think in that error and inconsistency can enter into measurement at many points. Consider the clinical situation in which two nurses obtain a blood pressure (BP) on a patient with a stable BP. Assume: (1) when the first nurse meets the patient, he is standing at the doorway to the room; (2) the measurements are separated by a 5-minute interval; (3) the second nurse does not know the value the first nurse obtained. Most likely the two BP values obtained will not be exactly the same, even with digital machines. The difference is probably attributable to variations in their measurement methods more than it is to changes in the patient's BP. Differences in cuff size, improper application of the cuff, inconsistent patient body position, use of a different arm, arm position, failure to wait before repeating the measurement, and the calibration of the device used can contribute to variation in BP values. In research, differences in readings caused by the difference in measurement technique are considered measurement error because the two readings are not identical because of measurement technique as opposed to an actual difference in BP.

To the extent that the BP measurements are obtained using the correct technique each time, they will have less error and will more consistently reflect actual BP. When a measurement method consistently captures the actual value, or close to it, the measuring method is considered reliable. To increase the reliability of blood pressure measurements in research studies, researchers spell out in great detail the procedure for obtaining and recording a blood pressure measurement to ensure that all persons collecting data do so in the same way.

Specific tests of instrument consistency will be explained in detail as they are used in the exemplar study of this chapter and later chapters.

Validity When measuring something across time and persons, low reliability is not the only problem. The measurement instrument or method may fail to fully capture the essence of the phenomenon of interest. In other words, the measure does not truly measure what it is supposed to measure. Often this is because the variable is difficult to define. For instance, coping with a stressful situation is difficult to define—in contrast to blood pressure, which is much easier to define.

Conceptually, blood pressure is the pressure generated by the ejection of blood from the left ventricle into the aorta and dispersed throughout the arteries and capillaries. So, blood pressure is a combination of left ventricular ejection force, the elastic properties of the arterial system, and the location of the measurement relative to the level of the heart. The most direct measurement of blood pressure is achieved by placing a small catheter in a peripheral artery and connecting it to a transducer, which senses the pressure, converts it into a waveform, and eventually into a number value. Of course, blood pressure can also be measured indirectly by a blood pressure cuff and sphygmomanometer or nonmercury device. In most situations, indirect BP measurement captures the totality that makes up blood pressure, which is to say that it is a valid measure of what is generally defined as "blood pressure."

In everyday usage, the word *valid* means "true." This is similar to the meaning of the word when used to describe a measurement instrument. It is a true (or valid) measure if there is data supporting that it captures in essence and in full the concept it claims to represent. Over the years, a great deal of data supports the high validity of direct blood pressure measurement and the slightly lower validity of indirect BP measurement. The lower validity of indirect BP measurement is due to the fact that direct BP measurement produces accurate values under a wide range of conditions, including low cardiac output, high peripheral resistance, and patient obesity. However, indirect measurement is either difficult or inaccurate under these conditions. Thus, indirect BP measurement may be valid with some patient populations but have less validity with other populations.

The essence and features of coping are much more difficult to capture than BP. In part this is because coping is a complex, psychological, subjective response of a person over time. It has many features, contextual interactions, and manifestations, whereas blood pressure is made up of fewer, readily identified determinants that are very similar in everyone. Also, our understanding of coping is considerably less than is our understanding of BP. The result of the complexity, subjective nature, and limited knowledge of coping is that capturing its attributes and diverse manifestations is illusive.

Study participants can be asked to report their level of coping but the word itself means different things to different persons. Alternatively, the researcher could ask participants to complete a questionnaire asking them to rate various aspects of their daily functioning, emotions, thought processes, sleeping, and eating. A total coping score for each participant could then be produced to reflect various levels of coping. This measurement process sounds comprehensive and straightforward, but the reality is that the questionnaire would have to be developed carefully over time to be sure that it truly captures the many features and manifestations of coping. It would also have to be tested in various populations because it could be valid with some groups of people and not with others. It could be valid with persons with chronic pain but not with persons in a stressful marriage. In short, the measurement of coping is much more complex and much less objective than is the measurement of blood pressure. In general, obtaining valid measurements of psychological states is more difficult than obtaining valid measurements of physiological states.

Reliability = Consistency of measurement
Validity = Accurate capture of underlying concept

Psychosocial Variables Measuring psychosocial variables is much trickier than measuring biophysical variables because psychosocial variables do not exist as physical realities. Rather, they exist in the minds, emotions, perceptions, experiences, and behaviors of individuals. They also exist conceptually as varying definitions that clinicians, researchers, and theorists assign to them. Thus, psychosocial variables are both subjective and intangible. Researchers develop questionnaires, scales, and observation scoring guides to get at the features specified by a particular definition of the concept. To make questionnaires and scales reliable and valid, researchers revise develop and refine them over time, just as the indirect measurement of blood pressure was refined over the years.

To make a long story short, it takes conceptual clarity, testing, revision, and retesting to produce a valid psychosocial instrument. It is all too easy for a questionnaire to include features of another psychosocial phenomenon that is similar to but slightly different from the phenomenon it is intended to measure. For example, self-confidence and optimism are concepts that have similarities to—even overlap with—coping. If the questionnaire items are not chosen correctly and the balance of items about various features of coping is not right, the questionnaire might capture self-confidence or optimism instead of coping. Sometimes a physiological measure can be used as an indicator of a psychological state or behavior. Thus, instead of measuring a psychosocial variable by participant self-report, a physiological, trace indicator of that variable can be measured. For instance, salivary cortisol level is used as an indicator of stress (Galvin, Benson, Deckro, Fricchione, & Dusek, 2006), and serum glycosylated hemoglobin (HbA1c), which reflects average blood sugar over the past 1 to 3 months (but is heavily weighted to the past 2–4 weeks), is used as an indicator of patient self-management of diabetes (Whittemore, D'Eramo Melkus, & Grey, 2005).

Rather than explain here how researchers report validity and reliability of instruments, I explain it in the commentaries about the exemplar studies throughout the book. It is much easier to understand with specific numbers in front of you. However, you now have enough information to understand what the researcher is writing about when you read the exemplar report in this chapter.

Appropriate choice of measurement instruments + Proven measurement instruments + Sound data collection procedures → Trustworthy data

Extraneous Variables

Before leaving the topic of variables, I want to point out that when designing a study, the researcher decides which variables will be studied. Other variables may have influence in the situation but are not of interest in the particular study, and these are referred to as extraneous variables—*extraneous* meaning outside the interest of the study. Even though they are not of interest, if they influence the data being collected, they can lead to wrong conclusions. To prevent this, researchers try to anticipate these variables in advance of doing the study by eliminating or controlling them. Controlling means to isolate, eliminate, or hold steady their influence in the situation.

Let us say that a researcher is interested in studying whether women of different income levels have different levels of receptivity to TV spots about osteoporosis prevention. If the study involves collecting data from a random sample of women ages 15 to 50, age could be lurking as an extraneous variable. Thus, even though the data may be analyzed so as to answer the questions about how income influences receptivity to TV health messages, any differences found could actually be from a combination of income and age (women with lower incomes might be younger than women with higher incomes). Thus, age is an extraneous variable. It is not of interest in the study, but it may be at work in the situation (e.g., younger women may watch more TV) and could confound the findings—meaning that it confuses, or muddies, the interpretation of the results.

Recognizing this problem in advance would allow the researcher to conduct the data analysis in a way that takes the effect of age into account. To do that, the researcher could control the age variable by studying only women in a narrower age range, say, 35 to 50 years. The research question would still be about income level and responsiveness to the TV spots, but the influence of age differences would be greatly reduced. However, in the process the researcher will obtain less information; depending on the research question, this may be okay. Alternatively, there are statistical methods of analysis that could be used to control the effect of age.

One extraneous factor that always must be kept in mind is that in most studies, the participants are aware of the fact that they are being studied or that their responses will be examined in detail by the researchers. This may make them think more about issues than they would ordinarily, thus they may report problems that persons who are not in the study are not consciously aware of. Another possibility is that the questions asked on a questionnaire influence the person's thinking and change how they answer subsequent questions. Researchers try to minimize the effect of participation in a study, sometimes referred to as the **Hawthorne effect**, by considering the order in which data are collected and/or by giving equal attention to all groups from whom data are collected.

Researchers design studies so as to gain control over extraneous variables and thereby produce findings regarding the variables that are of real interest. However, the world is complex and it is almost impossible to control all the extraneous variables that are operative in a situation. Therefore, researchers often point out in the discussion section of the report any extraneous variables that were not well controlled in their study and may have influenced the findings. Moreover, as clinicians read study reports, they often identify extraneous variables that may have influenced the results—and which the researcher was not aware of.

Target Population and Sampling

Ultimately, the aim of quantitative research is to create knowledge about a specified population of people, a population being a large group of persons with characteristics in common (e.g., they all have chronic bone pain after a complex fracture of a leg bone). However, data cannot be collected on all persons in the specified population—it is not possible for logistical and cost reasons. Instead, researchers collect data about the variables from a small group of people who are part of the larger population. This smaller group is the sample; the group to whom the researchers think their findings are applicable is the **target population**.

So, data are collected from the **sample** and statistics are calculated. Even though the statistical results are based on data from one sample, they are the best estimate of what the data might be in the target population. For instance, the mean of the sample is a single-point, best estimate of what the mean of the target population is. In research lingo, we say that the population mean is inferred from the sample mean (see **Figure 5-2**).

The flaw in this method of estimating the population mean is that it is based on just one sample. We know that if the researcher obtained other samples from that same population, the mean of each of those samples would not be exactly the same, but chances are they would not vary widely. But, given the fact that data from other samples are not available, the best single-point estimate of the population mean is the mean obtained in the study.

However . . . there is a statistical way of estimating what the means of those other samples from the population might be. It is called a confidence interval around the sample mean. It is an interval with defined endpoints between which the means of many other samples from the population are likely to lie. Although it is based on the data from the sample at hand, this interval is highly likely to capture the true population mean. Thus, in Figure 5-2, there is a +/- sign indicating that the inferred population mean is an estimate and the population mean probably is not exactly that value. That is all I will say about confidence intervals now.

Importantly, for an inference from a sample to a population to be legitimate, the sample must be representative of the population. This means that the sample must be like the population; the sample must match or accurately reflect the population. Any difference could make the inference to the population invalid.

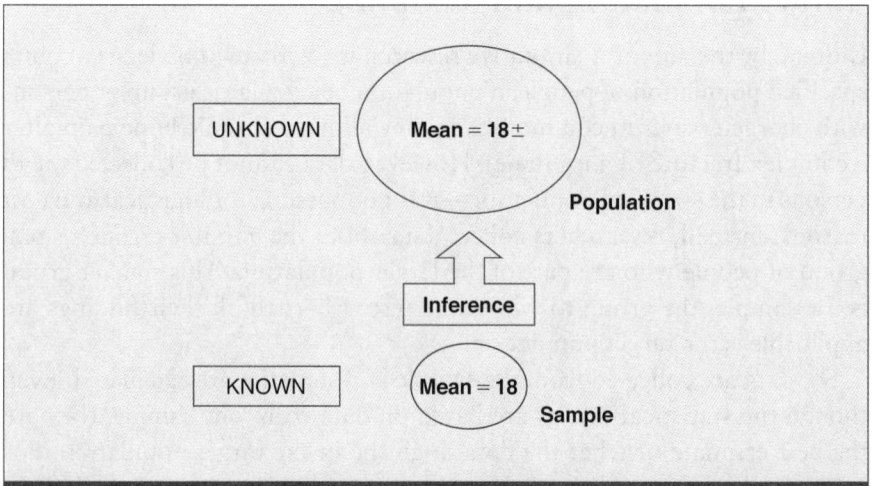

Figure 5-2 Example of Inference

Random Sampling

The very best way to ensure that a sample faithfully represents a population is to randomly select a specified number of persons from the entire population to be in the sample. *Randomly select* means that chance alone determines who is selected for the sample, thus every person in the population has the same chance of being in the sample. This is possible when a list of the entire membership of a defined population exists and a method that approximates drawing names out of a hat is used to select who will be in the sample; of course, computer programs, not names in a hat, are most often used to extract a random sample from a list. A sample that is randomly selected from a list of population members is known as a **simple random sample** and usually produces a sample whose profile is very similar to the characteristics of the actual population from which it was drawn. Generally speaking, however, the larger the sample size relative to the size of the population, the greater the likelihood that the sample will faithfully reflect the population. This method of obtaining a sample and inferring results to the population from which it was drawn is shown graphically in the top diagram of **Figure 5-3**.

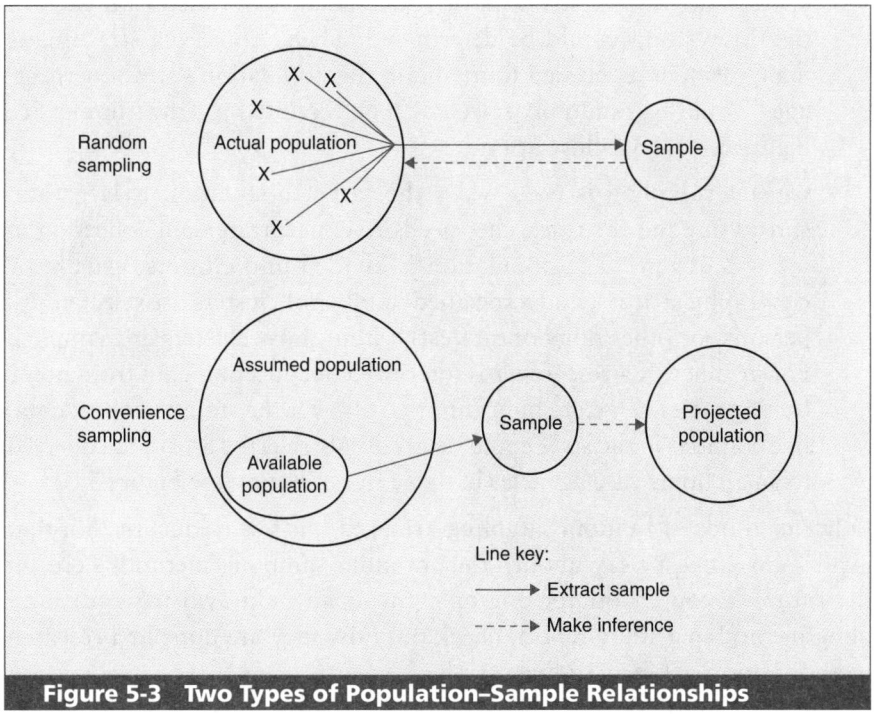

Figure 5-3 Two Types of Population–Sample Relationships

SIMPLE RANDOM SAMPLING

1. **Start with a list of all members of the actual population.**
2. **Randomly draw a sample of predetermined size.**
3. **Conduct the study with the sample.**
4. **Make statistical inferences and generalizations to the actual population.**

There are several more complicated ways of obtaining a random sample that is representative of a specified population.

- Stratified random sampling is used when the researcher wants to be sure to get data from subgroups of the population that are small and might be not be present in sufficient numbers in a simple random sample. The researcher first identifies the relevant strata and their actual percentages in the population. Those percentages determine how many persons are randomly selected from each stratum. Let us say a researcher is interested in studying psychosomatic thinking in diabetics, prediabetics, and nondiabetics and has access to a health center's list of patients. First, the percentages of persons in each of the three strata would be determined. Then, from each stratum, as many persons as needed to maintain the population's strata percentages would be randomly selected to be recruited for the sample. See **Figure 5-4** for an illustration.
- Cluster sampling is used when the target population is large and spread out and the researcher needs to concentrate data collection in a few locations. The population is divided into clusters, usually by geographical areas, and a specified number of clusters are selected. All persons (or other units of interest) within those clusters are sampled. For instance, if a researcher is interested in collecting data from home care agencies in a state but cannot go all over the state to collect data, five counties in the state could be randomly selected and data collected from all home care agencies in those five counties (see **Figure 5-5**).

Other methods of random sampling are used but less frequently. So, that is all I am going to say about other random sampling methods here. In the future if you encounter one of them or an unknown (to you) sampling method in a study report, check out how they are done in a research methods book or via an online search.

Population = 1,000 creatures

800  = 80%

200  = 20%

Sample = 120

96  = 80% (Randomly selected from the 800 mice)

24  = 20% (Randomly selected from the 200 birds)

Figure 5-4 Stratified Random Sampling

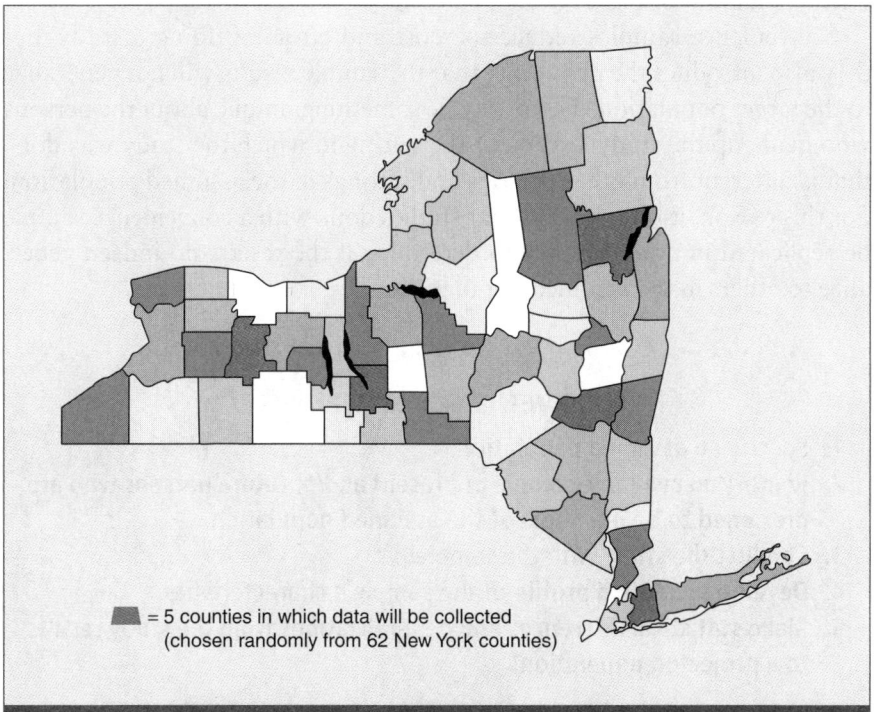

Figure 5-5 Cluster Sampling

Convenience Sampling

In healthcare research, complete lists of population members are quite rare; instead it is quite common to draw a sample from an available population. Many healthcare studies recruit participants from those available in one or two healthcare agencies. A sample extracted from an available population is referred to as a convenience sample. To avoid bias, recognized ways of selecting who from the available population will be asked to participate in the study are followed.

Convenience sampling starts with an assumed population that is defined by demographic, disease, functional, symptom, or wellness characteristics. Then, persons are identified who are (1) presumed to be in the assumed population and (2) accessible or available to the researcher; these persons may be accessible in the present or prospectively, i.e., going forward. When the study is reported, a detailed profile of the participants, i.e., the study sample, is provided; this profile becomes the basis for describing in detail the projected population to which statistical conclusions and generalizations can be inferred. Convenience sampling is graphically illustrated in the bottom diagram of Figure 5-3.

Convenience samples reduce the cost and effort of doing a study, but they also introduce the possibility that the sample results will not generalize to the target population. There may be something unique about the persons who made up the study sample or the setting in which the study was done that is different from other persons and settings in the assumed population. For this reason, it is important that studies done with a convenience sample be replicated in other settings to determine if the results do indeed generalize to others in the assumed population.

CONVENIENCE SAMPLING

1. **Specify an assumed population.**
2. **Identify an available sample of present and/or future persons who are presumed to be members of the assumed population.**
3. **Conduct the study with the sample.**
4. **Develop a detailed profile of the sample's characteristics.**
5. **Make statistical inferences and generalizations from the study results to a projected population.**

Erosion of Representativeness

An important caveat for both random sampling and convenience sampling is that even though the sample selected to be in the study may be representative of the target population, the representativeness of those who actually contribute data, i.e., the *actual* study sample, depends on a high level of consent to participate by those selected to participate and a low level of dropouts once the study is under way. Erosion of representativeness is particularly likely if those who were selected for the sample but decline participation or drop out have something in common, such as illegal immigration status, no childcare support, or language difficulties.

Finally, sampling is a broad and complex topic. The preceding explanations just touch on it. Rather than discuss it further here, various methods of obtaining samples and the consequences of those methods are discussed in the commentaries of the studies you will read in this and later chapters.

A target population can be

- **The actual population (with a random sample)**
  OR
- **A projected population (with a convenience sample)**

Sample Size

There is no easy rule for determining how many participants should be in a study. Earlier, you learned that researchers conducting qualitative studies do not predetermine their sample size; rather they stop recruiting participants when no new information is forthcoming. In contrast, researchers conducting quantitative studies predetermine their sample sizes taking into consideration several factors:

- Type of study
- The number of the variable being studied
- Statistics that will be used
- How much variability is expected in measurements
- How much difference between comparison groups is expected
- Resources available to conduct the study

Generally, the sample must be large enough that the statistics can precisely estimate the population values or determine whether differences between groups are likely to exist in the population.

Surveys

A common type of descriptive study is the survey. In surveys, self-reported data are collected by mail, Internet, telephone, or in person. Surveys are widely used because a lot of data can be collected from large numbers of people with minimal effort and expense. However, surveys are also widely misused—by persons who fail to recognize the various ways in which they can lead to erroneous conclusions (Dillman, Smyth, & Christian, 2009). The main problems in surveys are the following:

- Failure to obtain a sample that is representative of the target population right from the start
- Difficulty in constructing questionnaires and interview questions that are clear to everyone who will complete the survey
- Low response rates, which make the respondents not representative of the target population (Dillman et al., 2009)

The response rate difficulties of surveys are revealed in a study of the cardiovascular risk factors and lifestyle habits of preventive cardiovascular nurses (Fair, Gulanick, & Braun, 2009). E-mails (n = 5,163) were sent to all current and past members of the Preventive Cardiovascular Nurses Association using e-mail addresses from the membership database. A total of 1,358 surveys were completed in the Survey Monkey database, which is a response rate of 26%. The low response rate occurred in spite of the use of participation enhancement strategies such as early notification, reminders, and incentives. The authors' acknowledged the low response rate as a study limitation in their report. Unfortunately, the low response rate calls into question the generalizability of the findings to the larger population of preventive cardiovascular nurses. In fact, this level of response is not uncommon—it is even quite high—for mailed and e-mail online surveys. Surveys present considerable challenges, but when conducted properly, they provide useful information. When conducted by the inexperienced, they often produce misleading information.

Results

Percentages

Descriptive studies report results in a variety of ways. Perhaps the most common way is percentages. In a study of Australian cardiac patients' knowledge and use of sublingual glyceryl trinitrate (also called sublingual nitroglycerin), results included the following: (1) 82% of participants carried the medication with them at all times, and (2) 24.4% knew that taking the drug to prevent chest pain was an appropriate use (Fan, Mitchell, & Cooke, 2007).

Center and Spread of the Scores

To convey the typical or representative score, the mean or median may be reported. Remember, the mean is the numerical average of the scores and is the best description of group average when the scores are evenly distributed around the mean. Means are reported when most of the scores are near the mean with gradual decreases in frequency of scores on both sides further from the mean. The median, which is the variable value of the middle case, is more typical when the distribution of scores is skewed (i.e., there are a few scores strung out on *one side* toward the end of the score continuum—away from the majority).

In a study of why elderly people delay responding to heart failure symptoms (Jurgens, Hoke, Byrnes, & Riegel, 2009), the median duration of various symptoms before hospital admission was reported. The median delay reported by patients experiencing dyspnea was 3 days. The authors reported the median because there were several persons who delayed for up to 90 days, and this skewed the data toward longer delay; those few cases elevated the mean so it was not representative of average or typical persons, so the delay reported by the middle case provided a better sense of the middle of the data.

To convey the variability or spread in the data, researchers often report the range of scores (actual low score and high score) or the interquartile range, which indicates the spread of the middle 50% of scores (see **Figure 5-6**). Data with narrow ranges or interquartile ranges are less dispersed than are data with wide ranges. Sometimes data dispersion is of as much interest as is the average of the scores.

Case	1	2	3	4	5	6	7	8	9	10	11
Score	52	54	55	57	58	59	60	62	65	66	68
Quartile			Q1			Q2 Median			Q3		

[---------- IQR = 55–65 ----------]

Figure 5-6 Example of Interquartile Range (IQR)

Wrap-up: Percentages, means, medians, and ranges are widely used in reporting the results of descriptive studies. This, plus the natural conditions under which data is collected, makes descriptive studies generally easy to read and understand. Thus, a descriptive study serves as the first quantitative design to be considered.

Exemplar

Reading Tips

If you do not know what an endotracheal tube is, you will get more from this research article if you take a few minutes to obtain some basic information about it from a medical–surgical text, medical dictionary, or online search.

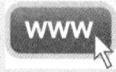

An Observational Study on the Open-System Endotracheal Suctioning Practices of Critical Care Nurses

SEAN KELLEHER AND TOM ANDREWS

JOURNAL OF CLINICAL NURSING (2008), *17*(3), 360–369.

Aim and objectives. The purpose of this study was to investigate open-system endotracheal suctioning (ETS) practices of critical care nurses. Specific objectives were to examine nurses' practices prior to, during, and post-ETS and to compare nurses' ETS practices with current research recommendations.

Background. ETS is a potentially harmful procedure that, if performed inappropriately or incorrectly, might result in life-threatening complications for patients. The literature suggests that critical care nurses vary in their suctioning practices; however, the evidence is predominantly based on retrospective studies that fail to address how ETS is practiced on a daily basis.

Design and method. In March 2005, a structured observational study was conducted using a piloted 20-item observational schedule on two adult intensive-care units to determine how critical care nurses ($n = 45$) perform ETS in their daily practice and to establish whether the current best practice recommendations for ETS are being adhered to.

Results. The findings indicate that participants varied in their ETS practices; did not adhere to best practice suctioning recommendations; and consequently provided lower-quality ETS treatment than expected. Significant discrepancies were observed in the participants' respiratory assessment techniques, hyperoxygenation and infection control practices, patient reassurance and the level of negative pressure used to clear secretions.

Conclusion. The findings suggest that critical care nurses do not adhere to best practice recommendations when performing ETS. The results of this study offer an Irish/European perspective on critical care nurses' daily suctioning practices.

Relevance to clinical practice. As a matter of urgency, institutional policies and guidelines, which are based on current best practice recommendations, need to be developed and/or reviewed and teaching interventions developed to improve nurses' ETS practices, particularly in regard to auscultation skills, hyperoxygenation practices, suctioning pressures and infection control measures.

Key Words

clinical significance, critical care, evidence-based practice, nursing practice, observation

* * *

Introduction

The ultimate goal of nursing is to provide evidence-based care that promotes quality outcomes for patients, families, health-care providers and the health-care system (Craig & Smyth 2002). While the literature has demonstrated that nurses are increasingly recognizing the role research has to play within modern health care (Hundley *et al*. 2000), it seems that many established nursing practices are not underpinned by sound evidence (Glacken & Chaney 2004). One area of nursing practice that has caused concern is the endotracheal suctioning (ETS) of intubated patients (Swartz *et al*. 1996, Thompson 2000, Sole *et al*. 2003). ETS is an important intervention in caring for patients with an artificial airway (Thompson 2000) and an essential aspect of effective airway management in the critically ill (Wood 1998b). It is an invasive, potentially harmful procedure, which when performed inappropriately or incorrectly can result in serious complications (Celik & Elbas 2000, Paul Allen & Ostrow 2000). It is important, therefore, that those carrying out such a procedure are aware of the potential risks and practice in a manner that ensures effectiveness and patient safety.

Literature Review

While ETS is an important intervention when caring for critically ill patients, the practice surrounding ETS can vary widely between institutions and practitioners (Swartz *et al*. 1996, Sole *et al*. 2003) with much of that practice based on anecdote and routine rather than research (Paul Allen & Ostrow 2000, Thompson 2000, Day *et al*. 2002b). This may partially have been influenced by a paucity of research evidence to guide practitioners in the care of a patient with an endotracheal tube (Thompson 2000). The last decade has seen a steady increase in the body of literature relating to how and when ETS should be performed (Glass & Grap 1995, Wainwright & Gould 1996, Wood 1998b, Thompson 2000, Day *et al*. 2002b, Moore 2003). Much of this evidence is in the form of succinct literature reviews (Wood 1998b, Day *et al*. 2002a) and systematic reviews (Thompson 2000) enabling practitioners quickly and easily to determine current research recommendations irrespective of their ability to interpret the research findings. Nonetheless, there is still some disparity in regard to what exactly constitutes the best ETS practice (Swartz *et al*. 1996) owing largely to a dearth of quality research on ETS techniques. While Thompson (2000), in a systematic review of the literature, isolated aspects of the ETS procedure that are generally accepted as being the most important, a lack of homogeneity and methodological flaws in some of the studies (Thompson 2000) resulted in 13 non-prescriptive recommendations for practice. Conversely, the more conventional literature reviews (Wood 1998a, Day *et al*. 2002a, Moore 2003), which are generally regarded as being less rigorous than systematic reviews (Dickson 2003), explicitly describe how ETS should be performed, but overlook the quality of the evidence from which they originate. Notwithstanding the lack of rigorous research concerning ETS practice, it is generally accepted that the ETS techniques, when used inappropriately or incorrectly can have deleterious effects on patients (Wood 1998b, Celik & Elbas 2000, Paul Allen & Ostrow 2000). It is important therefore to establish how critical care nurses perform ETS and establish how it compares with the current best practice recommendations.

Critical Care Nurses' ETS Practices

A study conducted by Swartz *et al.* (1996) used a quantitative, descriptive design using a survey method to examine 'national' suctioning practices on 80 paediatric intensive-care units (ICU) across the United States. The results indicated that suctioning techniques among critical care nurses varied and were based on a combination of nursing judgement and ward routine. Paul Allen and Ostrow (2000) report similar findings in a quantitative descriptive study which aimed to identify the closed-system ETS practices of 241 randomly selected critical care nurses. One hundred and twenty nurses (50%) responded to a mailed questionnaire. The findings indicated variations in nurses' suctioning techniques. While the results of both studies suggest that critical care nurses vary in their ETS practices, the '*ex-post facto*' focus of the studies may not necessarily be an accurate reflection of nurses' daily practice. Carter (1996), cited in Cormack and Benton (1996), suggests that the subjects' written responses to questionnaire items about how they carry out a procedure may bear little resemblance to how they actually perform it.

Day *et al.* (2002b) triangulated observation, interview and questionnaire methods to explore nurses' theoretical knowledge and practical competence in ETS. Using convenience sampling, 28 critical care nurses were recruited from three critical care wards in a large teaching hospital in the UK. The results indicated that many nurses failed to demonstrate an acceptable level of theoretical knowledge and competence in practice and that there was no significant relationship between nurses' theoretical knowledge and observed practice. Furthermore, many nurses were unaware of recommended practice and some demonstrated potentially unsafe practice. These findings are supported in the literature (Celik & Elbas 2000) and have considerable implications for the safety of critically ill patients.

The observational element of Day *et al*'s. (2002a) study ensures a more accurate reflection of what happens in practice than the descriptive retrospective studies discussed earlier (Swartz *et al.* 1996, Paul Allen & Ostrow 2000). This view is supported in the literature, which suggests that observational methods provide data on the realities of current practice from a firsthand perspective (Zeitz 2005). Day *et al*'s. (2002b) findings are, therefore, very significant as they support previous research that identified wide variations in nurses' ETS practices (Swartz et al. 1996, Paul Allen & Ostrow 2000) and that nurses are inclined to rely on personal experience and ward routine to inform practice over any other source (Sole *et al.* 2003).

Summary of the Literature

The literature search identified a paucity of empirical evidence relating to how well ETS is performed in the clinical area. The literature that does exist raises concerns about the standard of ETS practice among nurses (Paul Allen & Ostrow 2000, Day *et al*. 2002b). This evidence is predominantly American and based on descriptive, retrospective studies that focus on closed suctioning systems (Swartz *et al*. 1996, Paul Allen & Ostrow 2000, Sole *et al*. 2003). While such studies are important for describing and documenting the aspects of ETS practice, they have one primary limitation. Participants may have a tendency to misrepresent attitudes or traits by giving answers that are consistent with prevailing social views (Polit *et al*. 2001). A few observational studies addressing nurses' ETS practices are identifiable in the literature (Day *et al*. 2002b, McKillop 2004), with only one assessing how actual nursing practice is compared with the recommended practice (Day *et al*. 2002b).

The inconclusive literature relating to nurses' real ETS practices indicates the urgent need for more observational studies in this area. It is only by distinguishing between the real and perceived ETS practice that the degree of deviance, if any, from what the literature has established as being general best practice, can accurately be established.

Method

Aims

The purpose of the study was to investigate open-system ETS practices of critical care nurses. Specific objectives were to:

1. Examine critical care nurses' practices prior to, during and post ETS;
2. Compare nurses' ETS practices with current research recommendations.

Based on the evidence, it is hypothesized that critical care nurses do not adhere to the best practice recommendations when performing ETS.

Design

A non-participant structured observational design was used for this study to gain insight into what is happening in practice. Structured observational studies involve the collection of data that specify the behaviours or events selected for observation and are conducted in the participants' natural environments (Polit *et al*. 2001). Fitzpatrick *et al*. (1994) suggest that direct observation is potentially a more comprehensive method to ascertain how nurses perform in real situations and to identify differences, if any, in practice.

Sample and Setting

The study took place in March 2005 on two adult ICU in Ireland. At the time of the study, the general ICU (GICU) had nine beds with the facility to ventilate patients in all beds at any one time. The cardiac ICU (CICU) had six beds and could facilitate the mechanical ventilation of six patients. GICU employed 53 full-time equivalent nurses and CICU employed 34. The nurses were generally allocated to only one patient per shift. The targeted population of interest were critical-care nurses, as they predominantly perform ETS, while the sampling unit was the ETS event itself. Event sampling was deemed the most appropriate method of observation because of the erratic nature of the ETS procedure. By means of quota sampling, a total of 45 individual ETS events was observed, whereby each nurse performed only one event. Quota sampling is procedurally similar to convenience sampling; however, the researcher can guide the selection of subjects so that the sample includes an appropriate number of cases from each stratum (Polit *et al.* 2001), the strata in this instance being GITU nurses and CICU nurses. The sample size ($n = 45$) (51%) [was] to be a representative sample of a combined total of 87 nurses (GITU 53, CITU 34) working on both ICUs and compares favourably with previous observational studies addressing ETS, wherein sample sizes ranged from $n = 9$ (Blackwood 1998) to $n = 28$ (Day *et al.* 2002b) observations. Inclusion and exclusion criteria were maintained.

Inclusion Criteria

- Full-time ICU staff members;
- Nurses with a minimum of one-year ICU experience on the study ICU.

Participants were required to fulfil these inclusion criteria to be considered eligible for the study. This can be justified by the argument that an experienced ICU nurse from a different ICU, who has recently been appointed, may work from a different practice/knowledge base depending on the ICU he/she comes from. Equally, nurses who have minimal ICU experience may not have acquired/developed a satisfactory practice/knowledge base from which to work.

Data Collection

Data were collected using a 20-item structured observational schedule (Appendix) adapted from a previously validated survey tool (McKillop 2004), which was constructed to reflect the observable behaviours associated with best-practice suctioning of adults with an artificial airway (Thompson 2000). Aspects of ETS practice that were not specified in the observational schedule developed by McKillop (2004) but implied in a systematic review by Thompson (2000) and established elsewhere as best-practice recommendations (Day *et al.* 2002a, Wood 1998a) were added to the instrument on the recommendation of experts in critical care nursing. The observational schedule was piloted to identify practical or local problems that might potentially affect the research process. No changes were made to the instrument based on the pilot study.

All items on the observational schedule were weighted with the digits 0 and 1, or 0 and 2, respectively. The higher weighting (2) constituted adherence to the best ETS practice as recommended by Thompson (2000) following a systematic review of the literature. The lower weighting (1) represented adherence to what is marginally accepted as constituting best ETS practice as they emanate from traditional literature reviews (Day *et al*. 2002a, Moore 2003). The weighting of 0 represented non-adherence to either of the aforementioned. High observation scores represented closer adherence to recommended best practice.

Validity and Reliability

The observational schedule was distributed for appraisal to a range of experts in critical care nursing, including a university lecturer in critical care nursing, two senior nursing intensive care practitioners and the researcher who developed the original instrument. During the pilot study, the observational schedule was tested for interrater reliability using a second observer, and no significant discrepancies were identified.

Ethical Considerations

Ethical approval to conduct the study was obtained from the appropriate ethics committee, and all participants were informed that their participation was voluntary and that their right to withdraw from the study would be respected at all times. Measures to ensure confidentiality and anonymity were implemented.

Data Analysis

Descriptive statistics included frequency ratings and percentages for nominal-level data. A one-sample *t*-test was used to test the null hypothesis and compare participants' ETS practices to ideal ETS best-practice recommendations. Analysis was performed using the Statistical Package for the Social Scientists (SPSS, version 9.0) software.

Quality of Treatment

To assess how individual participants' performances and subsequently a group's performance compared with recommended best practice, a variable representing 'recommended best practice' had to be developed. This was developed by calculating the sum of the highest possible scores for each observation, which was established as being 35. Each of the 20 items on the schedule was weighted with 0 and 1, or 0 and 2 depending on the strength of supporting evidence for that particular aspect of ETS. The number 35 therefore represented perfect adherence to best-practice recommendations, or ideal treatment. The higher a participant's/group's observational score, the closer the participant/group adhered to best-practice recommendations. Similarly, the lower a participant's/group's score, the less likely was the adherence to best-practice recommendations. This additional variable was subsequently termed 'quality of treatment'. For analysis, the variable was further divided into four subscales to describe the different aspects of the quality of treatment: practices prior to suctioning, infection control practices, the suctioning event and postsuctioning practices.

Results

In accordance with the observational schedule, the results were divided into five sections: practices prior to suctioning, infection control practices, the suctioning event, postsuctioning practices and quality of treatment.

Practices Prior to Suctioning

When assessing the need for ETS, only two (12%) CICU and four (14%) GICU participants auscultated the patient's chest (Table 1). All CICU participants communicated in some form to patients about the imminent procedure; however, eight (28%) GICU participants failed to communicate in any form. Similarly, a greater number of CICU participants were observed to perform hyperoxygenation on patients prior to ETS (n = 16, 94%) compared with the GICU group (n = 22, 79%).

Table 1 Practices Prior to Suctioning

Variable	Cardiac ICU (*n* = 17)	General ICU (*n* = 28)
Patient assessment		
No	15 (88%)	24 (86%)
Yes	2 (12%)	4 (14%)
Patient preparation		
No	0	8 (28%)
Yes	17 (100%)	20 (72%)
Prehyperoxygenation/hyperinflation		
Not given	1 (6%)	6 (21%)
Given	16 (94%)	22 (79%)
NaCl (sodium chloride)		
No	17 (100%)	28 (100%)
Yes	0	0

ICU, Intensive-care unit; *n* = sample number.

Infection Control Practices

In relation to wearing gloves and an apron during the ETS procedure, there was no difference between the two groups as both were fully compliant with practice recommendations (Table 2). Disparities in practices were noted, however, in relation to hand washing prior to the procedure, maintaining the sterility of the suction catheter until its insertion into the airway and wearing goggles. Only nine (31%) GICU participants washed their hands before performing ETS in contrast to 11 (65%) from CICU. Ten (59%) CICU and eight (29%) GICU participants failed to maintain the sterility of the suction catheter prior to its insertion into the patient's airway. Only two (12%) CICU participants and one (3%) GICU participant wore goggles during the ETS procedure.

Table 2 Infection Control Practices

Variable	Cardiac ICU (n = 17)	General ICU (n = 28)
Hand washing		
No	6 (35%)	19 (69%)
Yes	11 (65%)	9 (31%)
Gloves wearing		
No	0	0
Yes	17 (100%)	28 (100%)
Apron wearing		
No	0	0
Yes	17 (100%)	17 (100%)
Catheter sterility		
No	10 (59%)	8 (28%)
Yes	7 (41%)	20 (72%)
Goggles		
No	14 (88%)	27 (97%)
Yes	2 (12%)	1 (3%)

ICU, Intensive-care unit; n = sample number.

The Suctioning Event

Both groups complied fully with best-practice recommendations in relation to suctioning time and application of pressure; however, all participants in both groups exceeded the recommended suctioning pressure of 80 and 150 mmHg (Table 3). Seven (40%) of the CICU group and eight (28%) of the GICU group selected a catheter that was larger than the recommended size for suctioning, and six (21%) GICU participants required more than the maximum number of recommended suction passes.

Table 3 The Suctioning Event

Variable	Cardiac ICU (n = 17)	General ICU (n = 28)
Catheter size		
> Half internal diameter of ETT	7 (40%)	8 (28%)
≤ Half internal diameter of ETT	10 (60%)	20 (72%)
Number of suctioning passes		
More than two	0	6 (21%)
Two or less	17 (100%)	22 (79%)
Suction time		
> 15 seconds	0	0
≤ 15 seconds	17 (100%)	28 (100%)
Suction pressure		
80–150 mmHg	0	0
> 150 mmHg	17 (100%)	28 (100%)
Suction applied during		
Withdrawal	17 (100%)	28 (100%)
Insertion	0	0

ETT, endotracheal tube; ICU, Intensive-care unit; n = sample number.

Postsuctioning Practices

Two (12%) participants from CICU and seven (24%) from GICU failed to provide post-ETS hyperoxygenation (Table 4). Only one (6%) CICU participant and two (7%) GICU participants auscultated the patients' chest to evaluate the effectiveness of the ETS procedure. The main differences between the groups were in relation to hand washing and providing reassurance, with four (23%) CICU participants failing to wash their hands after the ETS procedure in comparison to 11 (38%) GICU participants. Patients were reassured by 15 (88%) CICU participants in contrast to 11 (38%) from GICU.

Table 4 Postsuctioning Practices

Factor	Cardiac ICU (n = 17)	General ICU (n = 28)
Oxygen reconnection		
>10 seconds	0	1 (3%)
<10 seconds	17 (100%)	27 (97%)
Postsuctioning hyperoxygenation		
No	2 (12%)	7 (24%)
Yes	15 (88%)	21 (76%)
Post-ETS assessment		
No	16 (94%)	26 (93%)
Yes	1 (6%)	2 (7%)
Patient reassured		
No	2 (12%)	17 (62%)
Yes	15 (88%)	11 (38%)
Hand washing postsuctioning		
No	4 (23%)	11 (38%)
Yes	13 (77%)	17 (62%)
Safety		
No	0	0
Yes	17 (100%)	17 (100%)

ICU, Intensive-care unit; n = sample number.

Quality of Treatment

Using a frequency distribution, the average treatment quality across both groups was 22·62 (SD = 3·10) (Table 5). The quality of treatment scores ranged from 14–30. Within the subscales, the highest average score was found in postsuctioning practices (mean = 6·47, SD = 1·53) and the lowest average score was found in infection control measures (mean = 4·67, SD = 1·17). A symmetric distribution was identified in the variable 'treatment quality' and its subscales.

Testing the Null Hypothesis

To compare participants' ETS practices with best-practice recommendations, a one-sample t-test was conducted, which compared the treatment quality observed with the ideal treatment quality score (Table 6). The test identified significant differences between the quality of treatment and its subscales (representing the combined ETS practices on both units) and the perfect score (representing recommended best practice). In all categories, the quality of treatment observed was significantly lower than the quality of treatment required ($p = 0{\cdot}01$). This indicates that our study's sample group only partially adhered to best-practice recommendations when performing ETS and hence rejects the null hypothesis.

Table 5 Quality of Treatment

	Practices Prior to Suctioning	Infection Control Practices	Suctioning Event Practices	Post Suctioning	Quality of Treatment
N	45·00	45·00	45·00	45·00	45·00
Mean	5·56	4·67	5·93	6·47	22·62
Median	6·00	5·00	6·00	7·00	23·00
Mode	6·00	5·00	7·00	8·00	25·00
Standard Deviation (S·D)	1·27	1·17	1·12	1·53	3·10
Range	6·00	5·00	5·00	6·00	16·00
Minimum	2·00	3·00	2·00	3·00	14·00
Maximum	8·00	8·00	7·00	9·00	30·00

Table 6 A Comparison Between Current Practice and Best-Practice Recommendations

Variable	Maximum Potential Score (representing best practice)	Mean (actual score)	SD	*T*	DF
Quality of treatment	35	22·62	3·10	−24·63*	44
Practices prior to suctioning	8	5·56	1·27	−12·90*	44
Infection control practices	9	4·67	1·17	−19·15*	44
The suctioning event	9	5·93	1·11	−18·43*	44
Postsuctioning practices	9	6·47	1·53	−11·10*	44

*$p < 0{\cdot}01$.

Discussion

The findings from this study have raised some interesting issues relating to the current ETS practice of critical care nurses. Best-practice ETS recommendations suggest that, when performing a respiratory assessment, nurses should auscultate the patient's chest to verify the need for ETS (Thompson 2000, Day *et al*. 2002a, Wood 1998a). Our findings show that the participants generally failed to do this. Day *et al*. (2002b) reported similar findings in a study of acute and high-dependency ward nurses. Their findings showed that only two nurses were observed to have performed auscultation. Given that the majority of participants failed to auscultate lung sounds prior to ETS, it is possible that they were working from a combination of clinical signs that indicated the necessity for ETS, such as noisy breathing or visible secretions in the airway (Thompson 2000). A limitation of observational methods, however, meant that there was no way of establishing whether participants' decision to perform ETS was informed by such indicators or whether they were working from some other perspective, such as unit routine, as is suggested in the literature (Swartz *et al*. 1996, Day *et al*. 2002a). Despite abundant evidence on the negative consequences of suctioning induced hypoxemia (Wood 1998a, Thompson 2000, Day *et al*. 2002a) 17 participants still failed to provide hyperoxygenation/hyperinflation either before and/or after ETS. Day *et al*. (2002b) reported similar findings, where only two out of 10 subjects in their study were observed to provide hyperoxygenation/hyperinflation in practice. Such findings are important as they have direct implications for patient safety and reflect poorly on a vital aspect of nursing care.

Nosocomial infections are among the most common complications affecting hospitalized patients (Burke 2003). Consequently, the importance of aseptic technique in suctioning practices and hand washing before and after such procedures is strongly emphasized in the literature (Thompson 2000, Wood 1998a, Day *et al*. 2002a). Twenty-five participants in our study were not observed to wash their hands prior to the ETS procedure. Boyce and Pittet (2003) suggest that nurses do not wash their hands as expected because of the time it takes out of a busy work schedule, particularly, in high-demand situations, such as critical care units, under busy working conditions and at times of overcrowding or understaffing. One study conducted in an ICU demonstrated that it took nurses an average of 62 seconds to leave a patient's bedside, walk to a sink, wash their hands and return to patient care (Boyce & Pittet 2003). Notably, however, all participants in our study were observed to wear gloves and an apron during ETS. This may suggest a perception among nurses that wearing gloves and using a 'non-touch' aseptic technique when inserting the suction catheter negates the need for frequent hand washing. However, the literature clearly suggests that gloves do not replace the need for hand washing (Pratt *et al*. 2001). These findings support earlier studies that report modest and even low levels of adherence to recommended hand-hygiene practices (Thompson 2000, Boyce & Pittet 2003).

Another area of particular concern is the suction pressure used when performing ETS. High negative pressure can cause mucosal trauma, which in turn predisposes the bronchial tree to a higher risk of infection (Wood 1998a). Using high negative pressures does not necessarily mean that more secretions will be aspirated; therefore, limiting pressures to between 80–150 mmHg is recommended (Wood 1998a, Thompson 2000, Day *et al*. 2002a). The results indicated that participants used suction pressures outside the recommend levels for safe practice with suction pressures ranging from 230 to 450 mmHg. Participants on GICU generally used lower suctioning pressures, ranging from 230–380 mmHg, which still exceeded the recommended pressures for safe practice. Again these findings support the study by Day *et al*. (2002b) which found nurses to be generally unaware of recommended best ETS practice.

Recommendations for Education, Practice and Research

- As a matter of urgency, institutional policies and guidelines, which are not based on current best-practice recommendations, need to be developed and/or reviewed.
- Teaching interventions to improve nurses' knowledge and competence in the care of patients requiring ETS is indicated particularly with regard to auscultation skills, hyperoxygenation practices, suctioning pressures and infection control measures.
- The orchestration and implementation of effective educational interventions to change practice may be time consuming. Therefore, in the interim, it is recommended that nurses become familiar with the clinical indicators for ETS and how to perform a simple respiratory assessment on ventilated patients.
- Infection control guidelines need to be reinforced and monitored to ensure compliance.
- A regular audit of ETS practice is recommended to ensure that patient safety is being assured.

This observational study was successful in achieving its objectives; however, further observational studies need to be conducted to substantiate the findings. Observation coupled with a form of 'think-aloud' methodology may uncover the reasons behind nurses' decisions (in 'think-aloud' techniques, subjects are questioned and asked to 'think aloud' in regard to a particular aspect of their ETS practice). Such methodologies are recognized as a useful source of data collection in observational studies (Yang 2003).

Limitations

Observation, like other methods has its own limitations and ethical implications (Parahoo 1997). One of the main problems is the effect of the 'observer' on the 'observed'. This is referred to as the Hawthorne effect and is an important threat to the validity of observational research, whereby participants' knowledge of being in a study may cause them to change their behaviour (Polit *et al.* 2001). In our study, the Hawthorne effect may have resulted in participants rehearsing ETS according to evidence-based recommendations prior to the observations. This being the case, it could be suggested that participants' practice is normally of a poorer quality than the results of our study suggest.

Given the observational nature of the study, there were several aspects of the ETS procedure that could not be assessed. It was not possible to determine participants' reasons for their practice, for example, the only observable aspect of patient assessment was the practice of auscultation, and even then, it was not possible to determine what participants heard and how it was interpreted. This may have resulted in an inaccurate interpretation of some of the data.

The sample size was not assessed for statistical significance. A power analysis would have established accurate sample size requirements for the study and consequently enhanced the representativeness of the findings (Polit *et al.* 2001). The evidence used to develop the observational tool for this study derived from what might be regarded as the best evidence available at the time of conducting the study; however, there is still some disparity in regard to what exactly constitutes best practice owing to the paucity of empirical research regarding ETS.

Finally, while the study was conducted on two different ICUs, they were both part of one institution. The findings therefore may not be representative of the general population of ICU nurses and threatens the external validity of the findings. This could have been enhanced by spreading observations over a range of sites, in different geographical locations.

Conclusion

This study supports the general finding in the literature that nurses adhere only partially to best-practice recommendations in relation to ETS (Celik & Elbas 2000, Paul Allen & Ostrow 2000, Day et al. 2002b). Under the code of professional practice, nurses are obliged to ensure patient safety and expected by the public and their employer to provide high-quality, efficient, well-executed and appropriate care of individuals (Huber 2000). By failing to adhere to what the literature has established as best ETS practice, nurses fall short of fulfilling any of the aforementioned expectations.

Despite an increased uptake in postregistration education among critical care nurses and a heightened interest in the expansion of their role, the literature indicates that they remain poor at many of the aspects of care that might be considered basic. Nurses need to assess and improve their current practices continually to guarantee that evidence-based practice recommendations are being adhered to and patient safety is being assured. This can only be achieved when nurses become more aware of their professional responsibilities and receive adequate support in practice.

Acknowledgement

We would like to acknowledge the advice of a statistician Itai Beerei, University College Cork.

Contributions

Study design: SK and manuscript preparation; SK, TA.

References

1. Blackwood B (1998) The practice and perception of intensive care staff using the closed suctioning system. *Journal of Advanced Nursing* **28**, 1020–1029.
2. Boyce J & Pittet D (2003) Guideline for hand hygiene in health-care settings. Recommendations of the Healthcare Infection Control Practices Advisory Committee and the HICPAC/SHEA/ APIC/IDSA Hand Hygiene Task Force Morbidity and Mortality Weekly Report. *Centers for Disease Control and Prevention* **51**(RR16), 1–44.
3. Burke J (2003) Infection control—a problem for patient safety. *The New England Journal of Medicine* **348**, 651–656.
4. Celik S & Elbas N (2000) The standard of suction for patients undergoing endotracheal intubation. *Intensive and Critical Care Nursing* **16**, 191–198.
5. Cormack D & Benton D (1996) (ed) *The Research Process in Nursing*, 3rd edn. Oxford Blackwell Science, pp. 357–372.
6. Craig J & Smyth R (2002) *The Evidence based Practice Manual for Nurses*. Churchill Livingstone, London.
7. Day T, Farnell S & Wilson-Barnett J (2002a) Suctioning: a review of current research recommendations. *Intensive and Critical Care Nursing* **18**, 79–89.
8. Day T, Farnell S, Haynes S, Wainwright S & Wilson-Barnett J (2002b) Tracheal suctioning: an exploration of nurses' knowledge and competence in acute and high dependency ward areas. *Journal of Advanced Nursing* **39**, 35–45.
9. Dickson R (2003) Systematic reviews. In *Achieving Evidence Based Practice. A Handbook for Practitioners* (Hamer S & Collinson G eds.). Balliere Tindall, London.
10. Fitzpatrick JM, While AE & Roberts JD (1994) The measurement of nurse performance and its differentiation by course of preparation. *Journal of Advanced Nursing* **20**, 761–768.
11. Glacken M & Chaney D (2004) Perceived barriers and facilitators to implementing research findings in the Irish practice setting. *Journal of Clinical Nursing* **13**, 731–740.
12. Glass CA & Grap MJ (1995) Ten tips for safer suctioning. *American Journal of Nursing* **5**, 51–53.

13. Huber D (2000) Leadership and Nursing Care Management, 2nd edn. Saunders, Philadelphia.
14. Hundley V, Milne J, Leighton-Beck L, Graham W & Fitzmaurice A (2000) Raising research awareness among midwives and nurses: does it work? *Journal of Advanced Nursing* **31**, 78–88.
15. McKillop A (2004) Evaluation of the implementation of a best practice information sheet: tracheal suctioning of adults with an artificial airway. *Joanna Briggs Institute Reports* **2**, 293–308.
16. Moore T (2003) Suctioning techniques for the removal of respiratory secretions. *Nursing Standard* **18**, 47–53.
17. Parahoo K (1997) Nursing research, principles, process and issues, Palgrave Macmillan: London.
18. Paul Allen J & Ostrow L (2000) Survey of nursing practices with closed system suctioning. *American Journal of Critical Care* **9**, 9–17.
19. Polit D, Beck C & Hungler B (2001) *Essentials of Nursing Research. Methods, Appraisal and Utilization*, 5th edn. Lippincott, Williams and Wilkins, Philadelphia.
20. Pratt RJ, Pellowe C, Loveday HP, Robinson N & Smith GW (2001) The epic project: developing national evidence based guidelines for preventing health care associated infections. Phase 1: guidelines for preventing hospital acquired infections. *Journal of Hospital Infection* **47**, S1–S82.
21. Sole M, Byers J, Ludy J, Zhang Y, Banta C & Brummel K (2003) A multisite survey of suctioning techniques and airway management practices. *American Journal of Critical Care* **12**, 220–232.
22. Swartz K, Noonan D & Edwards-Beckett J (1996) A national survey of endotracheal suctioning techniques in the pediatric population. *Heart and Lung: The Journal of Acute and Critical Care* **25**, 52–60.
23. Thompson L (2000) Suctioning adults with an artificial airway. A systematic review. *The Joanna Briggs Institute for Evidence Based Nursing and Midwifery*. Systematic Review No. 9.
24. Wainwright S & Gould D (1996) Endotracheal suctioning in adults with severe head injury: a literature review. *Intensive and Critical Care Nursing* **12**, 303–308.
25. Wood C (1998a) Can nurses safely assess the need for endotracheal suction in short term ventilated patients, instead of using routine techniques? *Intensive and Critical Care Nursing* **14**, 170–178.
26. Wood C (1998b) Endotracheal suctioning: a literature review. *Intensive and Critical Care Nursing* **14**, 124–136.
27. Yang SC (2003) Reconceptualizing think aloud methodology: refining the encoding and categorizing techniques via contextualized perspectives. *Computers in Human Behaviour* **19**, 95–115. Available at: http://www.elsevier.com/locate/comphumbeh (accessed 11 January 2005).
28. Zeitz, K (2005) Nursing observations during the first 24 hours after a surgical procedure: what do we do? *Journal of Clinical Nursing 14*, 334–343.

Appendix: Observational Schedule

Practices Prior to Suctioning

1: Patient assessment
Did the nurse auscultate the patient's chest before ETS?
0 = No
2 = Yes (Wood 1998a, Thompson 2000, Day *et al.* 2000)

2: Patient preparation
Did the nurse explain to/communicate with the patient about the procedure?
0 = No
2 = Yes (Wood 1998a, Thompson 2000, Day *et al.* 2000)

3: Presuctioning hyperoxygenation/hyperinflation
0 = Not given
2 = Given by means of manual resuscitation bag/given by ventilator (Thompson 2000, Day *et al.* 2000)

4: Sodium chloride instillation
0 = Yes
2 = No (Wood 1998a, Thompson 2000, Day *et al.* 2000)

Injection Control Practices

5: Hands are washed prior to suctioning
0 = No
2 = Yes (Wood 1998b, Thompson 2000, Day *et al.* 2000)

6: Gloves are worn
0 = No
2 = Yes (Wood 1998a, Thompson 2000, Day *et al.* 2000)

7: Apron is worn
0 = No
1 = Yes (Wood 1998a, Day *et al.* 2000)

8: Sterility of suction catheter maintained until inserted into airway
0 = No
2 = Yes (Wood 1998a, Thompson 2000, Day *et al.* 2000)

9: Goggles/face mask worn
0 = No
2 = Yes (Wood 1998a, Thompson 2000, Day *et al.* 2000)

The Suctioning Event

10: Size of suction catheter .....
Size of ETT .....
0 = > Half of the internal diameter of ETT

2 = ≤ Half of the internal diameter of ETT (Wood 1998a, Thompson 2000, Day *et al.* 1998)

11: Number of suction passes .....
0 = > 2
1 = < 2 (Thompson 2000)

12: Length of time suction applied to airway
0 = More than 15 seconds
2 = Less than 15 seconds (Wood 1998a, Thompson 2000, Day *et al.* 2000)

13: Level of suction pressure
0 = < 80 mmHg/ > 150 mmHg
2 = 80–150 mmHg (10·6–20 kPa) (Thompson 2000, Day *et al.* 2000)

14: Position of catheter when suction applied
0 = suction applied during insertion
2 = suction applied during withdrawal from airway only (Thompson 2000, Day *et al.* 2000)

Postsuctioning Practices

15: Patient reconnected to oxygen
0 = > 10 seconds post suctioning
1 = within 10 seconds post suctioning (Day *et al.* 2000)

16: Postsuctioning hyperoxygenation/hyperinflation
0 = Not given
2 = Given by means of manual resuscitation bag/ventilator (Wood 1998a, Thompson 2000, Day *et al.* 2000)

17: Post-ETS assessment
Did the nurse auscultate the patient's chest?
0 = No
1 = Yes (Day *et al.* 2000)

18: Patient reassured
0 = No
1 = Yes (Day *et al.* 2000)

19: Hands washed postsuctioning
0 = No
2 = Yes (Wood 1998a, Thompson 2000, Day *et al.* 2000)

20: Used catheter and gloves are disposed of in a manner that prevents contamination from secretions
0 = No
2 = Yes (Thompson 2000)

Profile & Commentary

STUDY PURPOSE

Two specific objectives are stated. The one that dominates the report is to compare critical care nurses' ETS practices with current research recommendations. The researchers go a step beyond comparative description to hypothesize that critical care nurses do not adhere to a high level of best-practice recommendations for open-system ETS.

The adjective "open-system" is important because there are two different systems for suctioning the ET tubes of patients on mechanical ventilators: open and closed systems. Briefly, open systems require disconnecting the ET tube from the ventilator to allow suctioning, whereas closed systems allow the ET tube to stay connected to the ventilator during suctioning. Even as of 2012, neither system has been demonstrated to be superior to the other. There are clinical advantages and disadvantages to both systems. This study examined only open-system practices.

In the review of research that was done (studies prior to 2005), the authors note that most of the studies asked nurses about their ETS practices, as opposed to actually observing them perform ETS. The lack of reference to more recent studies is due in part to the lag in bringing this study to print. The data for this study were collected in 2005, the article was submitted in 2006, and the article was published in 2008. Unfortunately, lag is not uncommon. However, nurses practicing in critical care tell me that today's standards for ETS suctioning adults have not changed appreciably from those used in the study.

DESIGN

"A non-participant structured observational design was used . . ." Structured observation means they used a set of prespecified action statements to structure what they would observe; the actions either were or were not performed. The word *nonparticipant* indicates that the researcher did not participate in any of the nursing care actions and did not intervene in any way (unless of course there was a distinct danger posed to the patient) but simply assumed the role of an onlooker (Kelleher, Sean, personal communication, February 25, 2010).

Sample

The projected target population could be considered the suctioning practices of nurses working in general ICUs and cardiac ICUs who work full time and have a minimum of 1 year of experience in the ICU. More narrowly, it could be considered the practices of full-time nurses with a minimum of 1 year of experience working in the general ICUs and cardiac ICUs of Irish hospitals. Even more narrowly, the target population could be considered other experienced nurses working in the GICU and CICU of one hospital. Using the middle definition of the projected population, the suction practices found in this study would be expected to generalize to, i.e., be true of, other experienced nurses working in critical care units in Ireland.

The 45 nurses who were observed performing an ET suctioning event for the study were selected using quota sampling, which is a form of convenience sampling; it has a goal of obtaining a sample with characteristics that are in proportion to how the characteristics exist in the population. Thus, the percentages of nurses observed from each of the two units were similar to their actual percentages in the setting. Quota sampling starts like stratified sampling, which was described earlier, but after the percentage needed from each group is determined, the actual participants are selected by convenience, not by random sampling as is the case with stratified sampling. The characteristics of the setting are described, which helps envision the projected population to whom the results could apply.

ASSUMED POPULATION: ET open-system practices of critical care nurses in Ireland

SAMPLE: ET open-system actions of 45 full-time nurses with at least 1 year of ICU experience in a general and a cardiac ICU in one hospital in Ireland

PROJECTED POPULATION: ET open-system action of experienced, critical care, Irish nurses who are assigned to only one patient during their shifts

Measurement

The observation instrument used to observe and record observed events was an adaptation of a previously validated survey tool. The adaptation involved adding several actions not in the original tool; the added actions were based on more recent research findings and best-practice recommendations. A pilot study of the observational schedule was conducted and the interrater reliability of the instrument was checked: "no significant discrepancies were identified." Presumably, this means that the level of agreement between two raters in scoring was at least 80%. When two or more observers are using a scoring instrument, it is important that they are in sync; that is, they score the same events in the same way. If they do not, the data will not be good because it is inconsistent, i.e., it is dependent on who did the scoring. Eighty percent is considered the minimally acceptable level of agreement that must be established between two raters.

Looking at the tool itself (in *Appendix: Observation Schedule* of the exemplar), you can see that the 20 specific actions observed were grouped in four sequentially ordered categories. In observing an ETS event, the rater marked *Yes* or *No* (or another choice of two answers) for each action, thus indicating whether or not the action was performed according to the best practice standard; the higher number represents best practice. Note that the actual numerical value associated with a Yes or No answer varied from zero to two; the authors provide a rationale for assigning the numerical values they did to actions. In addition to calculating scores for each of the four categories, an overall quality score was calculated by summing the scores from all the items.

Ethical Considerations

The study was reviewed and approved by the ethics committee at the hospital where the study was conducted. Written consents were most likely obtained from the participating nurses. This study could be viewed as sensitive as the nurses asked to participate might worry that their suctioning technique might be reported to their nurse manager; steps would have to be put in place to prevent this and assurances provided to the nurses asked to participate.

Descriptive Results Descriptive statistic results for the four sections of actions by the two groups of nurses are reported first in Tables 1 through 4. To those familiar with suctioning standards, these tables may be quite straightforward, but for those who are not familiar with them, it may not be obvious whether Yes or No represents the standard. For instance, for most answers, Yes represents the best practice standard, but for NaCl instillation, No represents the standard. Also, the answer representing the standard for catheter size, suction time, and suction pressure may not be obvious to all readers (including me). To make the answer representing the standard clear in Tables 1 through 4, I went through and put an asterisk beside each answer that represented the standard; I determined the standard from the scoring provided in *Appendix: Observation Schedule*. This made it easy to identify practice standards that were met at low levels. Sizeable discrepancies between best practice and actual actions occurred for many actions, particularly presuctioning assessment, pre–hand washing, catheter sterility, goggles, catheter size, postassessment, and post–hand washing.

In Table 5 the data of the two groups of nurses are combined and descriptive statistics for the overall quality of treatment and the four sections are set forth. For explanatory purposes, I want to focus just on the overall Quality of Treatment results. The mean Quality of Treatment was 22.6 out of an ideal of 35. Right off you know that the practice of the sample observed in this study fell considerably short of best practice. You can see that the highest total quality score was 30 and the lowest was 14. The fact that the mean, median, and mode for overall quality are close to one another indicates that the scores were approximately normally distributed around the mean. Note that you have to be careful in comparing the mean scores for the four section mean scores because in the appendix you will note that the section *Practices Prior to Suctioning* had eight possible points, whereas the other three sections had nine possible points. (This is a good illustration of how you have to read data quite carefully; superficial reading can lead to wrong conclusions.)

Hypothesis Testing Results In Table 6, we see that the researchers went a step further than just providing descriptive statistics about the data; they tested the hypothesis that they stated earlier: critical care nurses do not adhere to the best practice recommendations when performing ETS. They compared Best Practice scores to the actual scores in their sample. They were interested in determining if the actual scores attained could just be the means of this sample of suction events, even though the target population mean actually is 35 for the overall Quality of Treatment, and 8, 9, 9, and 9 for the sections, respectively. In other words, could the sample scores just be expected variations from 35, 8, 9, and 9?

T-tests were run comparing each sample score to the maximum possible. For instance, a *t*-test was run to determine if the sample Quality of

Treatment mean of 22.62 is just a sampling variation on a population mean of 35; the result was $t = -24.63$, $p < 0.01$.[1]

P-value Interpretation Because this is your first introduction to *p*-value results in this book, a few words of review might be helpful. Remember from your statistics course that when comparing the means of two samples drawn from the same population, it is not expected that the means will be identical—some variation is expected because the data are not from identical samples. But both means would be expected to be reasonably close to the population mean but not identical to it. When comparing two means, the question is: Are they truly different or is the difference what we would expect from different samples around the same mean? Statistical analysis answers this question.

To illustrate expected variation, if you selected two simple **random samples** (n = 50 in each group) from a list of 200 healthy 28–34-year-old soccer players, one sample might have a mean heart rate of 68.1, the other sample a mean heart rate of 66.9. A *t*-test run to determine if the two means are just chance variation or a true difference in the heart rates of the two groups might produce results of $t = 1.5$, $p = 0.137$. (The **p value** is what is important, not the *t*-value by itself.) This result means that there are about 14 chances in 100 that the difference between these means is just a chance variation. From a statistical perspective that is a high probability and would lead the researcher to conclude that there is a higher than acceptable probability that the difference is not a true difference between the two groups; it very well could be due to expected variation from sample to sample.

p value = probability that the difference in the means being compared is just chance variation

[1]An aside for the observant reader: You might wonder what it means that the *t*-tests were negative. A *t*-test's sign indicates the direction of the difference found; that is, which group had the higher score. It is determined by how the calculation was set up, but we do not need to know how it was set up because the table clearly indicates what the Best Practice scores and the mean scores of the sample are for each variable—we know which was higher. Most often, *t*-values are reported as the absolute value of the *t*-value given by the statistical program and the scores being compared are explicitly indicated.

When the researcher wants to decide if a difference found between two means is a true difference, not a chance one, the researcher wants to have confidence in his conclusion. So he sets a cap on his chances of making a wrong conclusion when he calls the difference a true difference. He does this by prespecifying the probability of being wrong that he is willing to accept; this prespecified cap is called the level of significance and is expressed as a *p*-level (often at $p = 0.05$ or $p = 0.01$). It is also referred to as ((alpha). By setting the maximally acceptable *p*-level at 0.05, the researchers is saying that when calling the difference a true difference, he is willing to accept up to 5 chances in 100 (or 1 in 20) of being wrong. A probability over that carries too high a chance that the difference is just due to random variation.

If a data-based *p*-value is equal to or less than the prespecified *p*-level, it indicates that the difference found has a low probability of being just a chance difference. Such a result is considered statistically significant and will lead the researcher to conclude that the two means are most likely truly different. In contrast, a *p*-value higher than the prespecified *p*-level indicates a high probability that the difference found is just a chance variation. This statistical result will lead the researcher to conclude that the difference found in the two means could be chance variation, and therefore he concludes that the difference found is probably not a true difference. For a graphical display of this explanation, see **Figure 5-7**.

Importantly, a true difference means that a difference is likely to be found in the target population. Ultimately, learning whether a difference is likely in the target population is why research is conducted. It is conducted using sample data, but the end goal is knowledge about how things are or what would happen in the target population.

In the *t*-test result in the exemplar study, for overall quality of the treatment, $t = -24.63$, $p < 0.01$. This is a statistically significant result because

***p*-level result**	<.001	.01	.025	**.05**	.08	.15	.59>
Finding	Significant difference				Nonsignificant difference		
Conclusion	A difference would likely be found in the population.				A difference would *not* likely be found in the population.		

Figure 5-7 Interpretation of p-values by t-tests

the data-based p-value is lower than the level of significance p-level (it is not clear if that is 0.05 or 0.01). This result indicates that the best practice score and the mean of the sample are truly different. The sample score of 22.62 is not a sample variation on the best practice score of 35. The hypothesis that critical care nurses do not adhere to best practice recommendations when performing ETS was supported (for overall quality and all four subcategories of practice). The conclusion is that in the population, the overall quality of ET open-system suctioning most likely falls short of best practice standards; this is also true for each of the section practices. Intuitively, we probably knew when we looked at the descriptive statistics what the finding and the conclusion regarding the hypothesis testing would be because the difference between the sample mean and the ideal mean was so large. The p-value obtained, < 0.01, confirmed our intuition.

Discussion

In this section, the researchers discuss the shortcomings in practice that are likely to have serious ramifications for patients' well-being. Recommendations based on the findings are also offered. Among the limitations of the study is the fact that the nurses knew they were being observed, so they may have used their best technique (the Hawthorne effect); this led the researchers to the inference that unobserved technique may be of even lower quality.

Another limitation is that the 45 observed events of ETS practice were made in one hospital and therefore may not represent practice in other settings. This limitation is called limited **generalizability**. It reflects that one cannot be confident that the findings can be viewed as representing settings that are dissimilar from the one in which the study was done. However, other studies in other countries have also found only partial adherence to best-practice recommendations for ETS. Thus, although these findings are from one particular setting, they contribute to a larger body of knowledge about ETS practice.

http://go.jblearning.com/brown3e

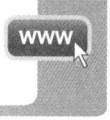

References

Dillman, D. A., Smyth, J. D., & Christian, L. M. (2009). *Internet, mail, and mixed-mode surveys: The tailored design method* (3rd ed.). New York, NY: John Wiley.

Fair, J. M., Gulanick, M., & Braun, L. T. (2009). Cardiovascular risk factors and lifestyle habits among preventive cardiovascular nurses. *Journal of Cardiovascular Nursing, 24*, 272–286.

Fan, M. I., Mitchell, M., & Cooke, M. (2007). Cardiac patients' knowledge and use of sublingual glyceryl trinitrate (SLGTN). *Australian Journal of Advanced Nursing, 26*(3), 32–38.

Galvin, J. A., Benson, H., Deckro, G. R., Fricchione, G. L., & Dusek, J. A. (2006). The relaxation response: Reducing stress and improving cognition in healthy aging adults. *Complimentary Therapies in Clinical Practice, 12*(3), 186–191.

Jurgens, C. Y., Hoke, L., Byrnes, J., & Riegel, B. (2009). Why do elders delay responding to heart failure symptoms? *Nursing Research, 58*(4), 274–282.

Kelleher, S., & Andrews, T. (2008). An observational study on the open-system endotracheal suctioning practices of critical care nurses. *Journal of Clinical Nursing, 17*(3), 360–369.

Maze, L. M., & Bakas, T. (2004). Factors associated with hospital arrival time for stroke patients. *Journal of Neuroscience Nursing, 36*(3), 136–141.

Whittemore, R., D'Eramo Melkus, G., & Grey, M. (2005). Metabolic control, self-management and psychosocial adjustment in women with type 2 diabetes. *Journal of Clinical Nursing, 14*(2), 195–203.

CHAPTER SIX

Correlational Research

Once qualitative and descriptive studies have provided knowledge about the variables at work in a health situation, researchers and clinicians naturally start asking questions about how the variables are related and how they influence one another. Questions such as: Is there a relationship between size of a family's social support network and their teenagers' emotional and social development? Is spousal or partner support associated with diabetics' self-care practices and blood sugar control? Are hearing loss and osteoporosis related? Do lung capacity levels predict exercise capacity? In general terms, these questions ask, "Are variable *X* and variable *Y* related?" These questions go beyond description of each variable separately to examine the relationship between them. They are the kinds of questions that can be answered by **correlational research**.

Relationship

Just what does this word *relationship* mean in the research context? In simplest terms, relationship describes a connection between variables—two variables are connected when a change in one is associated with a change in the other. The change has two dimensions—direction and strength. The direction of change can be in the same direction or in opposite directions. In a positive relationship, as one variable's values increase, the other's values also increase. In a negative relationship, as one variable's values increase, the other's values decrease.

A relationship can also be characterized as strong, moderate, or weak, indicating the strength of the relationship between the two variables. A relationship is strong when (1) persons who score high on variable *A* also score high on variable *B*, (2) persons who score low on variable *A* also score low on variable *B*, and (3) those who score intermediate on variable *A* also score intermediate on variable *B*. By contrast, a weak relationship exists when (1) persons who score high on variable *A* have assorted scores (high, medium, and low) on variable *B*, and (2) persons who score low on variable *A* have assorted scores on variable *B*. In other words, the relationship is weak when there is very little connection between scores on *A* and scores on *B*. The opposite of relationship is *independence*, meaning that there is no connection between scores on the two variables.

Measuring Relationship

Statistical Perspectives on Relationship

The direction and strength of a relationship between two variables are quantified using one of several statistical tests. The actual statistic used depends on the scale that was used to quantify the variables. When both variables were measured on an interval level scale, the Pearson *r* coefficient is used; it is the most widely used **correlation** statistic (Burns & Grove, 2009). An interval level scale is a measurement scale with a range of numerical values having equal distance between them, such as degrees on a thermometer or pounds on a weight scale. If either or both of the variables are measured using an ordered set of categories, for example, low, medium, or high, the Pearson *r* coefficient is not used; rather another correlation coefficient would be used. There are several, but they all are interpreted similarly to how the Pearson *r* is interpreted.

The value of the Pearson *r* statistic varies from −1 to +1, which means that it can be −1, a negative decimal, zero, a positive decimal, or +1. The sign indicates whether the two variables have a positive or negative relationship; if positive, they move in the same direction (as one goes up, the other goes up); if negative, they move in opposite directions (as one goes up, the other goes down). The closer the value is to −1 or +1, the stronger the relationship between the two variables. Zero means the two variables are completely independent of one another, and a value close to zero indicates a very weak relationship.

	Interpretation of *r*						
***r* Value**	- 1	-0.8	-0.5	0	+0.6	+0.8	+1
Relationship	perfect negative	strong neg	moderate neg	none	moderate positive	strong pos	perfect pos

Graph Perspectives on Relationship

To illustrate relationship in the concrete, a hypothetical study (**Box 6–1**) and five possible data sets for the study are presented in the following figures (**Figures 6-1 through 6-5**). Each data set is accompanied by a scatter plot for the data, the Pearson *r* coefficient for the data, and explanations about what these two analytical tools tell us. The samples in the data sets were limited to five to make it easier to see the relationship between the two variables, although a real study would not have as few as five cases. If you are not up to speed regarding scatter plots, also called scatter diagrams, you should go back and read about them in your statistics reference text. You will not see many scatterplots in journal reports because they take up too much room, but they are helpful in acquiring an understanding of what Pearson *r* correlation coefficients mean.

BOX 6–1 Hypothetical Correlational Study

STUDY PURPOSE: To examine the relationship between hope and adaptation in persons who have had multiple sclerosis for at least 3 years.

MEASUREMENT: Hope is measured on a 1 to 5 scale, 1 = barely present hope, 5 = an abundance of hope. Adaptation is measured on a 1 to 10 scale, 1 = not adapting, 10 = adapting without problems. Note that both variables are scored on continuous scales; this is a key requirement for using the Pearson *r* correlation coefficient to portray the relationship between the two variables. If one variable is a categorical variable (e.g., gender) and the other is a continuous variable (e.g., adaptation), the Pearson *r* statistic could not be used.

SAMPLE: 5 persons

RESULTS: Several possible sets of scores are presented in Figures 6–1 through 6–5. To make the relationship between the variables stand out, the Hope scores are the same from dataset to dataset, but the Adaptation scores are different.

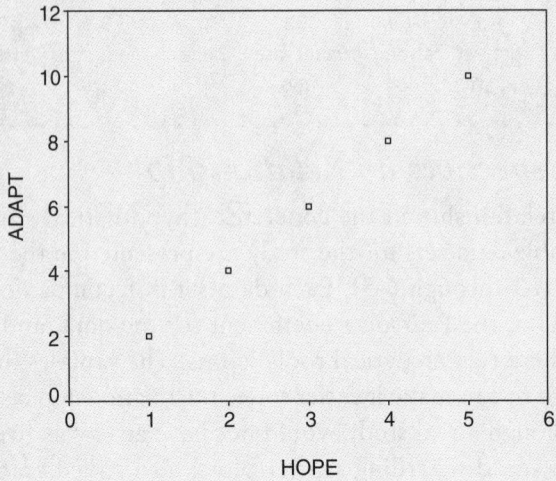

Note that for each increase of 1 point in Hope scores, there is a 2-point increase in the Adaptation scores. If you know a person's Hope score, you can accurately predict that person's Adaptation score; similarly if you know the person's Adaptation score, you can accurately predict his or her Hope score. When two variables change in lockstep with one another, we say that they have a perfect positive correlation. There is nothing magical about the 1-point Hope score to 2-point Adaptation score relationship. It could just as easily be that a 1-point change in Hope is related to a 4-point change in Adaptation.

Note that scatterplots provide the same information as the dataset table. Each point on the scatterplot represents one score. For example, the person who scored 1 on Hope scored 2 on Adaptation and has a point on the scatterplot as does the person who scored 4 on Hope and 8 on Adaptation. Because the relationship between the two variables is in lockstep, a line drawn between all the data points is a straight line.

The Pearson r statistic for this dataset is $r = +1$, which indicates a perfect positive relationship. The two variables move in lockstep with one another with high scores on one being paired with high scores on the other and low scores on one being paired with low scores on the other. The Pearson r statistic has possible values between +1 and –1.

Figure 6-1 Hypothetical Dataset 1

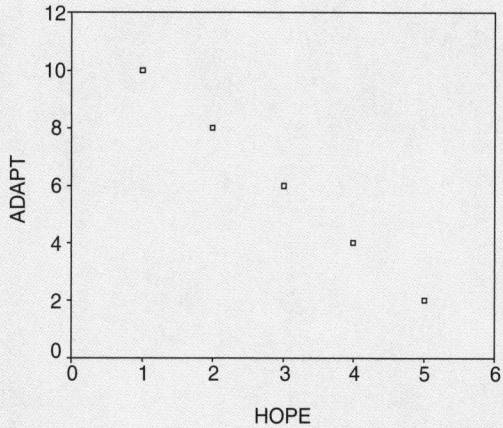

Note that for each increase of 1 point in Hope score there is a 2-point decrease in Adaptation score. Just as in dataset 1, if you know a person's Hope score, you can accurately predict that person's Adaptation score; similarly if you know the person's Adaptation score, you can accurately predict his or her Hope score. However, instead of moving in the same direction as they did in dataset #1, they move in the opposite direction. The variables in this dataset have a perfect negative relationship: As one variable goes up, the other goes down in lockstep a specific amount. Again, a line drawn between all the data points is a straight line. The Pearson r value for this dataset is $r = -1$, indicating a perfect negative relationship.

Figure 6-2 Hypothetical Dataset 2

Perfect correlations are, of course, a rare happening in the real world where variation and multiple influences are characteristic of reality, especially in the social, psychological, and behavioral realms. Instead, weak, moderate, and moderately strong correlations occur more often. These kinds of relationships are illustrated in the next three hypothetical data sets (Figures 6-3, 6-4, and 6-5).

Dataset 3

Person	Hope Score	Adaptation Score
1	1	2
2	2	3
3	3	6
4	4	9
5	5	8

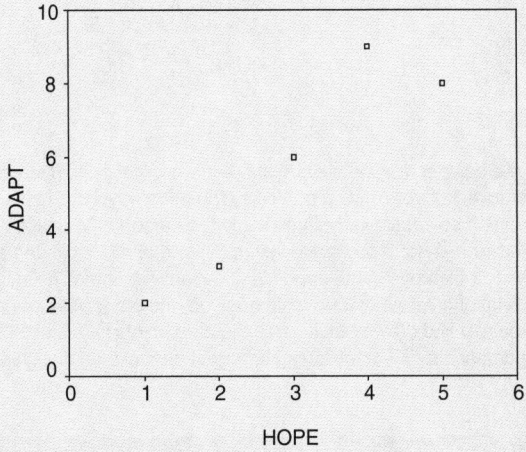

Note that an increase in Hope is roughly related to an increase in Adaptation. The two variables are strongly but not perfectly correlated. If you know a person's score on one variable, you can make a pretty good estimate of the person's score on the other variable.

A trend in the data is quite obvious, but all the data points are not in a straight line. If a straight line were drawn through the middle of the data, three data points would be on or very close to that line and two would be a bit farther away. The line is called the *trend line* and represents the middle of the data. Take a straight edge and add a trend line to this graph.

The Pearson *r* for this dataset is + .93, a strong, positive correlation.

Figure 6-3 Hypothetical Dataset 3

Dataset 4

Person	Hope Score	Adaptation Score
1	1	2
2	2	10
3	3	6
4	4	4
5	5	8

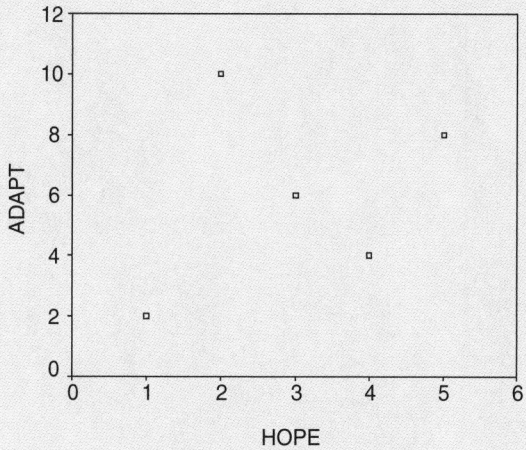

There is a bit of a linear trend in the relationship between Hope and Adaptation; as Hope scores go up, there is a bit of a trend for the Adaptation score to go up, but the relationship is weak. Any effort to base one score on the other score would have a low likelihood of being accurate.

A trend line drawn through the middle of the data would show that three data points are on or close to the trend line, but two are quite far from it. Thus, there is a trend, but a weak one. The Pearson *r* for this dataset is +.30, indicating a weak positive correlation.

Figure 6-4 Hypothetical Dataset 4

Dataset 5

Person	Hope Score	Adaptation Score
1	1	7
2	2	3
3	3	10
4	4	5
5	5	6

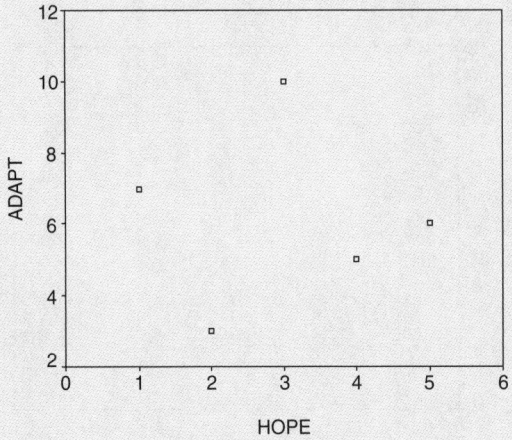

In this dataset, there is no relationship between the Hope score and the Adaptation score; the two scores are independent of one another. Knowing one score will not enable you to predict the other one.

All data points are quite far from a trend line drawn through the data. The Pearson *r* for this dataset is 0, indicating no relationship between the two variables.

Figure 6-5 Hypothetical Dataset 5

In summary, a correlation coefficient indicates the direction (positive or negative) and strength (perfect, strong, moderate, weak, or none) of a relationship.

Caveat

Importantly, a strong relationship between two variables says nothing about the underlying dynamic that produces the relationship. Even a very high correlation (near −1 or +1) does not mean there is a cause-and-effect relationship between the variables. High correlation only conveys that there is a pattern in the relationship between the two variables. The relationship between the two variables could be much more complex than straightforward cause and effect.

For instance, look at Figure 6-3 again. At first glance, the scatter plot and the Pearson r of 0.93 may seem to suggest that level of hope determines level of adaptation. However, identical data could be found if the reverse were true; that is, successful adaptation generates hope. Another possibility is that the relationship between the two variables is not a direct one. There could be another lurking variable in the background that has a strong effect on both hope and adaptation and causes them to move in concert with one another; that lurking variable could be something like prognosis or response to treatment. In any of these three dynamics, the data and the Pearson r value could be the same as in Figure 6-3. The point is this: Correlation sheds no light on the dynamic underlying the relationship—even when one precedes the other in time. Correlation only detects a relationship. The dynamics of that relationship need to be ferreted out by further research using other research designs or justified by other knowledge about the two phenomena.

Correlation ≠ Cause
(Huck, 2011)

When the relationship between ratings of perceived exertion and heart rates of young African Americans was studied in treadmill tests (Karavatas & Tavakol, 2005), the overall Pearson r was 0.58. The authors interpreted this result as a moderately strong relationship in which heart rate influences perceived exertion. This directional interpretation is justified by physiological knowledge, not by the statistical result itself.

Outliers

When looking at scatter plots, the researcher looks for outliers, which are cases that have very atypical pairings. An outlier's data point will lie very far from the trend line. Importantly, with small sample sizes, a single outlier can lower the Pearson *r* considerably. Consider the scatter plot in **Figure 6-6**. Note that most of the scores lie close to the positive correlation trend line, except for the person who scored 4 on hope and 1 on adaptation. This person's data is an outlier because it is very different from the other scores. The Pearson *r* for this data set is 0.50, which is a modest correlation. However, when this outlier is removed, reanalysis produces a Pearson *r* of 0.99 for the other four scores. The Pearson *r* calculated with the outlier in is greatly influenced because the sample size is so small; still, studies with larger sample sizes can be moderately influenced by a single outlier.

An outlier can either understate or exaggerate the strength of the relationship between the two variables, depending on the values that make up the outlier. Removing an outlier or even several in a data set, can uncover a trend that would be less clear if the outliers were left in. When researchers remove data for an analysis, they should do so with good rationale, and they should acknowledge that they did so. Removing data could be a form

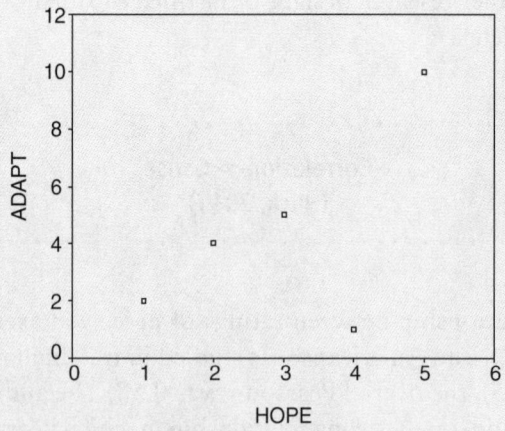

Pearson *r* for this dataset is .50, indicating a modest association.

Figure 6-6 Example of Outlier

of bias, particularly when the study has a small sample size. Sometimes, a researcher will examine outlier cases in great depth because doing so can yield valuable insights that set the agenda for future research.

Practical Perspectives on r

Even though an r of 1.00 indicates a perfect positive relationship between hope and adaptation in which the variables move in lockstep with one another, an r-value of 0.70 *does not mean* that 70% of the values of hope move in lockstep with adaptation; rather the r-value indicates the relative strength of the relationship on a scale from −1 to +1.

Huck (2011) points out that r exaggerates how strong the relationship really is between two variables. A more realistic and practical perspective is gained by squaring the value of r to produce r^2, which is called the **coefficient of determination**. The r^2 value indicates the percentage of variation in hope that is related to adaptation and the percentage of variation in adaptation that is related to hope. When an r of 0.70 is squared, yielding an r^2 of 0.49, this tells us that about half the variation in hope is related to adaptation, and half of the variation in adaptation is related to hope (see **Figure 6-7**). The other 51% of both variables is attributable to other influences. In short, r^2 provides a more practical sense of the strength of the relationship between the two variables than r itself does.

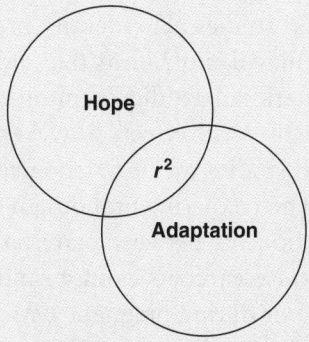

r^2 indicates the amount of variability in each variable that is explained by the other variable. The rest is explained by other, often unknown, influences.

Figure 6-7 r^2

Correlational Design

Purposes

The most straightforward correlational design is when the relationship between several variables is studied in a single group of people. The researcher measures the participants on each of the variables of interest using instruments that have been established as reliable and valid with the population under study (Brink & Wood, 1998), but no attempt is made to control or manipulate the situation. As with descriptive studies, good data are key to a good study; thus most researchers report information about the reliability and validity of the instruments they use. Analysis of the data consists of running correlational tests to determine if and how the variables are related. The analysis consists of measuring the correlation between various combinations of two variables, which is called *bivariate correlational analysis*. If there are three variables in the study, *A*, *B*, and *C*, bivariate analysis could be run on the relationship between *A* and *B*, *A* and *C*, and *B* and *C*, thus producing three correlation coefficients.

Often, researchers conduct correlational studies to explore clinical issues that are murky, such as:

- What factors influence young women's positive adaptation to having human papilloma virus (HPV)?
- What factors influence a double amputee's motivation in rehabilitation?

Some of the variables included in a study come from the hunches of clinicians practicing in the area; others come from theory or related academic work. Correlational studies help identify promising ideas for future research, whereas others may demote ideas that did not hold up.

As said earlier, correlational studies cannot by themselves establish a connection between cause and effect; however, there are times when results from correlational studies make a strong case for cause and effect. This would be the case when experimental design cannot be used, such as studying the possible relationship between maternal gum disease and infant preterm low birth weight. Researchers cannot randomly assign mothers to have gum disease prior to or during pregnancy. Moreover, if a study found a high correlation between gum disease and low birth weight, it is possible that a third factor may have influenced the development of both conditions—such as poor diet, smoking, or alcohol consumption. It would also be prudent to keep in mind that most health conditions are not caused by a single determinant and that several determinants often interact with each other to cause a condition. To make a claim that maternal gum disease causes infant low birth weight would require **cohort studies** and a credible theory regarding the causative mechanism—but a correlational study could be a starting point for examining the issue.

More Complex Designs

Most of this chapter has focused on the simplest type of correlational study, but there are more powerful ones. Complex correlational designs collect data on quite a few variables to determine the combination of variables that best *predict* an outcome variable of interest. One such design uses multiple regression analysis to determine which *set* of predictor variables best predicts the level of an outcome variable. Using a statistical program, predictor variable values are entered into the analysis one at a time until the combination of variables that best predicts levels of the outcome variable is found. The amount of variance in the outcome variable explained by the best set of variables is quantified as the R^2 statistic.

For example, a study examined five variables that might predict functional recovery after a stroke (Hinkle, 2006). The major finding was that age, cognitive status, and initial function had the highest correlations with recovery and were the best set of predictors of motor recovery. $R^2 = 42\%$, meaning that together these three variables predicted 42% of the variability in functional recovery. Adding the variables lesion volume and motor strength to the analysis did not increase the R^2.

Other studies involve using predictor variables to predict group membership (e.g., quit smoking/did not quit smoking); this statistical technique is called discriminate analysis. Both multiple regression analysis and discriminate analysis are advanced forms of correlation in which the relationships among sets of predictor variables and an outcome variable are examined. The exemplar you will read examines bivariate correlations and includes a multiple regression analysis, so you will become familiar with the two most frequently used types of correlation firsthand.

Exemplar

Reading Tips

The only aspects of this research report that could be difficult are the physiological variables that comprise cardiac function. To make the reading easier, the following list defines those variables. Still, there are references to medications with which you may be unfamiliar; I leave it to you to look those up.

- Ejection fraction: Using one of several imaging techniques (cardiac catheterization, MRI, or CT scan), the percentage of blood that is pumped out of the left ventricle with each heartbeat is measured; a normal ejection fraction is 55–70%.
- Peak VO_2 (also called maximal oxygen uptake): During cardiopulmonary exercise testing (bicycle or treadmill), breathing exchange is measured. Peak VO_2 is the oxygen consumption per minute when the patient is exercising at a maximum level. An expected level is predicted based on age and gender. Generally, a value below 14 ml/kg/minute indicates a poor prognosis.
- Maximal workload: During exercise testing, the heart's work output at the safe target heart rate or when the test has to be stopped because of symptoms, exhaustion, or EKG changes is the maximal workload; it is expressed in watts per minute.
- Systolic heart failure: Inadequate pumping of blood from the left ventricle during contraction due to weakness of the ventricle walls results in systolic heart failure.

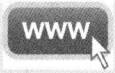

Correlates of Fatigue in Patients with Heart Failure

Lorraine S. Evangelista, Debra K. Moser, Cheryl Westlake, Nancy Pike, Alvina Ter-Galstanyan, and Kathleen Dracup

Progress in Cardiovascular Nursing (2008), *23*(1), 12–17.

This study was conducted to determine the prevalence of fatigue and identify its demographic, clinical, and psychological correlates in 150 heart failure (HF) patients (73% men, 66% Caucasian, mean age 55.0 years, mean ejection fraction 26.7% ± 11%), from a single HF center, using the Profile of Mood States-Fatigue Subscale, the Minnesota Living With Heart Failure Questionnaire, and the Beck Depression Inventory. Sociodemographic and clinical data were obtained through self-report and chart abstraction. High levels of fatigue were reported in 50.4% of men and 51.2% of women. In a multivariate model, maximal workload, physical health, emotional health, and depression explained 51% of the variance in fatigue ($P < .001$).

Fatigue in patients with HF is associated with both clinical and psychosocial variables, offering a number of targets for intervention. These findings suggest the need for multiple risk factor intervention strategies that improve physical and emotional health to decrease fatigue. Patients with depression warrant particular scrutiny. Prog Cardiovasc Nurs. 2008;23:12–17. (c)2008 Le Jacq

Fatigue accompanies many illnesses and can be an incapacitating symptom that interferes with return to work, activities of daily living, and social or family responsibilities.[1] Factors underlying fatigue have been examined extensively in patients with cancer[2] and multiple sclerosis,[3] and findings strongly support an association between fatigue, depression, and quality of life (QOL). Fatigue in these conditions is multifactorial and involves complex pathophysiologic and psychological processes that reflect both disease conditions. Interest in the impact of fatigue in cancer patients has led to the development of a treatment algorithm in which patients are evaluated regularly for fatigue, and treatment is targeted to their fatigue level.[2] In addition, treatment strategies including exercise programs, cooling, dietary changes, and energy conservation have also been developed to ameliorate fatigue in these patient populations.[2,3]

Fatigue is one of the 2 most common symptoms (along with dyspnea) reported by patients with heart failure (HF).[4–7] Also commonly referred to as activity intolerance, fatigue in patients with HF is defined as persistent tiredness and the perception of difficulty performing daily activities because of this persistent tiredness. Fatigue is often one of the first symptoms of HF and is commonly overlooked because it is viewed by both lay people and health care providers as a vague complaint. Indeed, as many as one-third of patients with HF view fatigue as an unimportant symptom and up to 50% report having difficulty recognizing it as a symptom of worsening HF.[8] The origins of fatigue in HF are unclear and are likely to be multifactorial. Probable pathophysiologic causes of fatigue in HF include low cardiac output and poor tissue perfusion, muscle metabolic abnormalities, autonomic nervous system abnormalities, deconditioning effects, and endothelial dysfunction.

Investigators have examined the relative contribution of psychological factors and physical symptoms to the variance in fatigue in older women with HF and demonstrated that fatigue was related more to physical symptoms than to psychological factors.[4] In another study, both men and women with HF were examined during hospitalization to assess relationships among physical symptoms, functional limitations, and depression.[5] Depression was strongly related to physical symptoms but not functional limitations. Ekman and Ehrenberg[9] explored sex differences in experiences of fatigue and found that there was an agreement in fatigue prevalence between men and women with HF, but the rating for fatigue severity differed by sex. When describing the character and intensity of fatigue, women described their fatigue as severe, whereas men described their fatigue as mild.[9] Despite earlier studies examining the nature of fatigue in patients with HF, this symptom continues to be poorly understood by clinicians and researchers. The purpose of the current investigation was to examine the prevalence of fatigue and identify its demographic, clinical, and psychological correlates in patients with systolic HF. Knowledge of the patterns and mechanisms of fatigue experienced by HF patients may provide information about the type and nature of interventions needed to cope with this distressing symptom and the challenges related to living with the chronic illness of HF.

Study Design and Patients

A cross-sectional, correlational design was used. A convenience sample of 150 patients with HF was recruited from a single outpatient HF clinic located within a tertiary, university-affiliated medical center on the US West Coast. Patients were included in the study if they were aged 18 years or older; able to read, write, and speak English; had a left ventricular ejection fraction < 40% documented by echocardiography or ventriculography; and had symptoms of HF for 6 months or longer.

Procedures

Institutional Review Board approval was received before study initiation. Patients who expressed an interest in participating in the study signed an informed consent during their routine clinic visit and received a battery of paper and pencil instruments to complete. Sociodemographic (ie, sex, age, race, income, education, marital status, and employment status) and clinical data (ie, etiology of HF, left ventricular ejection fraction, current medications, maximal oxygen uptake [peak VO_2], and maximal workload) were obtained from patient self-reports and verified through most current (within 3 months of study participation) diagnostic tests obtained during medical records abstraction.

Instruments

The questionnaires took 10 to 15 minutes to complete and included the following:

Profile of Mood States-Fatigue (POMS-F). The POMS-F, used to measure fatigue, is a 7-item subscale obtained from the 65-item Profile of Mood States instrument that was developed to assess transient distinct mood states specific to fatigue-inertia.[10] Participants were asked to rate their feelings related to being "worn out," "listless," "fatigued," "exhausted," "sluggish," "weary," and "bushed" on a 0 (not at all) to 4 (extremely) scale. Summative scores range from 0 to 28, with a higher score denoting greater fatigue. The standardized POMS-F scores were established in a sample of adult patients (N = 400) between the ages of 18 and 94 years with a mean age of 44 ± 18.4 years. Sixty-four percent of the patients in the normative sample were married, 48% were men, and the average years of education was 14.3 ± 2.7 years. The mean scores for men and women in the sample were 7.3 ± 5.7 and 8.7 ± 6.1, respectively.[11] These mean values were used in the current study to determine the presence of low (ie, below norm) and high (ie, above norm) levels of fatigue. The POMS Total Mood Disturbance score correlated highly ($r = 0.79$) with a Visual Analog Composite score.[2] Reliability of the POMS-F was 0.91 in a sample of 428 cancer patients.[12] Internal consistency of the POMS-F was acceptable with a Cronbach's α of 0.88.

Quality of Life. Quality of life was measured using the Minnesota Living With Heart Failure Questionnaire (LHFQ), a 21-item disease-specific tool that asks participants to indicate the extent to which various symptoms they have experienced in the previous month have prevented them from living as they wanted to. The items can be combined to form an overall QOL score as well as scores for physical health (8 items) and emotional health (5 items). The physical subscale contains items associated with the fatigue and dyspnea of HF. The emotional subscale consists of items such as being worried or feeling depressed. The remaining 8 items include questions about other areas of life affected by HF and are used to compute the overall QOL score.[13] Response options are presented as 6-point ordinal scales ranging from 0 (no) to 5 (very much), with a total maximum score of 105 (40 for physical and 25 for emotional health); a lower LHFQ score indicates better QOL.

Beck Depression Inventory (BDI). Depression was measured using the BDI, which is widely used in chronically ill populations and is well validated.[14] The BDI is a self-reported inventory designed to measure severity of depressive mood or symptoms. The 21-item inventory consists of a Likert-type scale from 0 (absence of symptom) to 3 (severe or persistent presence of the symptom). Five of the BDI items pertain to somatic symptoms of depression (eg, loss of appetite and sleep disturbance) and 16 of the items reflect nonsomatic symptoms of depression (eg, hopelessness and social withdrawal). Scores on the BDI range from 0 to 63. Patients with BDI scores 0 to 9 are considered as having minimal symptoms of depression, scores 10 to 16 mild, scores 17 to 29 moderate, and scores 30 to 63 as having severe symptoms of depression.[15]

Data Analyses

Data were analyzed using SPSS for Windows (version 11.0; SPSS, Inc, Chicago, IL). Descriptive statistics were used to characterize the study population and analyze mean fatigue scores. Sex differences in fatigue scores were compared using the independent *t* test. Fatigue was dichotomized using validated cutoff points; a score > 7.3 for men and > 8.7 in women was indicative of moderate to high levels of fatigue.[11]

Univariate analyses were conducted to assess the impact of sociodemographic, clinical, and psychosocial factors on fatigue. Group comparisons of patients with low vs moderate to high fatigue levels were conducted using chi-square statistics or *t* test, depending on the level of measurement. Multivariate stepwise regression analyses were then used to identify which combination of variables provided the most predictive power for overall fatigue. Variables significant at an $\alpha < .10$ in the univariate analysis were included in the regression model.

To reflect the context variables, age and sex of patients were the first variables added to the model. Next, to depict the impact of clinical variables (peak VO_2, maximal workload, use of lipid-lowering medications [statins]) were added as a second set. Psychological factors including QOL, physical and emotional health, and depression were added last. Criteria for entry and removal of variables were based on the likelihood ratio test, with enter and remove limits set at $P \leq .05$ and $P \geq .10$, respectively.

Results

Mean age of the patients in the sample was 55.0 ± 12.1 years (range, 20–72 years). No significant differences were found in the sociodemographic characteristics and most clinical characteristics between patients who reported low vs high levels of fatigue (Table I). Ejection fraction was similar in both groups; however, peak VO_2 and maximal workload were significantly lower in patients who reported high levels of fatigue compared with those reporting lower levels of fatigue. This finding validates the measure of fatigue used in this study.

Fatigue scores for men and women were higher than the category scores for moderate-severe fatigue in a healthy adult population; men scored 9.5 (SD ± 7.5) and women scored 10.4 (SD ± 7.0). These scores reflect high levels of fatigue reported in 55 (50.4%) men and 21 (51.2%) women. The QOL, physical and emotional health, and depression scores are listed in Table II. No differences were found between men and women in the variables studied. Depression was detected in > 28% of the sample by the BDI questionnaire; 29 (19%) had mild depressive symptoms and 14 (9%) had moderate to severe depressive symptoms.

Table I Demographic and Clinical Characteristics of HF Patients With Low or High Fatigue Levels

	Total (N=150)	Low Fatigue (N=74)	High Fatigue (N=76)
Age, y	55.0 ± 12.1	56.8 ± 2.2	54.7 ± 13.0
Years with HF	5.9 ± 6.1	5.8 ± 5.0	6.2 ± 7.1
Ejection fraction, %	26.7 ± 11.5	26.1 ± 11.7	27.3 ± 11.6
Maximal oxygen uptake (peak VO_2), mL/kg/min	15.8 ± 5.3	16.4 ± 5.3	13.2 ± 4.3[a]
Maximal workload, watts	96 ± 53	102 ± 52	72 ± 46[b]
Men, %	72.7	73.0	72.4
Race, %			
White	65.6	62.5	68.8
Black	26.9	28.8	25.0
Asians	7.5	8.7	6.2
Married, %	65.6	68.8	62.5
Education, %			
Some high school	12.5	12.5	12.5
High school graduate	21.9	25.0	18.8
Some college	37.5	25.0	50.0
College graduate	28.1	37.5	18.7
Not employed, %	78.0	72.0	75.0
Heart failure etiology, %			
Idiopathic	57.5	58.8	56.3
Ischemic	42.5	41.2	43.7
NYHA class, %			
II	44.8	46.3	43.3
III	42.7	41.2	44.2
IV	12.5	12.5	12.5
Medications, %			
ACE inhibitors	78.7	75.7	78.9
β-Blockers	73.3	68.9	68.4
Diuretics	96.0	93.2	93.4
Digoxin	57.3	58.1	48.7
Statins	64.0	63.5	68.4[a]

Abbreviations: ACE, angiotensin-converting enzyme; HF, heart failure; NYHA, New York Heart Association.
Values are expressed as mean ± SD unless otherwise indicated. [a]$P < .05$. [b]$P < .001$.

Table II Quality of Life, Physical and Emotional Health, and Depression Scores (N = 150)

Characteristic	Mean	SD	Range[a]
Quality of life-total, sum score	42.2	26.7	0–100
Quality of life-physical health, sum score	18.0	12.0	0–40
Quality of life-emotional health, sum score	8.4	7.1	0–25
Depression, sum score	9.9	8.2	0–50

[a]These values reflect the actual range of scores for the sample.

In a univariate analysis, age and sex were not correlated with fatigue; however, a strong correlation existed between fatigue, total QOL, physical and emotional health, and depression (Table III). Clinical and physiological variables associated with higher levels of fatigue were use of statins, lower peak VO_2, and lower maximal workload. Cardiac factors including HF etiology, New York Heart Association (NYHA) functional class, and left ventricular ejection fraction were not related to fatigue.

Table III Correlational Matrix for the Key Variables (N = 150)

Variable	1	2	3	4	5	6	7	8	9
Fatigue									
Age	−.067								
EF%	.095	.032							
Peak VO_2	−.227[a]	−.116	−.155						
Maximal workload	−.354[b]	−.178	.103	.203[a]					
Use of statins	.204[a]	−.230[b]	.010	.100	−.065				
QOL (total)	.596[b]	−.071	−.056	−.177[a]	−.318[b]	.182[a]			
Physical health	.595[b]	.002	−.039	−.167[a]	−.419[b]	.077	.945[b]		
Emotional health	.627[b]	−.069	−.056	−.172[a]	−.402[b]	.134	.807[b]	.638[b]	
Depression	.576[b]	−.166[a]	−.042	−.226[a]	−.249[b]	.239[b]	.511[b]	.367[b]	.684[b]

Abbreviations: EF, ejection fraction; QOL, quality of life; VO_2, maximal oxygen uptake. [a]$P < .05$. [b]$P < .001$.

In a multiple regression model, lower maximal workload, physical and emotional health scores, and depression were found to be independent predictors of fatigue (Table IV). These 4 predictors accounted for 51% of variance in the fatigue scores of patients. There was evidence of a linear fit for each variable in the final model. Post hoc analysis, done to test for multicollinearity among variables, demonstrated that each of the predictors had unique effects on fatigue.

Table IV Predictors of Fatigue (N = 150)

Variable	Adjusted R^2	F	P Value
Maximal workload, watts	.114	14.66	< .0001
Emotional health	.415	38.53	< .0001
Physical health	.466	31.8	< .0001
Depression	.506	28.13	< .0001

Discussion

Despite the pervasiveness of fatigue in patients with HF, little research has concentrated on this phenomenon. Given the importance of symptom status to patients and the value of symptom status as an indicator of the effectiveness of clinical therapies to clinicians, it is vital that research efforts are directed toward understanding fatigue. The current study is novel in that we used a multivariate model to determine correlates of fatigue and demonstrated the multifactorial nature of fatigue in this population. Both clinical and psychological variables were important correlates of fatigue: maximal workload, physical and emotional health scores, and depression were independent correlates of fatigue. In addition, we found that approximately one-half of the study participants experienced fatigue when compared with a healthy adult population utilizing the same measure.[11] Similar prevalence was also reported in a cohort of older women with HF in the United States[4] and in an elderly cohort of men and women with HF in Sweden.[16,17]

Lower peak VO_2 and maximal workload both correlated with higher fatigue; however, only lower maximal workload was found to independently predict higher fatigue in this sample. Peak VO_2 is traditionally used for risk stratification in HF; the impact it has on mortality is well supported in the literature.[18] Peak VO_2 has also been used to predict limitations ($VO_2 \leq 14$ mL/kg/min) in daily activities as a result of poor exercise tolerance.[19] Intuitively, patients with high levels of fatigue are less tolerant to increasing maximum workloads and experience decreased levels of peak VO_2. Although the mechanisms for these physiological responses are not well understood, our findings indicate that HF patients with lower maximal workload thresholds and peak VO_2 indices are at high risk for fatigue.

Higher fatigue correlated with poorer physical health. Our findings are consistent with previous study results that showed an association between fatigue and restrictions in physical activity and limitations in self-care.[7,16,17] Additionally, fatigue in older women with HF was related more to other concurrent physical symptoms than to psychological factors.[4] Investigators examined plausible explanations that link fatigue with higher functional limitations and identified impaired peripheral circulatory perfusion with reduced oxygen delivery and impaired muscle strength as potential confounders.[20] Fatigue and physical health warrant further investigation including what comes first, fatigue or physical health limitations. Our findings support the need to assess for ongoing physical symptoms (ie, dyspnea, edema) that may increase susceptibility to increased fatigue. At the current time, the best method of assessing for fatigue may be the most direct and simple, ie, asking patients about the presence of the symptom and helping patients to identify fatigue by specific questioning directed at uncovering fatigue in the context of daily activities. Patients who report a chronic physical symptom pattern should be screened for concomitant fatigue that may merit intervention. Finally, the need to consider interventions that focus on physical symptoms as a first step to managing fatigue in HF patients is vital.

Specific interventions to combat fatigue have not yet been tested in patients with HF, but data to date on the impact of exercise suggest that fatigue may be managed best by assisting patients to increase their activity levels. Given the relationship between depression and fatigue found in this and other studies, interventions to treat depression will likely have a beneficial impact on fatigue also. Exercise has a positive influence on depression. Assisting patients to increase their activity levels, which has been shown to be safe in the management of HF, can be recommended for the management of fatigue in patients with HF. It is also appropriate to teach HF patients energy conservation techniques for the management of fatigue, so their activity efforts are efficient and not exhausting.

The study supports previous reports that poor QOL and emotional health are common in patients with HF and that higher fatigue was related to poorer QOL.[17] Women who scored high on fatigue also scored high on stress related to illness and were less satisfied with life.[4] Our findings were similar and also showed that more than a fourth of the participants reported depressive symptoms, which is higher than depression rates reported among patients hospitalized with HF.[5] Both studies, however, consistently showed that higher depressive symptoms were associated with higher fatigue. The relationship between fatigue and depression has also been reported in women with breast cancer. Women reporting high levels of fatigue also reported greater symptom distress, lower activity, and poorer physical and social health status.[2] Hence, treatment strategies that help patients manage symptoms, relax, and obtain adequate sleep, especially patients experiencing greater emotional distress and depressive symptoms, may modify fatigue. Complementary therapies (eg, yoga, meditation, massage) and self-care strategies that promote sleep and exercise may also help patients cope with the emotional impact of fatigue.[5]

It may seem counterintuitive that we failed to find an association between fatigue and NYHA functional class or ejection fraction. However, given the nature of measurement of fatigue and the aspects of HF pathophysiology captured by NYHA functional class or ejection fraction, these findings are not unexpected. Given its subjective nature, fatigue is difficult to measure with precision. The NYHA classification also suffers from lack of precision in its measurement; at each of the 3 indicators at which symptoms are present (ie, classes II, III, and IV), the assessment seeks only whether any symptom is present, not specifically whether fatigue is present. Ejection fraction is likely not associated with fatigue because all patients with HF, regardless of ejection fraction, are expected to have symptoms such as fatigue, and symptom status has never correlated well with ejection fraction. This lack of correlation is one reason HF guidelines do not recommend using ejection fraction to reflect effectiveness of drug therapy, but they do recommend that symptom improvement be a major indicator.

Of interest, fatigue in HF was associated with the use of statins, which has been shown to increase the risk of myopathy, resulting in symptoms of fatigue, weakness, and pain. Although statin-related side effects were originally identified as affecting only 1% to 5% of patients,[21] some investigators have indicated that these effects may be common and often go unreported.[22] The risk of these adverse effects with statin use can be exacerbated by several factors, including compromised hepatic and renal function, hypothyroidism, diabetes, and use of concomitant medications, but the mechanisms causing statin-induced myopathy have not been elucidated and warrant further study.[23] Our finding, however, that statin use was not independently associated with fatigue suggests that discontinuation of statins to treat fatigue in patients with HF may not be warranted.

Some limitations must be considered when interpreting the results from our study. First, causation cannot be inferred; thus, we cannot say that low QOL, poor physical and emotional health, or depression leads to high levels of fatigue, nor can we comment on the direction of the hypothesized causality. The experience of severe fatigue may lead to low QOL, poor physical and emotional health, or depression. Our findings merely support the association between fatigue and several clinical and psychosocial variables. Next, the sample that was used for the study was fairly homogeneous; patients were all being seen at a single transplant referral center and their mean age was lower than the typical mean age for HF in the general community, thus limiting our ability to generalize to all patients with HF. Finally, the use of a convenience sample from a single center limits the utility of any estimate of prevalence of fatigue and could also introduce a bias in the ascertainment of correlates of fatigue.

Conclusions

Our data demonstrate that fatigue levels were moderately intense and highly prevalent in our sample of patients with systolic HF. We found that fatigue has predictable clinical dimensions and psychosocial correlates and is an important symptom to consider. Fatigue may influence patients' adherence to the medical regimen, their social relationships, and general QOL. Early identification of fatigue could facilitate the initiation of interventions to reduce the cost of associated health care.

Evaluation and treatment of fatigue in HF patients requires a multidisciplinary approach because the fatigue has many possible etiologies and several contributing factors. A comprehensive approach is required, especially for patients with moderate to severe fatigue, so that all possible contributing factors can be determined and an appropriate treatment plan created. The short- and long-term effects of various treatment strategies on the fatigue in HF patients should be assessed in future studies.

Disclosure: This research was partially supported by a grant from the American Heart Association Western Division (NCR, 133–09, PI, K. Dracup) and by a University of California School of Nursing Intramural Research Grant.

References

1. Solano JP, Gomes B, Higginson IJ. A comparison of symptom prevalence in far advanced cancer, AIDS, heart disease, chronic obstructive pulmonary disease and renal disease. *J Pain Symptom Manage*. 2006;31:58–69.
2. Payne J, Piper B, Rabinowitz I, et al. Biomarkers, fatigue, sleep, and depressive symptoms in women with breast cancer. *Oncol Nurs Forum*. 2006;33:775–783.
3. MacAllister WS, Krupp LB. Multiple sclerosis-related fatigue. *Phys Med Rehabil Clin N Am*. 2005;16:483–502.
4. Friedman MM, King KB. Correlates of fatigue in older women with heart failure. *Heart Lung*. 1995;24:512–518.
5. Friedman MM, Griffin JA. Relationship of physical symptoms and physical functioning to depression in patients with heart failure. *Heart Lung*. 2001;30:98–104.

6. Nordgren L, Sorensen S. Symptoms experienced in the last six months of life in patients with end-stage heart failure. *Eur J Cardiovasc Nurs*. 2003;2:213–217.
7. Mayou R, Blackwood R, Bryant B, et al. Cardiac failure: symptoms and functional status. *J Psychosom Res*. 1991;35:399–407.
8. Carlson B, Riegel B, Moser D. Self-care abilities of patients with heart failure. *Heart Lung*. 2001;30:351–359.
9. Ekman I, Ehrenberg A. Fatigue in chronic heart failure—does gender make a difference? *Eur J Cardiovasc Nurs*. 2002;1:77–82.
10. McNair D, Loir M, Droppleman L. *Profile of Mood States*. San Diego, CA: Educational and Testing Services; 1971.
11. Nyenhuis DL, Yamamoto C, Luchetta T, et al. Adult and geriatric normative data and validation of the profile of mood states. *J Clin Psychol*. 1999;55:79–86.
12. Baker F, Denniston M, Zabora J, et al. POMS short form for cancer patients: psychometric and structural evaluation. *Psychooncology*. 2002;11:273–281.
13. Rector TS, Johnson G, Dunkman WB. Evaluation by patients with heart failure of the effects of enalapril compared with hydralazine plus isosorbide dinitrate on quality of life. V-HeFT II. The V-HeFT VA Cooperative Studies Group. *Circulation*. 1993;87:VI71–VI77.
14. Beck AT. *Depression: Clinical, Experimental and Theoretical Aspects*. New York, NY: Hoeber; 1967.
15. Beck AT, Rial W, Rickels K. Short form of depression inventory: cross validation. *Psychol Rep*. 1974;34:1184–1186.
16. Falk K, Swedberg K, Gaston-Johansson F, et al. Fatigue is a prevalent and severe symptom associated with uncertainty and sense of coherence in patients with chronic heart failure. *Eur J Cardiovasc Nurs*. 2007;6:99–104.
17. Falk K, Swedberg K, Gaston-Johansson F, et al. Fatigue and anaemia in patients with chronic heart failure. *Eur J Heart Fail*. 2006;8:744–749.
18. Corra U, Mezzani A, Bosimini E, et al. Limited predictive value of cardiopulmonary exercise indices in patients with moderate chronic heart failure treated with carvedilol. *Am Heart J*. 2004;147:553–560.
19. Gitt AK, Wasserman K, Kilkowski C, et al. Exercise anaerobic threshold and ventilatory efficiency identify heart failure patients for high risk of early death. *Circulation*. 2002;106:3079–3084.
20. Drexler H, Coats AJS. Explaining fatigue in congestive heart failure. *Annu Rev Med*. 1996;47:241–256.
21. Dirks AJ, Jones KM. Statin-induced apoptosis and skeletal myopathy. *Am J Physiol Cell Physiol*. 2006;291:C1208–C1212.
22. Langsjoen PH, Langsjoen JO, Langsjoen AM, et al. Treatment of statin adverse effects with supplemental Coenzyme Q10 and statin drug discontinuation. *Biofactors*. 2005;25:147–152.
23. Thompson PD, Clarkson P, Karas RH. Statin-associated myopathy. *JAMA*. 2003;289:1681–1690.

Profile & Commentary

STUDY PURPOSE

The stated purpose of this study is twofold: (1) to determine how prevalent fatigue is in patients with systolic heart failure (HF), and (2) to identify clinical and psychological states associated with HF. In the opening paragraphs, the researchers define fatigue and summarize research that has been done about the topic.

STUDY DESIGN

"A cross-sectional, correlational design was used." Cross-sectional means data were collected once from each participant; no effort was made to study change over time. The study used correlational design because data were collected about 10 variables and the relationships among them were of interest.

Sample

The 150 patients who made up the sample were drawn from persons who attended an outpatient clinic for HF patients at a transplant referral medical center in the United States. A detailed profile of the patients in the sample is provided in Table I. This information provides a detailed portrayal of the projected target population as a whole and of two subgroups (i.e., a low-fatigue subgroup and a high-fatigue subgroup). Notice how cutoff values were used to categorize sample patients into the subgroups.

Several pieces of information in this table are particularly noteworthy. First, the average age is quite young for persons with HF. This is puzzling until you read on the last page of the article that they were "being seen at a single transplant referral center." This explains the younger than expected age although it is not clear how many were actually awaiting transplant. Still, the low average age and the setting in which they were seen means that the population to whom the results would apply are not the typical population of older persons with heart failure.

ASSUMED POPULATION: Heart failure patients

SAMPLE: 150 patients with heart failure in an outpatient clinic at a large city transplant referral center

PROJECTED POPULATION: patients with heart failure for approximately 6 years, now rated at NYHA class II–IV, 20–72 years of age (average 55 years), who are taking usual medications for treating heart failure.

The researchers were interested in knowing whether persons in the high- and low-fatigue level groups had similar or different characteristics. The superscript *a* and *b* designations to the right of the right column help do this. They tell us about the results of the *t*-tests used to compare characteristics of the high- and low-level fatigue groups. Only the characteristics with an [a] or [b] beside them were different enough to be considered a real difference, meaning that it is likely that a different level of the characteristic would exist in high- and low-fatigue groups from the larger population of patients, not just in this sample. The [a] designation means that the difference in the two groups on that particular characteristic is large enough that there are only 5 chances in 100 that a difference that large would occur just by chance if the two groups in the population really had the same level of that characteristic. The [b] designation means that the difference between the two groups on that characteristic is large enough that it would occur just by chance 1 time out of 1,000—a rare occurrence indeed.

As the researchers tell us in the first paragraph under Results, the two groups were essentially similar on all variables except mean peak VO_2, mean maximal workload, and the proportion of participants who took statin drugs. This information suggests an association between two indicators of heart physiology and fatigue.

Measurement

Three questionnaire-type instruments were used to measure fatigue, quality of life, and depression. The descriptions of these instruments are quite good, so I will not repeat that information other than to make a few points.

The response scales of the three instruments are different (0–4, 0–5, and 0–3, respectively). Also note the direction of the scoring. A high number on the fatigue scale denotes greater fatigue (↑ ↑); a high number on the QOL scales indicates poorer quality of life (↑ ↓); and a high number on the depression scale denotes more severe depression (↑ ↑). All three instruments are widely used.

Regarding the POMS-F, first note that this instrument is made up of a seven-item subscale extracted from a larger instrument; the seven items get specifically at mood related to fatigue, not mood more generally. Normative values for the POMS-F instrument were established previously by having 400 healthy persons complete the instrument. We are also informed that the reliability of the POMS-F was 0.91 and its internal consistency was 0.88 in a sample of cancer patients.

What Does This Mean? Well, there are several types of reliability. In a study previously in this text, ratings were done by two observers and interrater reliability was reported. However, in this study there were no observers; rather participants self-reported by completing questionnaires. Thus **interrater reliability** is not an issue. Although the specific type of reliability done on the POMS-F that was done is not named, I assume that it was test-retest reliability. Remember reliability refers to an instrument's consistency. **Test-retest reliability** evaluates the consistency with which persons score themselves similarly on the questionnaire at two completions of the questionnaire separated by an appropriate period of time. If a person scored exactly the same both times, the instrument would have a test-retest reliability of 1. If a person had quite different answers on the two questionnaires, the test-retest reliability would be very low, say 0.30. Generally, a reliability score of 0.80 or greater indicates that the instrument consistency elicits similar answers, so there is not a lot of uncertainty about how to answer the questions. The reported reliability of 0.91 in this report indicates the meaning of the questions is clear to the responders so the answers do not fluctuate a lot.

Another type of reliability—**internal consistency**—is reported. This refers to the extent to which the items/questions that make up the questionnaire hang together to measure the underlying characteristic concept. A commonly used measure of internal consistency is Cronbach's α. You do not need to know how it is calculated; rather you should know that the calculated values, like other measures of reliability, will be between 0 and +1.0.

A high value indicates that all of the items of the questionnaire are getting at the same concept, albeit at slightly different aspects of it. The internal consistency of the POMS-F is reported as 0.88, which is a high level.

THREE FORMS OF RELIABILITY/CONSISTENCY

1. **Interrater reliability (observers' consistency)**
2. **Test-retest reliability (stability over time)**
3. **Internal consistency (items hang together)**

Data Analysis

Mean scores of sociodemographic, clinical, and quality of life variables were calculated for the patients with high versus and low levels of fatigue. Correlations statistics (Pearson *r*) were run on all different bivariate combinations of the 10 variables listed in Table III. And finally, a multiple regression statistical analysis was run to determine the best set of predictors of fatigue. The results in the first paragraph of the article are explained earlier in this commentary, where the sample was discussed.

Analyses of Fatigue In the second paragraph, we learn that women, on average, reported more fatigue than men; women's mean level of fatigue was 10.4, whereas the mean for men was 9.5. Both levels are higher than the normative mean of 8.7 and 7.3, respectively. Thus both women and men have, on average, moderate to severe fatigue. Reported differently, about half the total sample had high levels of fatigue.

Analyses of Other Predictor Variables Table II provides summary data for the total group scores of QOL total, physical health, emotional health, and depression. To put them in perspective, it might help to write the maximum possible score to the right of Table II, and note in the text that lower depression scores indicate fewer symptoms of depression but lower QOL scores indicate better QOL, and. The mean/average QOL-total, QOL–physical, and QOL–emotional scores are low, which means that the respondents on average reported a good quality of life. The mean level of depression (9.9) is in the mild depression range based on normative ranges. Also note the rather high standard deviations for all the scores; they indicate a wide spread in the data, i.e., large variability in the scores. I consider these results a bit of a surprise because, given that they were seen at a heart transplant center, I would have expected these persons to have lower QOL and more depression. However, looking at the range of depression scores reminds us that at least one person, and maybe more, did have a very high level of depression; also the text tells us that 28% of the sample had mild or moderate depression. So, even though the mean depression score is rather modest, a sizeable percentage did have appreciable symptoms of depression.

Correlational Analyses Now we get to the correlations. To make Table III (the correlation matrix) more easily readable, I suggest that you put the variable numbers 1–10 down the left side of the table beside each variable respectively. So variable 1 is fatigue, 2 is age, 3 is EF%, and so on to variable 10, depression. The column numbers across the top then correspond with the now numbered variables listed in the left column.

The numbers at each cross point of column and row are Pearson *r* correlation statistics for combinations of two variables. For instance, the correlation between fatigue (column 1) and physical health (row 8) is 0.595. Note the small ^{b} beside this value indicating that this is a **statistically significant** result; there is less than a 1 in 1,000 (0.001) probability that the correlation between these two variables is actually 0 in the target population. It may not be 0.595, but it is not 0 (see **Figure 6-8**).

The most interesting findings are in column 1 because these indicate how the various factors correlate with fatigue. Essentially, fatigue has a statistically significant correlation with all the other variables except age and ejection fraction. The highest correlations are between fatigue and emotional health, QOL, physical health, and depression

To obtain perspective on the *r*-values, do as suggested in the introduction to this chapter, and square *r* to get r^2. In doing so, the *r* for emotional health and fatigue ($r = 0.627$) informs us that emotional health and fatigue have a moderately large overlap, 39% to be precise ($0.627^2 = 0.393$). Therefore, when looking just at emotional health and fatigue, 39% of the variation in fatigue is explained by its relationship with emotional health, and 39% of the variation in emotional health is explained by its relationship with

Data-based *p*-value	<.001	.01	.025	**.05**	.08	.15	.42>
Finding	Significant correlation				Nonsignificant correlation		
Conclusion	The variables probably are related in the population.				The variables probably are not related in the population.		

*Using a .05 level of significance decision-point

Figure 6-8 Interpretations of *p*-values associated with Pearson *r*

fatigue—a moderate relationship. Clearly, other factors also influence both fatigue and emotional health.

Other correlations in the table may also be of interest to you. For instance, physical health is highly correlated with QOL total (column 7) with a Pearson r of 0.945. As a check on your ability to read a correlation matrix, what is the correlation between depression and Quality of Life (QOL total)? The answer is in the footnote at the bottom of this page.

Multiple Tests of Significance One final point needs to be made about correlation matrices, such as the one found in this report. Whenever a large number of statistical tests are conducted in a study, there is an increased chance that one or more of them will be statistically significant just by chance (Huck, 2011). To avoid accepting a correlation result resulting from multiple comparisons/tests, some experts advise that the level of significance required for each statistical test to be considered statistically significant should be raised. That is done using a procedure called **Bonferroni correction.** However if the Bonferroni correction were applied to the results of this study, all of the correlations that were significant at the $p < .001$ level (those indicated by the [b] designation) will still qualify as statistically significant, albeit with less confidence that the relationship is not a chance result; the results that were significant at the $p < .05$ level (indicated by the [a] designation) would no longer be deemed statistically significant.

*0.511 Read depression row across to column 7 which is QOL

Multiple Regression Analysis Multiple regression analysis is done using a statistical program to find the set of predictor variables that best predicts an outcome. As a new reader of research reports, do not get hung up on the technical details regarding what and how variables are entered into the analysis, but rather focus on the predictor variables that make up the model.

Looking at Table IV, we see that maximal workload was entered into the analysis first, and it predicted 11.4% of the variance in fatigue. When emotional health was also added, the two variables together predicted 41.5% of the variance in fatigue. Then physical health was added; it produced a 5% bump in explained variance to 46.6%. When depression was added, another 5% boost was achieved to arrive at the total variance in fatigue that was explained by the four variables of 50.6%. Adding other variables did not appreciably increase the amount of variance explained. The four best predictors are referred to as "the model." Predicting almost 51% of the variance in an outcome with just four predictor variables is a fairly high level of prediction. (Note: The last two sentences in the Results section pertain to advanced aspects of the analysis that relate to the confidence in the model—you can ignore them.)

Discussion

The discussion is long and a bit technical, but some of the takeaway points are as follows:

1. Fatigue is associated with quite a few physical, psychological, and treatment factors
2. Approximately one half of participants experienced moderate to severe fatigue.
3. The discussion of peak VO_2 and maximal workload, and later ejection fraction, convey that only maximal workload was found to independently predict fatigue in the sample.
4. The best method of assessing fatigue is to directly ask the patient about it.
5. Interventions to control fatigue have not been tested, but based on the findings of this study, they could include help with getting good sleep, control of other sources of pain (e.g., arthritis), pacing activity to conserve energy, exercise to maintain conditioning, and relaxation therapies.
6. The authors issue a cautionary note about using the findings of this study in planning the care of other heart failure populations. The

sample of this study is unique, not typical of the larger population of heart failure patients. Not only are they younger, they are at least being considered by a transplant program. They have some hope out in front of them. This makes them different from the typical population that will be managed by medications for the rest of their lives. In research language, the generalizability, or external validity, of the findings of this study is limited to heart failure patients being considered or awaiting heart transplant. (This is not as clear as it might be in the article, so I may be making an assumption.)The extent to which older persons with heart failure have the same experience profile as those in this study is not known.

7. The authors close with the mantra set forth in the introduction to this chapter: association/relationship does not confer causation. When you think about it, it makes sense that emotional health and fatigue are related, but which way is the direction of influence? Most likely it is a bidirectional relationship; the experience of fatigue influences emotional health while at the same time emotional health influences the experience of fatigue.

In summary, this correlation study provides insights regarding the complex nature of fatigue in heart failure patients. It reminds us that fatigue is not just a physiological symptom of poor heart function; rather it is influenced by and influences life perspectives.

http://go.jblearning.com/brown3e

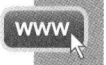

References

Brink, P. J., & Wood, M. J. (1998). Correlational designs. In P. J. Brink & M. J. Wood (Eds.), *Advanced designs in nursing research* (2nd ed., pp. 235–282). Newbury Park, CA: Sage.

Burns, N., & Grove, S. K. (2009). *Practice of nursing research: Conduct, critique, and utilization* (6th ed.). St. Louis, MO: Elsevier Saunders.

Evangelista, L. S., Moser, D. K., Westlake, C., Pike, N., Ter-Galstanyan, A., & Dracup, K. (2008). Correlates of fatigue in patients with heart failure. *Progress in Cardiovascular Nursing, 23*(1), 12–17.

Hinkle, J. L. (2006). Variables explaining functional recovery following motor stroke. *Journal of Neuroscience Nursing, 38*(1), 6–12.

Huck, S. W. (2011). *Reading statistics and research* (6th ed.). Boston, MA: Pearson.

Karavatas, S. G., & Tavakol, K. (2005). Concurrent validity of Borg's rating of perceived exertion in African-American young adults, employing heart rate as the standard. *Internet Journal of Allied Health Sciences and Practice, 3*(1). Retrieved from http://ijahsp.nova.edu/articles/vol3num1/karavatas.htm

Kim, J. I., Oh, K. O., Li, C. Y., Min, H. S., Chang, E. S., & Song, R. (2011). Breast cancer screening practice and health-promoting behavior among Chinese women. *Asian Nursing Research, 5*(3), 157–163.

CHAPTER SEVEN

Experimental Research

Chapter Layout

This is a very long chapter; therefore it is divided into two sections. The first section focuses on the methods used to conduct experimental studies testing the effectiveness of nursing interventions. The second section delves into the ways results of experimental studies are reported.

In the first section, the methodological characteristics of experimental studies are explained, followed by the exemplar study reprint. You should read only the Introduction and Methods sections of the exemplar study, then read the Profile & Commentary about its methods.

The second section of the chapter opens with an explanation of the results of experimental studies. After reading that, you should read the Results section of the exemplar study and then the Profile & Commentary about its results. In other words, rather than have you ingest the whole research article at once, you will first consider the *why* and the *how*. Then you will delve into the *what*. When you see the amount of information in this chapter, you will understand why it is divided into two portions.

The explanations in this chapter will be limited to the classic two-group experiment, which is widely used in nursing research. Although in the future you will undoubtedly read three-group experimental studies, you should be able to understand them using what you know about two-group studies and reference to your statistics book. Other experimental designs that are used less often are not addressed in this book.

The classic experimental study discussed in this chapter is also referred to in healthcare research as a randomized clinical trial (RCT). Having said that, some people view an RCT more narrowly—in particular, as a definitive, late-stage test of an intervention's effectiveness, often in a large, diverse sample (Burns & Grove, 2009).

CHAPTER LAYOUT

SECTION 1

- **Methods explained**
- **Exemplar study: Read introduction and Methods sections only**
- **Profile & Commentary on methods**

SECTION 2

- **Results explained**
- **Exemplar study: Read Results & Discussion sections**
- **Profile & Commentary on results**

Section 1: Understanding Experimental Methods

Determining the effectiveness of nursing interventions and treatments requires carefully designed studies. Assembling a group of willing participants and measuring them on a physiologic condition, psychological state, or knowledge level before and after receiving the intervention of interest is considered a weak design (Kerlinger & Lee, 2000). It is weak because if an improvement is found, the researcher cannot claim with certainty that the intervention produced the improvement. Natural recovery, natural fluctuations in condition, or influences in the environment may have caused the observed improvements.

Key Features of Experimental Studies

When researchers want to test the effects of a nursing intervention on patient outcomes, the ideal research design is an experiment. A sample is drawn from a target population, and participants are randomly assigned to one of two groups. One group receives the test intervention and the other group receives no intervention or another intervention. At an appropriate time after the intervention, the researcher measures an outcome variable, or several, to determine whether one group did better than the other (see **Figure 7–1**). In designing an experimental study, the researcher tries to create conditions in which all influences on the outcome of interest, other than the effects of the different interventions, are the same for both groups. This sameness is necessary to be certain that any difference found in the outcomes of the two groups can be attributed to the fact that they received different interventions, not to some other influence.

The classic experimental study has six key features:

1. A well-defined target population
2. Adequate sample size
3. Random assignment of participants to intervention and comparison groups
4. Control of extraneous influences and bias
5. Consistent delivery of interventions
6. Low level of missing data

These features are key because they: (1) control error, bias, and unwanted influences; and (2) specify to whom the results will apply. In so doing, they bolster confidence in the credibility and applicability of the findings.

Before explaining each of these key features, I want to say something about the terminology used in reports of experimental studies. The new intervention (frequently the intervention of greatest interest) may be called the *experimental intervention* or *test intervention*; however, the terms *experimental treatment* and independent variable are also used. When referring to both interventions, the terms *interventions* and *treatment groups* may be used. The researcher's control over the design and delivery of the interventions may be referred to as *manipulation of the intervention*. I will use all these terms to help you get accustomed to them.

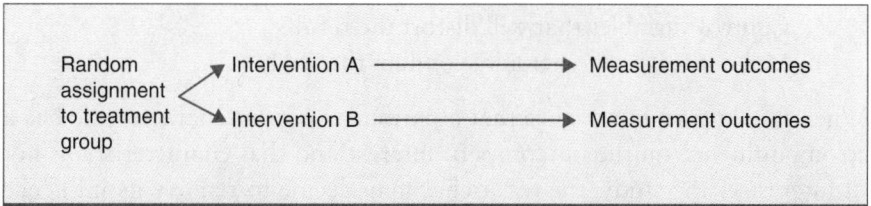

Figure 7-1 Classic 2-Group Experimental Study Sequence

Well-Defined Target Population

When researchers first think about doing a study, they have a target population in mind. As study design proceeds, they need to get very clear about the criteria that define the target population, and in so doing they produce a list of inclusion criteria (also called eligibility criteria). Commonly used inclusion criteria are age range, gender, ethnic group, medical diagnosis, clinical or functional status, care setting, and geographical location. Sometimes, in addition to inclusion criteria, the researcher will also specify exclusion criteria. A common exclusion criterion in U.S. studies is people who cannot speak English. Other examples of exclusions would be persons with physical conditions that would make it inadvisable for them to receive the intervention or to participate in the requirements of the study. (See example in text box.)

In a study testing the effects of music on postoperative pain relief after open-heart surgery during chair rest on the first postoperative day (Shu, 2010), the following eligibility criteria were used:

1. **First postoperative day after an open-heart surgery.**
2. **Stable condition and oriented.**
3. **Absence of hearing impairment.**
4. **Ability to follow commands and understand and read English.**

Patients with a femoral artery sheath in place after surgery were excluded because 6–8 hours bed rest is necessary to prevent hemorrhage after removal.

Inclusion and exclusion criteria serve four purposes:

1. Define the population to whom the findings will be generalizable.
2. Identify characteristics that must be present for a person to be included in the sample.
3. Control variables that will distort the results.
4. Make it feasible to actually conduct the study.

When it is known in advance that a particular patient characteristic has a strong influence on the outcomes of interest and that characteristic is not of interest in the study, the researcher may decide to remove its influence completely. This is done even though random sampling would even out the variable's influence across the two groups, because removing it allows the effect of the treatment being tested to stand out. One way to remove a very strong patient characteristic influence that is not of interest in the study is to include in the study only persons who do not have that characteristic.

To illustrate: If a study of persons with mild congestive heart failure examines the effects of two rehabilitation approaches on ability to walk for 6 minutes without stopping to catch their breath or rest, the researcher might exclude persons whose walking is affected by conditions other than their cardiac conditioning. This could be done by excluding all persons with preexisting physical disabilities that affect mobility, such as stroke, severe hip and knee arthritis, peripheral arterial disease, Parkinson's disease, and neurological disease. From the research point of view of, these exclusions make sense in that they control extraneous variables affecting mobility, and thereby increase the likelihood that the analysis will identify differences in walking outcomes resulting from the two different rehab approaches. However, a long list of exclusion criteria can also create problems in finding eligible participants for the study.

From the clinical perspective many persons who have mild congestive heart failure also have arthritis and other conditions affecting mobility. So, a study conducted with this many exclusions would apply only to a very narrow portion of the patients clinicians are likely to see, and we would say the study has limited generalizability in real-world practice. Thus, researchers have to use exclusion criteria with awareness regarding how they will affect the clinical usefulness of the findings.

Adequate Sample Size

An experimental study's sample size must be large enough to detect a difference in the outcomes of the two groups if it actually occurs. Determining "large enough" requires taking into account several aspects of the expected results; these expectations are based on findings from similar previous studies. Foremost among the aspects taken into account are (1) the strength of the experimental intervention's impact vis-à-vis the impact of the comparison intervention, and (2) the desired level of significance (i.e., the p value that will be used as a decision point for statistical significance). These values are entered into a calculation called a power analysis, which produces an estimate of the sample size required. You do not need to know how to do a power analysis, but you do need to know that doing a power analysis is the right way to determine sample size for correlational and experimental studies (Burns & Grove, 2009).

Power analysis should be done when designing an experimental study to avoid doing a study that has a very low capacity for finding a difference in the outcomes of the two groups. Insufficient sample size weakens the statistical calculations used to detect a significant difference in the outcomes of the two groups. It is like using a microscope with weak magnification—it just cannot see everything that is there. Researchers use the terms *low statistical power* and *underpowered* to refer to a study with low capacity to detect a difference in the outcomes of the two groups. A common reason for low statistical power is small sample size.

When there is good reason to expect that the intervention will have a very strong impact on the study outcomes, the power analysis may indicate that a small sample size will be adequate. However, nursing interventions typically have modest impacts. The reality is that many nursing studies done with 30 persons in each group that find no difference in the outcomes of the two groups would find a significant difference had they been done with 100 persons in each group. If the purpose of a study is to determine if one intervention is more effective than another, doing a study with too small a sample is a waste of time, effort, and resources on everyone's part (Burns & Grove, 2009).

Random Assignment to Treatment Groups

Random assignment of enrolled participants to treatment groups is a defining feature of experimental studies. It is accomplished by assigning each person in the sample to either the **experimental group** or to the **comparison group** *based on chance determination*—not on the basis of patient preference for one treatment approach over the other, on physician request, or on the convenience of the research staff. Chance assignment requires that each participant have an equal chance of being assigned to either group. A flip of a coin is one way of randomly assigning each participant to one of the two study groups; computers can also generate a list of random numbers that can be used to determine each person's group assignment.

The contribution of random assignment to experimental design is that it controls differences in participant characteristics by distributing them evenly across both treatment groups, thus producing two groups that are similar at the start. Equivalent groups at the start are necessary in experiments because at the end of the study the researcher wants to be confident that the results were not influenced by different group compositions. When random assignment is not used, the possibility exists that some difference between the two groups that was present prior to delivering the interventions may have produced the difference found in the outcomes. This possibility creates lack of confidence in the study findings.

The larger the sample size the greater the chances are that random assignment will create treatment groups that are equivalent at baseline on important demographic and clinical variables (e.g., age, body mass index, disease severity). Nevertheless, even in large studies, researchers run comparison statistics on important demographic and clinical variables to make sure that random assignment worked effectively. A table profiling the two groups helps answer questions such as:

- Did the groups have similar mean ages?
- Did the groups have approximately equal proportions of men to women?
- Was the health status of the persons in both groups about the same?

In short, random assignment to treatment groups, sometimes referred to as *randomization*, is the most powerful way of ensuring that the two treatment groups are similar at the onset of the study; it works by evening out the presence of participant characteristics across both groups. However, not all comparisons of treatment effectiveness can use randomization. It may be ethically or practically impossible to randomly assign persons to treatment groups. For instance, a comparison of the patient outcomes and costs associated with care of the frail elderly in home with support services versus nursing home living cannot create comparison groups by random assignment of persons to a care setting. The decision regarding how care will be provided to a frail elderly person is a highly personal one that hinges on many patient, family, and community factors. As a result, the research done on this issue consists of observational studies, i.e., comparisons of existing groups. Using a nonexperimental design to compare treatment effectiveness requires that researchers and readers of the study report make an effort to identify methodological risk of bias.

Do note that random assignment is different from random sampling, which was discussed earlier in Chapter 5. Briefly, random sampling is a way of obtaining a study sample that is representative of the target population, whereas random assignment is a way of determining the intervention each study participant will receive; what they share in common is the use of chance to control bias.

The important point here is that certain patient characteristics can influence the outcomes being studied and thereby complicate comparing the effects of the two treatments. Random assignment controls the influence of patient characteristics by ensuring that the patient characteristics are present to the same extent in both treatment groups.

Having said that patient characteristics create problems in detecting treatment effectiveness, it also must be noted that there are study designs that analyze how patient characteristics affect response to the intervention. These designs (called factorial designs) make important contributions to clinical knowledge because they provide valuable information about persons with whom the intervention is very effective, moderately effective, or not effective. We will not go there because factorial designs are complex and describing them here would lead us astray.

Control of Extraneous Variables and Bias

Even when patient characteristics have been controlled through random assignment and exclusion criteria, other sources of unwanted influence can affect the outcome data. Study activities and the settings in which the study is conducted can give rise to extraneous variables that influence the outcome variables directly. Steps must be taken to control them because they confound, that is, mix with, the situation and make it difficult to obtain a clear understanding of the relationship between the interventions and the outcomes. These influences can be persistent across the study setting or can influence one treatment group more than the other.

Sometimes the setting is the larger world of current events. For example, if during the time a study is being conducted to evaluate managing arthritis pain with the use of heat and cold, a new advertisement for a jazzy new whirlpool hits the TV waves big time, the advertisement could influence the results. Some persons in the heat group might be tempted to use the whirlpool instead of using heat according to the study protocol. In addition, some of those in the cold group might decide to abandon cold treatment all together. These changes in participant compliance with their assigned treatment method could result in persons in the treatment groups actually using different treatments than the study design indicates they are using. If the researcher is monitoring the study setting (immediate and more global), he may be able to detect such an extraneous influence and take steps to moderate it or check out its influence.

To control extraneous variables originating in the study activities, researchers develop very specific study procedures or protocols. In advance of starting the study, they specify:

- Characteristics of persons who are eligible for the study
- How participants are to be recruited
- How consent to participate in the study will be obtained
- How participants will be randomly assigned to treatment groups
- The activities that comprise each treatment
- The conditions under which the treatments will be delivered
- Training of data collectors
- How and when the outcomes will be measured

In studies where a research assistant observes and rates participants' responses, it is all too easy for well-intended data collectors to influence the **outcome measurement** even when they are trying to be neutral. **Blinding** the data collector controls this source of bias. Blinding is achieved by taking steps to ensure that the data collectors do not know which intervention the participant received. Obviously, blinding is not always possible. Consider a study comparing the effects of two positioning protocols on the comfort level of persons with fractured hips before they have surgery. It is almost impossible to blind data collectors as to which intervention the patient is receiving because the patient will be in a position associated with one or the other of the treatments when the data collectors obtain the comfort ratings.

Consistent Delivery of Interventions

Two-group experiments involve actively doing something to half of the participants and something else to the other half. In research language, one group receives the experimental intervention and the other group receives a comparison intervention. The experimental intervention is usually a somewhat "new" intervention in that its effectiveness has not been thoroughly evaluated; however, there should be good reason to believe that it is safe and will have a meaningful impact on the outcomes of interest. The comparison intervention can take one of five forms (Kerlinger & Lee, 2000):

- No intervention at all
- A placebo intervention
- A usual care intervention
- A different intervention
- Same intervention but of different dose (i.e., intensity, frequency, or timing)

Placebo interventions are designed to look and feel similar to the intervention being tested but to not really have an effect on the outcomes being studied. At the very least, placebo interventions provide an attention activity for the comparison group to nullify the attention the intervention group receives. This is done because by itself, the attention involved in delivering an intervention can have an impact on some outcomes. For this reason, studies of teaching or psychological support interventions often use a placebo group rather than a no intervention group.

Both the experimental and comparison interventions should be spelled out in considerable detail in advance of starting the study and consistently delivered throughout the study. If either intervention morphs during the course of the study, the contrast between them will be lost. This loss of contrast will invalidate the results because the comparison the researcher set out to make will no longer exist. Steps taken to ensure consistent delivery of the intervention include:

- Specific study protocols
- Training of those who will be delivering the intervention
- Checks on the delivery of the intervention to ensure compliance with study protocols

Low Level of Missing Data

Missing data can be a problem in clinical studies. There are a variety of reasons for not having complete data on all participants who were entered into the study and were randomized to a treatment group, including:

- Some participants dropped out of the study (e.g., moved from the area, did not want to continue in the study).
- The condition of some participants worsened so that they could not continue in the study (e.g., transfer to ICU, too sick to answer questions).
- Some participants were not available for measurement of the outcome variable at one or several data collection times (e.g., missed an appointment, could not contribute a specimen).
- The data collector failed to obtain some data (e.g., she was sick, she overlooked something).
- The burden of participating in the study was too great.

Generally, the reasons for missing data and the pattern of missing data are more important than the amount of missing data, although 20% missing data is clearly of more concern than 2% missing data. Also, random missing data is of less concern than is a pattern of missing data (Polit & Beck, 2012). Random missing data consists of values missing here and there throughout the data from both study groups. A pattern is present when more data is missing from one group than from the other, or when more data is missing from participants with a certain characteristic, such as the youngest or the oldest. Such a pattern can bias the findings.

In any case, the researcher is obligated to try to understand why the data is missing and decide how to analyze the results to prevent the missing data from distorting the statistical results. As a reader, you first suspect data is missing when you notice that the sample sizes of various analyses are different; there may be good reasons for this, but it could also be a result of problems in the way the study was conducted. Some researchers report and explain missing data, whereas others gloss over it.

Consider this description of missing data. If a randomized study evaluating the effectiveness of a smoking cessation method has a larger dropout rate in the test intervention group than in the comparison group, the results may be biased because only the people who found the test intervention agreeable would be included in the analysis. This would make the test intervention look better than it would have been had all the persons randomized to that group contributed outcome data. Also, the results are potentially biased because the even distribution of patient characteristics created by random assignment may have been destroyed; as a result the actual analysis may have been done on groups that do not have equivalent baseline characteristics. There are recognized ways of dealing with missing data—they will not be addressed here—but if there is considerable missing data, you should note if the researcher indicated how its influence was analyzed and managed.

Large numbers of dropouts and missing data also threaten the generalizability of the study's findings. For example, a randomized study of a new physical activity program for second- and third-grade inner-city children might find that the group who participated in the new program did better than those who received a placebo intervention. However, the study had a 26% dropout rate, which was evenly distributed across both treatment groups. Although the even distribution of dropouts may not have biased the study results, the benefit produced by the new program may not be realized if the program were given to all second- and third-grade inner-city kids. The high dropout rate could have produced a study sample that was not representative of the target population, and thus the generalizability of the study findings would be called into question.

Wrap-Up

In summary, an experimental study is usually sound when researchers do the following:

1. Specify the target population
2. Determine sample size by doing a power analysis
3. Use random assignment to ensure that groups are equivalent at the start of the study
4. Ensure that interventions are delivered consistently
5. Control extraneous influences and potential bias
6. Take steps to ensure that participants stay in the study and contribute data at all collection times

Use of these research strategies ensures that any significant differences detected in the outcomes of the groups studied can with confidence be attributed to the difference in treatments the groups received. And if no differences are found, use of these research strategies ensures that the lack of difference can be attributed to the fact that the two treatments truly do not have different impacts.

Measurement of the Outcome Variables

As described earlier in Chapter 5, an important standard for every quantitative study is good data. As this standard applies to experimental studies, the instruments used to measure the outcome variables should have high reliability and validity. The researcher should report the results of reliability and validity testing that has been done, particularly testing done in populations similar to the one being studied. Generally speaking, good data is produced by measurement instruments that have been rigorously developed through testing and thus have known reliability and validity levels. Instruments developed specifically for the study being reported often lack reliability and validity testing.

Limitations of Randomized Experiments

The randomized experiment is the gold standard study design for determining if a healthcare intervention brings about desired outcomes. However, when clinicians read a study report of a randomized study, they often want to decide if they should use the intervention with their patients; in this regard randomized studies have limitations. One problem is that the findings of many studies are reported as average outcomes of the two treatment groups. However, clinicians treat unique individuals, not average individuals, and thus the clinician does not know if the particular patient will respond like the average patient in the more effective study group or in a different way. Even if 80% of patients in a group respond favorably to an intervention, the clinician does not know if the patient he is treating will respond like the 80% or like the other 20%.

A second limitation of randomized controlled experiments is that they may have weak generalizability resulting from the exclusion of patients with conditions other than the one of interest—as described earlier. Exclusions control extraneous variables and thereby afford more certainty about the effectiveness of the intervention. However, they pose a dilemma for clinicians in that the patients in the study may have fewer health problems (i.e., comorbidities) than do patients seen in everyday practice. As a result, the intervention itself may be difficult to use, or similar results may not be realized.

A third limitation of randomized controlled experiments is that the interventions are delivered in a controlled manner, whereas in everyday practice an intervention is delivered by a diverse group of people. Often it is not clear how much variation can be introduced into the delivery of an intervention and still retain its effectiveness.

These limitations do not mean that randomized controlled experiments are not useful; however, they do point to the need for multiple studies regarding an intervention—under different conditions and with diverse groups of people. The limitations also require that researchers explore deeply why some people responded very positively to an intervention, others responded in a moderately positive manner, and still others responded negatively or poorly.

Quasi-Experimental Designs

Although experimental design is the gold standard for evaluating the cause–effect relationship between an intervention and an outcome, sometimes it is *not* possible to: (1) use random assignment to intervention groups; (2) have tight control over the delivery of the intervention; or (3) have a comparison group (Burns & Grove, 2009).

Studies that lack one or more of these features are described as quasi-experimental. They are enough like experiments to retain the word *experiment* in their description, but because they lack one of the important features of experiments, they leave open the door to uncontrolled extraneous variables and wrong conclusions to an extent that experimental designs do not.

To illustrate, if two methods for preventing heel pressure ulcers were studied on one unit of a long-term care facility, the staff might have difficulty keeping the two methods pure. So, the researchers might decide to use method A with at-risk patients on one unit and method B with at-risk patients on another similar unit. This would be a quasi-experimental study because individual participants are members of intact groups (patients on a particular unit) and the unit determines which intervention they receive, not random assignment. Even when the two patient groups seem similar, there is concern that they might be different in unidentified ways or that the quality of care on the two units is different. Any difference could act as an extraneous variable giving statistical results indicative of an intervention effect on the outcome, when in actuality it was a patient or unit difference that produced the results, not the intervention. The researcher conducting such a study could take steps to identify, control, or take into account extraneous influences. These steps would include comparing the characteristics of the patients on the two units and comparing the two units on variables such as staffing pattern, years of experience of the staff, and their educational levels. Taking any differences into account in the analysis would build confidence in study results, indicating that one intervention was more effective than the other in preventing heel ulcers. Another example of a quasi-experimental design is a study in which the first 100 participants receive treatment A and the second 100 receive treatment B. This would be a consecutive series method for assigning individuals to treatment groups; thus patient-participants are not randomly assigned to treatment groups. This design also raises concerns that the two treatment groups might not be equivalent at the start. Something may have changed in the environment during the time that lapsed between the beginning of one series and the beginning of the second series, such as a seasonal difference in patients, a change in staffing, or a change in work flow. Thus, an extraneous variable could be at work and produce a difference in patient outcomes.

Generally, quasi-experimental study designs are considered weaker than randomized experimental designs because there is lack of certainty that the two groups actually were equivalent at baseline or that they received exactly the same treatment. The reader of a report of a quasi-experimental study needs to be alert to nonequivalent groups, inconsistent treatment delivery, or the presence of extraneous variables because they could distort the results and study conclusions.

Exemplar

Reading Tips

One of the interventions evaluated in the exemplar study is the administration of promethazine, which is used to treat postoperative nausea and vomiting. If you are not familiar with this drug, you should look it up as it is widely used. Also, just to be clear: an alcohol prep pad is the little alcohol-impregnated piece of gauze used to cleanse skin prior to an injection or venipuncture.

At this point, read just the introductory and methods sections (up to *Results*).

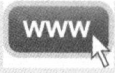

Comparison of Inhalation of Isopropyl Alcohol vs. Promethazine in the Treatment of Postoperative Nausea and Vomiting (PONV) in Patients Identified as at High Risk for Developing PONV.

Joseph Pellegrini, Jon DeLoge, John Bennett, and Joseph Kelly

AANA Journal (2009), *77*(4), 293–299.

Frequently, patients identified as high risk for postoperative nausea and vomiting (PONV) are treated prophylactically with intravenous (IV) ondansetron and postoperatively with IV promethazine. The purpose of this study was to determine if using an aromatic therapy of 70% isopropyl alcohol (IPA) would be more effective than promethazine in resolution of breakthrough PONV symptoms in groups of high-risk patients administered prophylactic ondansetron.

All subjects enrolled were identified as high risk for PONV, administered general anesthesia and a prophylactic antiemetic of 4 mg of IV ondansetron, and randomized to receive IPA or promethazine for treatment of breakthrough PONV. Demographics, verbal numeric rating scale (VNRS) scores for nausea, time to 50% reduction in VNRS scores, and overall antiemetic and incidence of PONV were measured.

The data for 85 subjects were included in analysis; no differences in demographic variables or baseline measurements were noted between groups. The IPA group reported a faster time to 50% reduction in VNRS scores and decreased overall antiemetic requirements. A similar incidence in PONV was noted between groups.

Based on these findings, we recommend that inhalation of 70% IPA is an option for treatment of PONV in high-risk patients who have received prophylactic ondansetron.

Key Words

Isopropyl alcohol, postoperative nausea and vomiting (PONV), promethazine, risk factors for PONV

* * *

In the general surgical population, the risk of postoperative nausea and vomiting (PONV) is between 16% and 30%; however, this risk ratio is increased even further when certain factors are present that predispose a patient to PONV.[1–5] These risk factors include general anesthesia of more than 60 minutes' duration, female gender, nonsmoker, history of PONV, and history of motion sickness.[1–7] In fact, it has been noted that the incidence of PONV increases exponentially from 16% when no risk factors are present to as high as 87% when all risk factors are present.[1–9] Therefore, it has become routine in many anesthesia practices to screen patients preoperatively to identify the patients at high risk for PONV so that an aggressive management plan can be implemented to prevent or decrease the severity of PONV symptoms.

Most typically, this aggressive management plan involves the prophylactic administration of an antiemetic agent that works specifically on an area of the brain called the chemotaxic trigger zone (CTZ).[1–5] The CTZ, located in the area postrema of the brain, lacks a blood–brain barrier, thereby making it highly receptive to stimulation from specific neurotransmitters that have been shown to be integral in eliciting an emetic response.[1–5] These neurotransmitters include serotonin, dopamine, histamine, and acetylcholine.[1–5] Although a variety of agents can be administered prophylactically to prevent PONV, the agent most often used is the serotonin antagonist ondansetron, an antiemetic agent that has been shown to be highly effective in preventing

PONV in a wide variety of patient populations, while still having a relatively low side-effect profile.[6–11]

Ondansetron, when used as a prophylactic agent, is routinely administered approximately 15 to 30 minutes before the conclusion of the surgical procedure. Studies have shown that the prophylactic administration of ondansetron results in a 50% to 80% reduction in PONV in groups of low-risk patients but only a 25% reduction in patients identified as high risk for PONV.[10–12] Because of this lack of effectiveness in preventing PONV in patients identified as high risk, the patients will often require a subsequent antiemetic for treatment, and one of the most common agents used to treat this breakthrough PONV is the antiemetic agent promethazine.[8,13]

Promethazine is a dopamine receptor blocking agent routinely administered because it has a rapid onset of action (within 3–5 minutes) and a relatively long duration of efficacy (approximately 2–6 hours).[8] However, unlike ondansetron, which has minimal side effects, promethazine is commonly associated with sedation, dry mouth, and, in rare cases, hypotension.[8,13] Despite these side effects, many practitioners prefer promethazine to other traditional antiemetic agents because it can be used in the inpatient and outpatient settings. Promethazine is routinely administered by the intravenous (IV) route to a patient while in the hospital but is also available in oral and suppository forms for outpatient administration.[8,13] However, some patients report hesitancy to taking an oral antiemetic when they are nauseous; therefore, many practitioners prescribe the suppository form to avoid oral administration and because it can be easily self-administered by a patient in the home setting. Despite this, many patients still report hesitancy toward self-administration of a promethazine suppository and often report that the side effects following administration are unacceptable.[9,14] Therefore, anesthesia practitioners are continually seeking alternative antiemetic treatments that are highly effective in treating PONV, can be easily self-administered in any setting, and have a low side-effect profile.

A PONV treatment that seems to meet all of these criteria is the aromatic treatment of 70% isopropyl alcohol (IPA) that is administered by simply using a single alcohol prep pad. Research has shown that inhalation of IPA from a simple alcohol prep pad is easy to administer in the inpatient and outpatient settings, is highly effective in treating PONV, and is associated with no side effects.[15–17] However, all of the studies to date using IPA have been done only with patients who are not classified as high risk for PONV, and IPA has never been used in a patient population that has been prophylactically treated with ondansetron. Therefore, the purpose of this study was to investigate the efficacy of IPA vs promethazine in treating breakthrough PONV in groups of high-risk patients who have received a perioperative prophylactic dose of ondansetron.

Methods

All patients scheduled for general anesthesia of more than 60 minutes' duration and having 2 of the 4 individual risk factors for PONV (female gender, nonsmoker, history of PONV or motion sickness) were approached for possible inclusion in this institutional review board–approved prospective study. Patients were excluded from participation if they reported a recent upper respiratory infection; documented allergy to IPA, ondansetron, promethazine, or metoclopramide; antiemetic or psychoactive drug use within 24 hours; inability to breathe through the nose; pregnancy; history of inner ear pathology; and/or taking disulfiram, cefoperazone, or metronidazole. Patients with a body mass index greater than 35 kg/m^2 also were excluded from the study. In addition, following enrollment, the data were excluded from analysis for subjects who required inpatient hospitalization for reasons not related to PONV.

Once inclusionary criteria were met, informed consent was obtained and demographic data were collected, including age, height, weight, gender, ASA class, body mass index, race, and surgical procedure. All subjects were then randomly assigned using a computer-generated random numbers process into a control or an experimental group. The control group was assigned to receive 12.5 to 25 mg IV promethazine for complaints of PONV in the postanesthesia care unit (PACU) and same-day surgery unit (SDSU) and by promethazine suppository self-administration following discharge to home. The experimental group was assigned to receive treatment of PONV by administration of inhaled 70% IPA.

In the preoperative holding area, all subjects received instruction on treatments, study requirements, and the home data collection tool. A baseline level of nausea was obtained on all subjects following informed consent using a 0 to 10 verbal numeric rating scale (VNRS) in which a score of "0" indicated "no nausea" and a score of "10" indicated the "worst imaginable nausea." Before transport to the operative suite, preoperative medications for anxiolysis and sedation were administered based on individual requirements and anesthesia providers' discretion using 0 to 5 mg of midazolam and/or 0 to 3 μg/kg of fentanyl IV. All preoperative medications administered were recorded.

On arrival to the operative suite, blood pressure, electrocardiographic, and pulse oximetry monitors were applied and a baseline set of vital signs was obtained and recorded. Anesthesia induction was facilitated with propofol, 1.5 to 2 mg/kg IV; lidocaine, 0 to 1 mg/kg IV; fentanyl, 0 to 5 μg/kg IV; and a neuromuscular blocking agent of the anesthesia provider's choice. Following induction, all subjects were endotracheally intubated, and, based on surgical requirements, an orogastric tube was inserted and stomach contents were evacuated. All orogastric tubes were removed immediately before extubation, and the use of an orogastric tube was recorded.

Maintenance of anesthesia was achieved with isoflurane, desflurane, or sevoflurane in combination with oxygen, 50% or 100%, and nitrous oxide, 0% or 50%. An opioid of provider choice was used for maintenance of analgesia. The doses of all opioids administered during the perioperative period were later converted to morphine equivalents for analysis.[18] Approximately 15 to 30 minutes before extubation, all subjects received ondansetron, 4 mg IV. Neuromuscular blockade was reversed, if necessary, using neostigmine, 0.05 mg/kg, and glycopyrrolate, 0.1 mg/kg IV. All medications administered intraoperatively were recorded on the data collection tool. Additional information collected and recorded included the type of surgery, use of laparoscopic technique, total estimated blood loss, total amount of IV fluids administered, estimated preoperative-postoperative fluid deficit, and anesthesia, surgical, and PACU times. All subjects were extubated before transfer to the PACU.

Following arrival to the PACU and SDSU, an admission VNRS for nausea was obtained and recorded. For the purposes of this study, nausea was defined as the subjective feeling of the urge to vomit, and vomiting was defined as the forceful expulsion of gastric contents. Each event had to be at least 60 seconds from any other event to be recorded as a separate event. In addition, VNRS scores were obtained and recorded at the first complaint of nausea, every 5 minutes following treatment for nausea for the first 30 minutes, and then every 15 minutes thereafter for 75 minutes after the event or until discharge from the PACU or SDSU. Nausea events were treated according to group assignment (IPA or promethazine).

Subjects in the control (promethazine) group received promethazine, 12.5 to 25 mg IV, at the first complaint of nausea in the PACU and SDSU; this dose could be repeated in 30 minutes for a maximum dose of 50 mg IV. For nausea that was refractory to promethazine, control subjects could receive metoclopramide, 10 mg IV every 15 minutes, not to exceed a total dose of 30 mg.

All subjects in the experimental (IPA) group received inhalation therapy using a commercially available 70% IPA pad (Webcol, Kendall Healthcare, Mansfield, Massachusetts). All subjects were instructed to remove the IPA pad from the protective covering, fold the IPA pad in half, hold the folded pad approximately 0.5 inches from their nares, and take 3 deep inhalations from the pad and discard it after use. This treatment could be administered by the PACU and SDSU nurses in the hospital setting or by the patient; however, subjects were instructed to self-administer their IPA treatments following discharge to home following the treatment regimen described above. The IPA treatments were ordered to be administered on an as-needed basis, up to a total of 3 separate applications (3 deep inhalations per application) every 15 minutes. For complaints of nausea refractory to IPA treatment (no resolution of PONV symptoms after 3 applications) or if a patient requested an antiemetic agent at any time, promethazine, 12.5 to 25 mg IV every 30 minutes was given, not to exceed a total dose of 50 mg IV, or metoclopramide, 10 mg IV every 15 minutes, not to exceed a total dose of 30 mg. These treatment protocols were the same in the PACU and SDSU settings. All pharmacologic treatments administered for nausea and VNRS score measurements were recorded.

Before discharge to home, all subjects were instructed to treat PONV symptoms based on their assigned group. The subjects in the promethazine group were instructed to treat any PONV using 25-mg promethazine suppositories every 6 hours on an as-needed basis. The subjects in the IPA group were instructed to use the folded IPA regimen as described in the hospital setting on an as-needed basis, up to a total of 3 separate applications. In addition, IPA subjects were also instructed that they could self-administer a 25-mg promethazine suppository for any PONV symptoms that were refractory to the IPA treatments or if they had exhausted the number of applications ordered and had not achieved resolution of PONV symptoms. All subjects were asked to record the time any antiemetic therapy was self-administered at home (IPA or promethazine), the number of nausea and emetic events, and the severity of nausea using the 0 to 10 VNRS scale before they self-administered any antiemetic therapy and every 15 minutes after initiation for a period of 30 minutes. Before discharge, all subjects were given a home data collection sheet to record these events and instructed that they would receive a telephone call by one of the investigators approximately 24 hours after surgery to obtain this information. In addition, during the telephone call, all subjects were asked to rate their level of satisfaction regarding their antiemetic therapy using the following scale: 1, totally dissatisfied; 2, somewhat dissatisfied; 3, somewhat satisfied; 4, satisfied; and 5, totally satisfied. All responses from the telephone interview were recorded on a data collection sheet.

Before initiation of this study, a power analysis was performed based on previous studies[15,16] that indicated that subjects in the IPA group would achieve a 50% reduction in their mean VNRS scores for nausea 15 minutes earlier than subjects randomized to receive promethazine treatment. By using an α of .05 and a β of .10, we determined that a sample size of 40 subjects per group would be required to determine if a difference between the groups existed. Factoring in a 20% attrition rate increased our sample size to 96 subjects (48 per group).

Statistical analysis was performed using SPSS software version 13.0 (SPSS Inc., Chicago, Illinois). Data analysis was accomplished using descriptive and inferential statistics. Demographic data and frequency data were analyzed using the χ^2 test and Pearson correlation. The VNRS scores and time to resolution were analyzed using a Student *t* test. Subject satisfaction scores, body mass index scores, and total promethazine requirements were analyzed using a Mann-Whitney *U* test. A *P* value of less than .05 was considered significant.

Results

A total of 96 subjects were enrolled, but 11 subjects were withdrawn, leaving a total of 85 subjects (IPA group, 42; promethazine group, 43) whose data would be included in the final analysis. Reasons for withdrawal included 4 subjects who received additional antiemetics intraoperatively (2 in each group), 1 subject inadvertently enrolled despite being scheduled for a nasal surgical procedure (IPA group), and 6 subjects who required postoperative inpatient hospitalization for reasons unrelated to PONV (3 in each group).

No differences were noted between the groups in relation to demographic variables, surgical times, anesthesia times, use of laparoscopy, orogastric tube use, time to first PONV event from PACU admission, history of motion sickness, primary volatile agent used, or the total number of PONV risk factors present. A noted difference was in the use of nitrous oxide between groups: 59% of the IPA group received 50% nitrous oxide compared with 37% in the promethazine group ($P = .049$). However when a separate analysis of nitrous oxide use and PONV was performed, no significance could be found to indicate that nitrous oxide administration increased the incidence of PONV. No differences in the amount of opioids administered during the perioperative period were noted between groups ($P > .05$) (Table 1). No differences in fluid deficit, estimated blood loss, type of surgical procedure performed, total amount of IV fluid administered, or total hours without oral intake were noted between groups.

The overall incidence of postoperative nausea was similar between groups, with 76% (n = 32) of the IPA group reporting postoperative nausea compared with 60% (n = 26) of the promethazine group ($P = .119$). Analysis of the incidence of nausea based on setting revealed that a higher incidence of PONV occurred in the IPA group in all settings but achieved significance only following discharge to home ($P = .019$). Promethazine was administered as the primary antiemetic agent in the promethazine group and as a rescue agent in the IPA group. Not surprisingly, the median dose of promethazine was higher in the promethazine group in all settings, achieving significance in the PACU and SDSU (Table 2). Analysis of the need for promethazine suppositories following discharge revealed that 23% (n = 10) of the promethazine group self-administered a promethazine suppository compared with only 7% (n = 3) of the IPA group ($P = .039$). No subject in either group required metoclopramide as a rescue agent in any setting. No differences in the VNRS scores were noted between groups on initial complaint of nausea in any setting (Figure 1). However, when time to 50% reduction in VNRS scores for nausea was analyzed, we noted a significantly faster time to a 50% reduction in VNRS scores in the IPA group compared with the promethazine group in the PACU ($P = .045$), SDSU ($P = .032$), and the home ($P = .017$) settings (Figure 2).

Table 1 Description of Demographic Data, Preoperative Risk Factors, and Perioperative Information[a]

	Isopropyl alcohol (n = 42)	Promethazine (n = 43)	*P*
Age (y)	33.98 ± 10.9	37.09 ± 11.0	.052
Weight (kg)	75.43 ± 17.4	74.84 ± 13.3	.939
Median (range) body mass index (kg/m^2)	27 (22–34)	27 (21–33)	.947
Laparoscopy			
Total	21	20	.748
Gynecologic	14	11	.433
Gender			.763
Female	30	33	
Male	12	10	
Surgical time (min)	50.57 ± 34.32	57.63 ± 44.3	.416
Anesthesia time (min)	90.45 ± 39.5	101.1 ± 48.7	.272
PONV risk factors			.676
3 risk factors	24	26	
4 risk factors	12	9	
5 risk factors	6	8	
Time from PACU admission to PONV event (min)	90.9 ± 101.8	78.8 ± 76.7	.664
History of motion sickness			.723
Yes	26	25	
No	16	18	
Primary volatile agent used			.326
Desflurane	18	25	
Sevoflurane	22	16	
Isoflurane	2	2	
Opioid morphine equivalent			
Perioperative	24.05 ± 16.4	21.5 ± 9.1	.375
PACU	8.8 ± 5.7	9.3 ± 5.6	.775
SDSU	4.4 ± 2.5	4.1 ± 1.9	.736
Nitrous oxide use			.049[b]
Yes	25	16	
No	17	27	
Orogastric tube use			.668
Yes	16	19	
No	26	24	

PONV indicates postoperative nausea and vomiting; PACU, postanesthesia care unit; SDSU, same-day surgical unit.

[a]Data are given as mean ± SD or number of cases unless otherwise indicated.

[b]Significant at $P < .05$.

Table 2. Incidence of Nausea Events and Median Doses of Promethazine Required Per Group Per Setting

	Isopropyl alcohol (n = 42)	Promethazine (n = 43)	*P*
No. (%) of nausea events			
PACU	7 (17)	10 (23)	.448
SDSU	17 (42)	10 (23)	.088
Home	19 (45)	10 (23)	.019[a]
Median (range) promethazine requirements (mg)			
PACU	0	12.5 (0–25)	.002[a]
SDSU	12.5 (0–25)	25.0 (0–50)	.033[a]
Home	12.5 (0–25)	12.5 (0–25)	.214

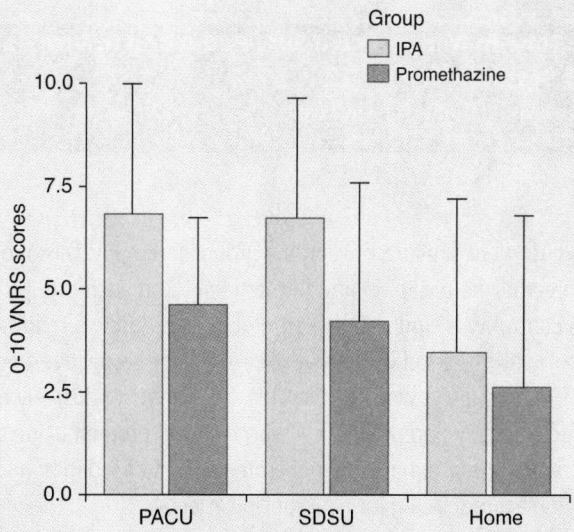

Figure 1 VNRS Scores on Initial Complaint Per Setting

VNRS indicates visual numeric rating scale; IPA, isopropyl alcohol; PACU, postanesthesia care unit; SDSU, same-day surgical unit.

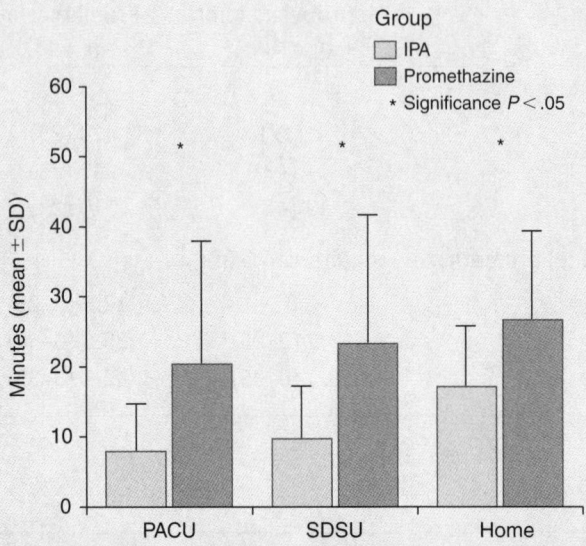

Figure 2 Time in Minutes to a 50% Reduction in VNRS Scores by Group Per Setting

VNRS indicates visual numeric rating scale; IPA, isopropyl alcohol; PACU, postanesthesia care unit; SDSU, same-day surgical unit.

Emetic events were similar between the groups in the PACU (none), SDSU (IPA group, 3; promethazine group, 2) and in the home (5 in each group). Satisfaction with nausea control was similar between groups: both groups reported a median of 4 (satisfied) with the level of nausea control for the respective treatment regimens ($P > .05$). No subject who received IPA treatments exclusively reported any untoward side effects, whereas subjects who received promethazine as a primary or rescue treatment reported mild to moderate degrees of sedation and dry mouth; however, no subject required treatment for side effects.

Discussion

Postoperative nausea and vomiting continue to be persistent problems following general anesthesia. In our study, we used the risk factors for PONV identified by Koivuranta et al.[1] that included the variables gender, smoking history, history of PONV, a history of motion sickness, and exposure to general anesthesia for more than 60 minutes to establish a risk of PONV. Koivuranta et al.[1] reported that the relative risk of PONV for someone with 3 risk factors is 54%, with 4 risk factors is 63%, and with all 5 risk factors is 87%.

Based on these findings, we anticipated the overall incidence of PONV to be approximately 60%, given that the number of risk factors ranged between 3 and 5 in both groups. We anticipated this number to be decreased by a ratio of 25% to 42% following ondansetron administration. We were surprised to find that the overall incidence of PONV ranged between 61% and 76%, thereby indicating that ondansetron prophylaxis was not as effective as we hypothesized. However, analysis of the incidence of nausea in the PACU and SDSU revealed that the overall incidence of nausea was approximately 45% in both groups, indicating that ondansetron is limited in providing prophylaxis for the first few hours after surgery. Because of this limited range of effectiveness, it is common for patients at high risk for PONV to require subsequent antiemetic agents for the treatment of breakthrough PONV, which can often result in some significant side effects such as sedation and hypotension.

Another problem with traditional antiemetic agents is that they often cannot be administered easily in the home setting. In addition, the potential for side effects may place postoperative patients at risk. We chose IPA aromatic therapy as an avenue for investigation because previous research showed that it is effective in treating the symptoms of nausea and can be easily administered in the home setting.[15,16] However, these earlier studies were not performed on a high-risk patient population or in groups of patients already given ondansetron. In this study, we showed that IPA is effective in alleviating the symptoms of PONV and works very well in concert with ondansetron.

There has been some research that found that IPA is no more effective than other aromatic therapies or having the patient take several deep breaths of ambient air. For example, Anderson and Gross[19] reported that no difference in nausea scores was found among groups of patients asked to inhale peppermint, IPA, or saline, and they concluded that it was the simple act of taking a deep inhalation of air that was the inducement to relieve PONV symptoms rather than any specific aromatic properties. However, it was noted that this study was done on a very small group of patients (33 subjects), and the researchers did not have control over subsequent antiemetics administered during the perioperative and postoperative periods; therefore, it is difficult to ascertain the specific agent that facilitated the relief of PONV symptoms in the study. The findings of Anderson and Gross are contradicted in an earlier study by Langevin and Brown,[17] who compared the inhalation of IPA with placebo (saline) in a double-blinded study (30 subjects; 15/group). These investigators reported that administration of IPA resulted in a complete resolution of PONV symptoms in 80% of patients treated with IPA and that deep inhalation from a saline-soaked pad was totally ineffective in resolution of PONV symptoms, indicating that simply performing deep inhalations through the nose is not effective in alleviating symptoms of PONV.

Our study had some limitations. The SDSU staff was required to record VNRS scores every 5 minutes on complaint of PONV; therefore, we were forced to limit our subject enrollment to 1 or 2 subjects per day to ensure quality data collection. Also, in the home setting, we found there was a social stigma associated with the insertion of suppositories, and some patients reported hesitancy to use the suppository. We specifically chose a suppository over oral medication because it has also been noted that many patients are also hesitant to orally ingest a medication when they are experiencing nausea. It is unknown what overall effect this hesitancy may have had on the number of subjects who reported that they did not use the promethazine suppository as a rescue medication in the home setting. In retrospect, perhaps a better choice of an antiemetic for use as a rescue agent following discharge to home may have been an agent that does not require oral ingestion or suppository insertion, for example, sublingual ondansetron.

Although this study was designed using a unimodal approach to PONV prophylaxis, many practitioners report that more clinical effectiveness is observed when a multimodal antiemetic approach is used. The multimodal approach is used in an effort to optimize coverage on different receptors in the CTZ. While using this approach has been shown to be more effective in preventing PONV than using a single modal approach, it usually results in an increase in side effects.[6–9] Because of this, we are planning a future study in which we plan to provide IPA prophylaxis immediately before induction of general anesthesia in addition to the standard ondansetron prophylaxis 15 to 30 minutes before the conclusion of the surgical procedure. It is unclear where IPA works in relation to blocking the receptors in the CTZ. We hypothesize that it may possibly work on several sites simultaneously in the CTZ; therefore, IPA pharmacokinetics may already use a multimodal approach. However, we note that the clinical duration of IPA is limited; therefore, we propose that in an effort to optimize this multimodal approach, it may be best tested by incorporating ondansetron prophylaxis into the design as well. To date, only 1 study has been performed in which IPA was administered prophylactically, and the investigators reported that the inhalation of IPA was no more effective than the administration of granisetron but was more effective than no prophylactic treatment.[20] This study indicated that IPA prophylaxis was effective in preventing PONV, but the study used a small sample and administered the IPA following extubation, a different method than the one we are planning.

We believe that we clearly showed that IPA is as effective in treating PONV as promethazine in patients who have been identified as high risk for PONV, but it works considerably faster, works well in concert with ondansetron, and can be easily administered in any setting. Therefore, we are confident in recommending that IPA be considered a viable option to conventional antiemetic therapy in treating breakthrough PONV in groups of patients identified as high risk for PONV who have received perioperative prophylactic ondansetron.

References

1. Koivuranta M, Lääräa E, Snåre L, Alahuhta S. A survey of postoperative nausea and vomiting. *Anaesthesia*. 1997;52(5):443–449.
2. Eberhart LH, Högel J, Seeling W, Staack M, Geldner G, Georgieff M. Evaluation of the three risk scores to predict postoperative nausea and vomiting. *Acta Anaesthesiol Scand*. 2000;44(4):480–488.
3. Cohen MM, Duncan PG, DeBoer DP, Tweed WA. The postoperative interview: assessing risk factors for nausea and vomiting. *Anesth Analg*. 1994;78(1):7–16.
4. Haigh CG, Kaplan LA, Durham JM, Dupeyron JP, Harmer M, Kenny GN. Nausea and vomiting after gynaecological surgery: a meta-analysis of factors affecting their incidence. *Br J Anaesth*. 1993;71:517–522.
5. Kenny GN. Risk factors for postoperative nausea and vomiting. *Anaesthesia*. 1994; 49(suppl):6–10.
6. Watcha MF, White PF. Postoperative nausea and vomiting: its etiology, treatment and prevention. *Anesthesiology*. 1992;77(1):162–184.
7. Apfel CC, Lääräa E, Koivuranta M, Greim CA, Roewer N. A simplified risk score for predicting postoperative nausea and vomiting: conclusions from cross-validations between two centers. *Anesthesiology*. 1999;91(3):693–700.
8. Kovac AL. Prevention and treatment of postoperative nausea and vomiting. *Drugs*. 2000;59(2):213–243.
9. Tong G. Postoperative nausea and vomiting: can it be eliminated? *JAMA*. 2002; 287(10):1233–1236.
10. Claybon L. Single dose intravenous ondansetron for the 24-hour treatment of postoperative nausea and vomiting. *Anaesthesia*. 1994;49 (suppl):24–29.
11. Kovac AL, O'Connor TA, Pearman MH, et al. Efficacy of repeat intravenous dosing of ondansetron in controlling postoperative nausea and vomiting: a randomized, double-blind, placebo-controlled multicenter trial. *J Clin Anesth*. 1999;11(6):453–459.
12. Jones S, Strobl R, Crosby D, Burkard JF, Maye J, Pellegrini JE. The effect of transdermal scopolamine on the incidence and severity of postoperative nausea and vomiting in a group of high-risk patients given prophylactic intravenous ondansetron. *AANA J*. 2006;74(2): 127–132.
13. Dillon GP Jr. Clinical evaluation of promethazine for prevention of postoperative vomiting. *Am Pract Dig Treat*. 1957;8(10):1571–1575.
14. Scuderi PE, James RL, Harris L, Mims GR III. Multimodal antiemetic management prevents early postoperative vomiting after outpatient laparoscopy. *Anesth Analg*. 2000;91(6):1408–1414.

15. Winston AW, Rinehart RS, Riley GP, Vacchiano CA, Pellegrini JE. Comparison of inhaled isopropyl alcohol and intravenous ondansetron for treatment of postoperative nausea. *AANA J*. 2003;71(2):127–132.
16. Cotton JW, Rowell LR, Hood RR, Pellegrini JE. A comparative analysis of isopropyl alcohol and ondansetron in the treatment of postoperative nausea and vomiting from the hospital setting to the home. *AANA J*. 2007;75(1):21–26.
17. Langevin P, Brown M. A simple, innocuous and inexpensive treatment for postoperative nausea and vomiting [abstract]. *Anesth Analg*. 1997; 84(suppl):S16.
18. Gordon DB, Stevenson KK, Griffie J, Muchka S, Rapp C, Ford-Roberts K. Opioid equianalgesic calculations. *J Palliat Med*. 1999;2(2):209–218.
19. Anderson LA, Gross JB. Aromatherapy with peppermint, isopropyl alcohol, or placebo is equally effective in relieving postoperative nausea. *J Perianesth Nurs*. 2004;19(1): 29–35.
20. Teran L, Hawkins JK. The effectiveness of inhalation isopropyl alcohol vs granisetron for the prevention of postoperative nausea and vomiting. *AANA J*. 2007;75(6):417–422.

Authors

Joseph Pellegrini, CRNA, PhD, CAPT(ret), NC, USN, is the former director of research, Navy Nurse Corps Anesthesia Program, Bethesda, Maryland. He is currently an associate professor, Nurse Anesthesia Program, University of Maryland, Baltimore, Maryland. Email: Pellegrini@son.umaryland.edu.

LT Jon DeLoge, CRNA, MSN, NC, USNR, is a staff nurse anesthetist at Naval Medical Center, Portsmouth, Virginia.

LCDR John Bennett, CRNA, MSN, NC, USNR, is a staff nurse anesthetist at Naval Medical Center, San Diego, California.

Joseph Kelly, CRNA, MS, CDR(ret), NC, USN, is a staff nurse anesthetist at University of Florida, Shands Medical Center, Jacksonville, Florida.

Disclaimer

The views expressed in this article are those of the authors and do not necessarily reflect the official policy or position of the Department of the Navy, Department of Defense, or the US Government. We are military service members. This work was prepared as part of our official duties. Title 17 U.S.C. 105 provides that 'Copyright protection under this title is not available for any work of the United States Government.' Title 17 U.S.C. 101 defines a United States Government work as a work prepared by a military service member or employee of the United States Government as part of that person's official duties.

Profile & Commentary: Introduction and Methods

STUDY PURPOSE

The purpose of this study was to compare the effectiveness of the inhalation of isopropyl alcohol (IPA) from a 70% prep pad to the drug promethazine in the treatment of postoperative nausea and vomiting (PONV) in patients who are at high risk for PONV. The researchers note that prior research that found IPA to be effective was done with patients who were not classified as high risk for PONV, which is why this study is needed. Information about the high prevalence of PONV and the risk factors for it is presented in the first several paragraphs.

STUDY DESIGN

This is a two-group experimental study in which participants were randomly assigned to one of two treatment groups, and the researchers had good control over the conditions under which treatments were given and data was collected. It is cross-sectional because data were collected for just one episode of care. Collecting data at several times that are close to one another (i.e., hospital then home) does not make it a longitudinal design as the intent was not to examine change over time.

Sample

Although the projected target population from a narrow perspective is the patients who have surgery in the one hospital, from a broader perspective the projected target population is patients similar to those described in Table 1 at similar hospitals. The absence of information about the setting precludes including those features in the characterization of the target population.

Persons included in the sample were those who: (1) had anesthesia that lasted longer than 60 minutes, (2) were identified as at high risk for PONV, (3) did not have one of the exclusion conditions, and (4) agreed to participate in the study. The reasons for exclusion are numerous; for the most part, these exclusions eliminated persons who should not be given one of the interventions. The 96 persons who qualified for the study were randomly assigned to a treatment group.

Eventually, data was available on 85 persons; 42 in the IPA group and 43 in the promethazine group. Note also that the reasons 11 persons were withdrawn from the study were given; the withdrawal rate and reasons for it were essentially the same in both groups group. Explicitly stating these facts eliminates concerns that uneven withdrawal could have undermined the equality of the two groups that was created by randomization.

The sample size was determined by a power analysis that took into account the expected effect of the IPA over the promethazine and the statistical certainty they wanted, as indicated by the *p*-level decision point (α) and by the level of power they wanted (β); they also took into account that 20% of those enrolled might not complete the study.

The sample is profiled in Table 1. The two groups were compared on demographic characteristics, risk factors, and perioperative information. The *p*-value column informs us that the only significant difference in the two groups at the start of the study was the proportions who received nitrous oxide during the operation; the researchers did some analysis of this difference and decided it did not increase the incidence of PONV. All the other differences were just chance variations expected in obtaining two samples from a population. From this table, we can conclude that randomization was very effective in creating two groups with similar profiles. In other words, we do not have to worry that the two groups were different in some way right at the start; thus when we look at the results, we will be able to eliminate initial differences in group composition as an explanation for the results.

You might wonder about the effects of different kinds of surgery. This was controlled to some extent by including only persons who would have general anesthesia of at least 60 minutes duration. Also, the fact that the two groups were not different in terms of surgical time, anesthesia time, laparoscopy cases, use of orogastric tubes, and gynecological cases assures us that the distribution of types of surgical procedures was probably also evenly distributed across both groups.

Interventions

Many details about how the interventions were delivered are provided in the report. It is clear from this description that every effort was made to control the consistency with which the interventions were delivered, thus controlling another source of extraneous influences. Importantly, in the hospital, if IPA was not effective, patients in that group would be given IV promethazine; however we are not told how many patients in the IPA group ended up being given IV promethazine. After discharge, the patients were to continue using the intervention they had in the hospital, although when promethazine was needed, it was to be taken via rectal suppositories (rather than given intravenously as in the hospital).

Outcome Measures

The outcomes studied were:

- Incidence of PONV
- Events of PONV
- Time to 50% reduction in the nausea
- Intensity of nausea
- Doses of promethazine required
- Satisfaction with nausea control

These outcomes were measured at various times.

The VNRS, which measured intensity of nausea, was obtained on admission to the PACU or SDCU, at the first complaint of nausea, and at defined intervals after the intervention was delivered. The VNRS is a 0 to 10 scale with 0 representing "no nausea" and 10 representing the "worst imaginable nausea." No information is provided about how well this scale captures gradations of nausea, but similar scales (visual analogue scales) are widely used in clinical practice and in symptom research. Reliability and validity of these scales are rarely discussed or provided.

At discharge, patients were given a home data collection sheet to record their events of nausea or vomiting and VNRS at intervals after an event. At the phone call 24 hours after discharge, patients were asked to rate their level of satisfaction with their treatment for nausea using a 5-point scale.

You should now have a sense of *how* this study was done. However, you may need to go back over it again to get some of the details fixed in your mind.

Section 2: Understanding Study Results

Was One Intervention More Effective Than the Other?

In most two-group experimental studies, the researcher's goal is to determine if one intervention is more effective than the other. Effectiveness is defined as impact or influence on the outcome variable, and more effectiveness is a greater degree of positive impact or influence.

There are two ways of thinking about effectiveness: from the clinical perspective and from the statistical perspective. At the center of both perspectives is a comparison of the amount of effect, or impact, each intervention had on the outcome variable. From the clinical perspective, the bottom line question is, "Is the difference in the outcomes of the two groups large enough to be clinically meaningful?" From the statistical perspective the bottom line question is, "Is the difference found a true difference or a chance difference?" When reading a report of an intervention study, too many people get hung up in the results of the statistical analysis (e.g., *p*-values, statistical significance). I suggest that you start by looking first at the results from a clinical perspective and then proceed to consider the meaning of the statistical tests of significance.

The Clinical Perspective

Generally speaking, the results of experimental studies are reported in one of two ways:

1. As the percentage of persons in each group who achieved a clinical outcome or milestone
2. As the mean scores of the two groups on the outcome variable

The term *scores* refers to the numerical values obtained by all forms of measurement, be it physiological measurement, questionnaires, or rating scales. When trying to get a read on the clinical significance of study results, percentages and mean scores require different analytical strategies.

Attainment of an Outcome When attainment of an outcome or milestone is reported as a "yes" or "no," it is called a dichotomous outcome. Examples of dichotomous variables are these:

- Rated pain control as good or better/ did not rate pain control as good or better
- Increased self-care knowledge/ did not increase self-care knowledge

- Gained the ability to walk 50 feet without assistance/ did not gain this ability
- Lived/ died
- Smoking at 1 year after intervention/ not smoking at 1 year

In experimental studies with dichotomous outcomes, the proportion of persons in each group who attained the yes/no outcome is determined. When the outcome is a good event, the difference in these two proportions is called the **absolute benefit increase (ABI)**. It is one of several measures of treatment effect used to portray the relative impact of two treatments (Sackett, Straus, Richardson, Rosenberg, & Haynes, 2000). The other one explained in this chapter is **number needed to treat (NNT)**.

Consider a fictional study in which a new program to encourage physical activity in second- and third-grade inner-city kids is evaluated. (Focus on the results, not the study design, and assume a low rate of dropout.) Two hundred children were randomly assigned to attend the new once-a-week after-school exercise program for 3 weeks or to receive a placebo treatment in which a study assistant played electronic, card, and board games with them once a week for 3 weeks. The milestone outcome being considered is actively exercising for 8 hours or more outside of school each week when measured 3 months after the program; this is a dichotomous outcome that is either achieved or not achieved. The results showed that 26% of the kids in the program attained the milestone outcome, whereas 12% of those in the placebo group attained it; stated as proportions these percentages are 0.26 and 0.12. So, the absolute difference between the proportion of those in the program who met the milestone and the proportion in the placebo group who met it is 0.14 (0.26–0.12); thus the absolute benefit increase (ABI) produced by the exercise intervention over the placebo intervention is 14%. The clinical ramifications of this measure of clinical significance should be considered: Is this a sizable enough difference to justify saying that the new program has a success rate that is clinically important?

The number needed to treat (NNT) provides another take on these results. It is the number of persons who would have to be given the more effective treatment rather than the less effective treatment for one additional person to achieve the milestone outcome—that is: one person more than the number that would have achieved the milestone outcome if the comparison treatment had been used. In our fictional study, the NNT is 8. This means that for every eight kids entered into the exercise program, rather than just getting attention, one additional kid will achieve the milestone exercise level than would have if all eight kids received just attention.

This provides a practical sense of how much benefit the exercise program would produce, which is actually pretty impressive.

Note that the NNT is easily calculated from the ABI; it is the inverse (reciprocal) of the ABI. That is: 1/ABI rounded up to a whole number—we do not treat 0.1 of a person. The treatment effect measures of the exercise program are portrayed in **Table 7–1**.

NNT is useful in considering whether to implement a similar program because it estimates in concrete terms the benefit that is likely to be realized from the program. The NNT is useful for two reasons. First, it provides a clinical perspective on how many more people are likely to benefit at a meaningful level from the program compared with no program. Second, the expected benefit can be considered in the context of the cost of the program, risks of exercise, and long-term risks of not developing an exercise habit.

Mean Level of an Outcome When the outcome variable of a study is measured on an interval level scale, a score is obtained for every patient, and group means are calculated. To make clinical sense of the results, you should first note the difference between the means of the two groups by subtracting one from the other—keeping in mind the range of the scale that was used to measure the variable. Then ask: Is this difference large enough to have clinical importance? For example:

- Is a 950 cc difference between the mean fluid intakes of two groups large enough to make a difference in patients' hydration status?
- Is an 8-mm difference between mean diastolic blood pressure levels of the two groups large enough to represent better blood pressure control and lowered risk of complications?

Consideration of the size of the difference between the means provides some clinical sense of whether the difference in the impact of the two treatments is large, small, or somewhere in between.

TABLE 7–1 Treatment Effect: Exercise Program for Kids

Measures of Clinical Effect (dichotomous data)	
Milestone attained with program	26% (.26)
Milestone attained without program	12% (.12)
Absolute benefit increase (ABI)	14% (.14)
Number needed to treat (NNT)	1 ÷ .14 = 7.1 rounded up to 8

The Statistical Perspective

When the outcome variable of a study is measured on an interval level scale and the results are reported as the means of each group, the statistical analysis provides information useful in answering the question: *Is the difference between the means of the two groups a true difference or a chance difference?* A true difference between the mean scores of the two groups is a difference that is robust enough that a difference is also likely to occur in the target population, not just in the study sample. Chance differences are caused by the normal variation in outcomes one would expect when measuring an outcome in two samples drawn from the same population.

In an experimental study, the two groups are treated differently; therefore a treatment effect is expected. A treatment effect is present when one treatment produces a larger effect on the outcome than the other treatment does. The larger the difference found between the outcome means of the two groups, the greater the chance that the difference is caused by one group receiving a treatment that was truly more effective than the other was. Moreover, the larger the difference in the means of the two groups, the greater the likelihood that a difference would be found if the whole population had been studied.

Note that even for the statistical question, your starting point is simple observation and common sense. Sometimes, just by looking at the mean outcome scores of the two groups and noting how different or close they are, you can get a first impression regarding whether the difference is caused by treatment effect or is just chance variation. If the difference is large, one treatment is most likely more effective than the other is and a benefit would probably be found beyond this one sample. If the difference in means is small, it is likely that it is just chance variation, which makes it unlikely that a benefit would be found in the target population. However, the definitive answer regarding whether the difference is a true difference or a chance difference is provided by inferential statistics. In the comparison of the scores of two groups, the *p*-value result produced by a *t*-test provides the definitive answer regarding interpretation of a difference in group mean scores.

The t-Test and *p*-Value The *t*-test is used to compare scores of two groups when the outcome variable is measured using an interval level scale; it cannot be used when the outcome variable is a dichotomous or categorical variable. The *t*-test analyzes the size of the difference between the means of two groups while taking into account the sample size and the spread of the scores across the possible range of scores (i.e., the standard deviation). It essentially asks: Even though a difference in means was found in this sample, what are the chances that in the target population *no* difference would be found?

The *t*-test analysis produces a *p*-value indicating the probability that the difference found between the means is just a chance occurrence. This data-based probability is then compared to a previously chosen level of significance *p*-level decision point. *P*-values below the decision point represent low probabilities that the difference found is just a chance difference; *p*-values higher that the decision point represent high levels of risk that the difference found is a chance difference. Thus, if the data-based *p*-value is equal to or lower than the decision point *p*-level, the researcher will conclude that the difference found is a true difference; i.e., a difference would likely be found in the population as well as in this sample. In contrast, if the data-based *p*-value is higher than the decision point *p*-level, the researcher will conclude that the difference found is a chance difference.

The researcher does not want to wrongly conclude that a difference is a true difference when in reality it is a chance difference; by only accepting a low level of probability that the difference is a chance difference, he can be quite confident when saying, "This is a true difference." Often, but not always, the level of significance decision point is set at 0.05. By setting it there, the researcher is accepting up to a 5% risk of being wrong when he says the difference found is a true difference.

So, let's say the researcher set the level of significance decision point at $p = .05$ and the data-based *p*-value comes in at .03. The researcher had decided in advance that she would be willing to accept a 5% chance of being wrong when concluding that the difference found is not just a chance occurrence. And the difference found only results in a 3% chance that she is wrong. So, the researcher says, "Okay, I'm confident in concluding that the difference found between the two groups is a true difference, meaning that a difference would likely be found in the population. I so conclude because there is only a 3% chance that I am wrong in doing so." In research lingo, a result like this would be reported as, "The difference found was statistically significant at the $p < .05$ level."

In contrast, consider the situation in which the researcher sets the level of significance decision point at $p = .05$ and the data-based *p*-value comes in at .08. This result means that the researcher was willing to accept a 5% chance of being wrong when concluding that the difference found was a true difference, but the difference found results in an 8% chance that she would be wrong in concluding that the difference found is a true difference.

In this situation, the researcher will think, "If I conclude this is a true difference, there is too high a probability of being wrong. Therefore, I am going to conclude that the difference found could be a chance occurrence and no difference would likely be found in the population." A result like this would be reported as not significant (ns).

The contrasting types of statistical results just described are portrayed graphically in **Figure 7–2.** Hopefully, it will make these complex issues a bit clearer. Also, I will provide a concrete example.

A hypothetical study tested the effects of two different methods of comforting babies during venipuncture (method A and method B); the infants' pain responses were measured 30 seconds after needle insertion using a scale with a value range of 0 to 10 (0 being no pain, 10 being a great deal of pain). Group A (n = 42) had a mean score of 3.6 and group B (n = 40) had a mean of 4.0, indicating that those in the method A group had on average less pain. A *t*-test was run on the difference between the means (0.4 points), and the result was $p = .02$. This is the data-based probability value; it indicates there are only 2 chances in 100 that a difference this large would occur because of chance variation. Said differently, if the researcher concluded that method A was more effective than method B, there would be 2 chances in 100 that his conclusion is wrong. When this data-based probability was compared to the decision point level of significance probability ($p \leq .05$), the conclusion was that it is a true difference in outcome, because there is an acceptably low probability that the difference is just chance variation. See Scenario No. 1 in **Table 7–2.**

Data-based *p*-value	<.001	.01	.025	**.05**	.08	.15	.59>
Finding	Significant difference				Not significant difference		
Conclusion	A difference would likely be found in the population.				A difference would *not* likely be found in the population.		

*Using a .05 level of significance decision-point

Figure 7-2 Interpretation of *p*-Values Produced by t-Tests*

TABLE 7–2 Statistical Conclusions

Scenario #1	Group A	Group B	
Mean pain level	3.6	40	
Difference in the means	.4		
Level of significance *p*-level			.05
Data-based *p*=			.02
Conclusion →			True difference
Probability that conclusion is wrong			2%

Scenario #2	Group A	Group B	
Mean pain level	3.6	3.8	
Difference in the means	.2		
Level of significance *p*-level			.05
Data-based *p*=			.10
Conclusion →			Chance difference
Probability that conclusion is wrong			Not easily calculated
If concluded that the difference is a true difference, probability that this conclusion is wrong			10%

Consider a different result for this same study: Group A had a mean of 3.6, group B had a mean of 3.8, and $p = .10$ (Scenario No. 2). Now, the difference is just 0.2 and there are 10 chances in 100 that the difference was a chance result. With this result, *if* the researcher concluded that the difference is a true difference, there would be 10 chances in 100 that his conclusion would be wrong. Based on the researcher's chosen level of significance decision point ($p \leq .05$), this is too high a chance of being wrong, so the researcher would conclude the two methods of comforting are essentially equivalent; i.e., a difference in effectiveness is doubtful, the difference found is not significant.

In summary, a difference in means associated with a low *p*-value (i.e., a data-based *p*-value that is equal to or below the decision point *p*-level) is considered statistically significant; it is a true difference in treatment effectiveness, meaning that a difference would likely be found in the population as well. A difference with a high *p*-value (i.e., a data-based *p*-value that is above the decision point *p*-level) is considered to be a not significant difference, meaning the probability that it is a chance difference is high; a difference would mostly likely not be found in the population. In study reports, the statistics just described are reported in a variety of ways. The absolute difference between the means of the two groups' outcomes may or may not be stated, but it can be easily calculated by subtracting the mean of one group from the mean of the other. The *t*-value may or may not be reported, but in and of itself, it is not of importance to the clinical reader. However, the *p*-value associated with a *t*-test or an indication of whether the difference is statistically significant will almost always be provided in the text or indicated by a symbol in a table.

Reporting of *p*-Values Researchers aim to present their results in ways that are both honest and favorable. For that reason, you will see a variety of adjectives used to describe the significance of results. When the researcher had preset the level of significance *p*-level at .05 and the data-based *p*-value comes in at .02 or .03, the researcher will connote this with a symbol or superscript letter indicating that the result was *significant at* $p \leq .05$. If, however the data-based *p*-value came in at .002, the researcher may describe the result as *highly significant*. This communicates that there is an even lower probability of the difference found being a chance event—much lower than the decision point he had set—thus he is very confident that the difference found is a true difference.

Another scenario is that the data-based *p*-value comes in just above the decision point *p*-level, with say $p = .06$ or .07. In this situation, the researcher might say that the result was "marginally significant" or "approached significance." This conveys that the *p*-value was close to the level of significance decision point; i.e., the difference in the two means was almost large enough to have confidence that it is a true difference. Reporting marginal results is justified when the study is an early test of an intervention because it may indicate a promising intervention that warrants another study. The examples in **Box 7–1** illustrate interpretations of *p*-values as they are expressed in two research articles.

BOX 7–1 Examples of *p*-Value Interpretations

1. **The effectiveness of a topical anesthetic in reducing the pain of subcutaneous measles–mumps–rubella vaccination in 1-year-old infants was studied in a double-blind, randomized, placebo-controlled trial (O'Brien, Taddio, Ipp, Goldbach, & Koren, 2004). The infants' pain levels were measured before the injection and after the injection; a high difference score from pre- to postinjection indicated more pain after the injection. Based on mean pre- to postinjection pain difference scores of 2.3 for the placebo group and 1.5 for the topical anesthesia group (p = .029), the researchers concluded that the topical anesthesia reduced the pain of vaccination. However, there is about a 3% chance that they are wrong in this conclusion, which is low enough that they are confident about their conclusion.**
2. **In a randomized controlled study evaluating the effects of a sliding-scale diuretic titration protocol for patients with heart failure in comparison to the usual method of set diuretic dosing, "There were significantly less ED visits in the diuretic titration group compared with the usual care group (3% vs 23%, p = .015)" (Prasun, Kocheril, Klass, Dunlap, & Piano, 2005). The researchers concluded that on average the diuretic titration protocol resulted in fewer ED visits because there is only between 1 and 2 chances in 100 that a 20% difference could have resulted from chance variation in sample groups. In other words, there is only a 1% to 2% chance that their conclusion that the titration method was more effective in reducing ED visits could be wrong.**

Recap If the statistical result is $p < .05$, the result is considered statistically significant. The researcher will conclude she can have confidence that a benefit/difference would be found in the population, not just in this sample. The fact that a difference is likely in the population justifies calling such a result a *true difference*. In contrast, if the data-based *p*-value is greater than .05, the result is considered not significant (ns). The researcher will conclude that she cannot have confidence that a difference benefit/difference would be found in the population. She so concludes because there is a high probability that the difference found between the groups in this sample is just expected variation from one sample to another from a population. This conclusion is justified when the study was well designed and the sample size was large enough to detect a difference.

Did I lose you in the last six to eight pages? If so, you need to go back to your statistics book and read about hypothesis testing and *p*-values. Even then, the concept may be less than clear to you—it is a tough topic. I offer the observation that the meaning of *p*-values will become clearer as you read more study reports. You will, however, have to pay attention to the *p*-values provided in reports and note how the researchers interpret them. This way, your understanding of them will increase over time. Understanding the meaning of *p*-values is crucial to understanding reports of quantitative studies. It is a concept that you must master.

Both Perspectives

Having explained both the clinical perspective and the statistical perspective on study results, I want to point out that statistical significance and clinical significance do not necessarily equate; rather, their relationship can take different forms:

1. The difference between the outcomes of the two treatment groups can be *clinically significant* and *statistically significant*. This would occur when the difference between means is large—of course, large is relative to the nature of the outcome being studied and to the scale used to measure it.
2. The difference can be *clinically not significant* and *statistically not significant*. This would occur when the difference between the means of the two groups is very small.
3. The difference between the two group means can be *clinically significant* but *statistically not significant*. This occurs most frequently in studies with small sample sizes, which are common in nursing. The clinician sees promise in the results, even though statistically they could be due to chance, and is of the opinion that the intervention needs to be studied with a larger sample.
4. The difference between two group means can be *clinically not significant* but *statistically significant*; that is, from a practical clinical perspective it is trivial or unimportant. Statistically significant but clinically not significant results occur most frequently in studies with very large sample sizes.

POSSIBLE RESULT COMBINATIONS

- **Clinically Significant and Statistically Significant (CS-SS)**
- **clinically not significant and statistically not significant (cs-ss)**
- **Clinically Significant and statistically not significant (CS-ss)**
- **clinically not significant and Statistically Significant (cs-SS)**

To illustrate some of the points made so far in this chapter, consider the results of a fictional randomized study comparing a new weight loss program to a program that has been around for a while. The results are displayed in **Table 7–3**.

First, note that the mean difference in weight lost by the two groups is 2.4 pounds and that this difference is statistically significant ($p = .02$). Do you think it is clinically significant? Note that the ABI and the NNT are more impressive than the mean difference. Based on the ABI and NNT for weight loss of 10 pounds or more, I am inclined to say that the new program achieves a weight loss that is clinically significant for more people than what the old program achieves. However, this is an opinion and others may look at these results and say that the effectiveness of the two programs is not different enough to make a meaningful change in weight over time. Ultimately, this call must be made with the details of the full report and

TABLE 7–3 Weight Loss Example

	New Program Group $n = 50$	Old Program Group $n = 50$
Mean lb lost at 6 months	13 lbs (sd = 4.9)	10.6 lbs (5.3)
Difference in the two means = 2.4 lbs		
95% CI of the difference: 0.37 to 4.4 lbs		
t-test *p*-value: 0.02		
% achieved a 10 lb loss or more	52%	30%
ABI = 20%		
ABI = 22%		
NNT = 5 (1 ÷ .22 = 4.5 rounded up)		

within the context of participants' feelings about the demands and expense of the two programs.

In many nursing studies, consideration of the clinical significance of the difference between outcomes is as important, if not more important, than consideration of whether the results are statistically significant. Unfortunately, the size of the clinical impact of the test intervention is not always discussed in a useful way in reports of nursing intervention studies—even though it should be. Once again, I would advise you not to obsess over the statistical results in a report; rather, think about the size of the difference between the outcomes of the two groups from a clinical perspective before moving on to thinking about them from the statistical perspective.

Opinion Regarding Reporting of Outcomes

Dichotomous clinical outcomes and their associated measures of effectiveness, ABI and NNT, are widely reported in the medical research literature but less often in the nursing literature. Hopefully, reporting dichotomous clinical outcomes will increase in nursing research because they add relevancy for clinicians. This is so because attainment of clinical outcomes and milestones are often important to patients—and memorable for clinicians. In contrast, mean scores on a scale or test are often indirect measures of outcomes important to patients and clinicians. I personally find that the reporting achievement of dichotomous patient outcomes adds clarity and clinical relevance to study reports.

Consider a fictional study in persons facing a risky medical procedure who were taught different ways of controlling anxiety in the days prior to the procedure; anxiety was measured on each of the 3 days before the procedure using a scale in which a low score indicated low anxiety and a high score indicated high anxiety. If the results reveal that the group taught method A had a mean anxiety score of 3 and group taught method B had a mean anxiety score of 7, we could say that clearly method A produced better anxiety prevention/relief, but we do not get a practical sense of how using method A actually improved patients' experiences of anxiety. In contrast, if the results were also reported as 11% of the persons in group A reported enough anxiety that it interfered with their sleep during one of the 3 nights before surgery and 24% of those in group B reported sleep disturbance during those nights, the difference in treatment effectiveness has immediate clinical relevance.

Exemplar

You should now reread the introduction and methods sections in the exemplar (Pellegrini, DeLoge, Bennett, & Kelly, 2009) and then carefully read the results and the discussion sections. The *Profile & Commentary: Results and Discussion* section that follows will focus on the results.

Profile & Commentary: Results and Discussion

The results section starts with a description of the sample, which has already been discussed in the commentary on methods. However, I would like to point out one more thing. In light of the earlier description of borderline results, consider this. The *t*-test run on the difference in the mean age of the two groups produced a *p*-value of .052, which was just above the level of significance decision cut point, and therefore was not interpreted as a significant difference. Some readers would conclude as the authors did, "The difference in average ages of the two groups is just a chance difference." However, other readers will think, "The difference in mean ages of the two groups was almost a true difference; I wonder if it *may* have influenced the different outcomes of the two groups." This dissimilarity in how the statistical result is viewed is inherent in the nature of using a decision cut point. In contrast, nitrous oxide use of the two groups was considered a statistically significant difference with a *p*-value of .049. Again, other readers may dismiss it as a chance difference because it is so close to the level of significance decision point. It is a bit like a racer winning by .003 of a second; even though the times of the first two racers were extremely close, a gold medal and a silver medal are awarded.

Incidence of PONV In Table 2 we see that the in-hospital incidence of nausea in the IPA and promethazine groups (17% versus 23% in PACU and 42% versus 23% in SDSU) was not statistically different, whereas the at-home incidence of nausea events was higher in the IPA group (45% versus 23%). Note that this home difference was statistically significant at the $p = .019$ level. The superscript *a* beside the *p*-value conveys this statistical significance by indicating that there are 5 or fewer chances in 100 that this difference is just due to chance.

Can you think of a reason why the incidence of nausea was higher at home in the IPA group than it was in the promethazine group? The reason that seems most likely to me is that IPA inhalation is shorter acting than is promethazine. Patients in the promethazine group may still have been getting benefits from the promethazine they received in the hospital.

In looking at Figure 1, focus on comparing the heights of the two bars in each setting. Doing so shows us the mean VNRS score of the IPA group at the time of the initial complaint of nausea in all three settings was higher than the mean score of the promethazine group. Although the bars make the differences in means look big, statistically they were not large enough to be considered a true difference, as stated in the text and as indicated by the absence of an asterisk over each comparison. In other words, the mean differences in initial VNRS score were in all three settings within what would be considered random variation around a mean common to both.

Comparative Effectiveness of the Treatments In the text and from Figure 2, we learn that the time to a 50% reduction in the VNRS scores after the treatments was shorter for the IPA patients in all settings. For example, in the PACU, a 50% reduction was achieved in approximately 8 minutes with IPA versus 20 minutes for the promethazine patients. You should think about whether or not you consider this a *clinically* significant difference. Would it be a benefit patients would value?

Statistically, the time to 50% reduction in VNRS score was significantly different in all three settings, as indicated by the *p*-values in the text and the asterisks in Figure 2. This leads the researcher to conclude that IPA would also give faster relief in the target population; the difference found is a true difference. In this regard, I call your attention to the reporting of these results in the text:

> However, when time to 50% reduction in VNRS scores for nausea was analyzed, we noted a significantly faster time to a 50% reduction in the IPA group compared to the promethazine group in the PACU ($P = .045$), SDSU ($P = .032$), and the home ($P = .017$) setting (Figure 2).

In Figure 2, each of these results is noted by an asterisk to be significant at the $P < .05$ level; indeed each *p*-value is below .05. However, I want to call your attention to the phrase "significantly faster time to a 50% reduction." The word *significant* is tricky because it has a statistical usage and an everyday usage. The authors are using it in the statistical sense

I described earlier. *It does not mean that the time to 50% reduction in nausea is clinically impressive or important.* It only means that a time difference (not exactly the one found in this study) would most likely be found in the target population also.

Continuing this thought, the fact that the *p*-value for home is smaller than the *p*-value for the PACU *does not mean* that the time to nausea reduction is greater in the home than in the PACU. Rather it means than when concluding that IPA produces faster relief, the author (and readers) can have slightly greater confidence in the conclusion that faster relief would be found in in the home setting than they could in the conclusion that faster relief would be found in the PACU setting.

Moving on, in the text we learn that vomiting (emetic events) was similar in both groups in all settings. So, too, were the median satisfaction with nausea control scores of the two groups (as indicated by $P > .05$. The report also informs us that no patients in the IPA group reported untoward side effects, whereas patients in the promethazine group did. Note how some results are found in both the tables and figures and the text, whereas other results are reported just in the text.

Dichotomous Outcome Although it is not addressed in the report, I was interested in knowing how effective IPA was in avoiding promethazine while in the hospital; taking or not taking promethazine is a dichotomous outcome. To get at this, I first needed to know the number of persons in each group who became nauseated and the number in each group who received promethazine. The number in each group who became nauseated is given in the article (32 in the IPA group and 26 in the promethazine group). I also knew that all the people in the promethazine group who became nauseated got the drug, according to the study protocol. The only missing piece was how many people in the IPA group who experienced nausea eventually had to be given promethazine. So I emailed the lead author, Pellegrini, who kindly responded with that information: 6 of the 32 persons in the IPA group who experienced nausea eventually required promethazine.

Now, to get at the outcome of interest (i.e., not requiring promethazine), I first determined the percentage in each group who experienced nausea but never had to take promethazine. That let me calculate the ABI and NNT for the benefit of IPA in achieving the outcome of not having to take promethazine at all. The calculation of the absolute benefit (AB) for both groups, the ABI achieved with IPA, and its NNT is as follows:

1. The number of persons in the IPA group who became nauseated and did *not* require promethazine was 26 (32 minus 6); in the promethazine group, the number who became nauseated and did *not* get the drug was 0 (26 minus 26) by study protocol.
2. In the IPA group, 81% of those who experienced nausea did not get promethazine (26 ÷ 32), so the AB of IPA was 0.81. In contrast, 0% of the promethazine group who experienced nausea did not get the drug, therefore the AB of promethazine was 0 (0 ÷ 26).
3. The absolute benefit increase (ABI) for IPA over promethazine was 0.81 (0.81 minus 0).
4. The NNT for IPA inhalation for the benefit of not requiring promethazine is 1 ÷ 0.81 = 1.23; this rounded up to an NNT of two persons.

This NNT means that just two persons would have to be treated with IPA as the first line of treatment in the hospital for PONV instead of giving promethazine as the first line of treatment to achieve one patient not having to receive promethazine at all. Thus, IPA inhalation has a strong clinical benefit in avoiding another drug at a time when patients already have several medications active in their body. Do you think this is a clinically significant result?

It may take you a couple of times through this calculation to get your head around NNT, but it is not higher mathematics. It involves some reasoning and simple subtraction and division. I think the perspective on clinical effect that is gained from the calculation is worth the effort because NNT provides a real-world sense of the benefit of one treatment vis-à-vis another in terms of an actual clinical event occurring or not occurring.

Discussion The section starts with a discussion about how the number of risk factors a person has increases his or her probability of PONV. The authors note that ondansetron, which is given in the operating room as the surgery is coming to a close to prevent postoperative nausea, is not as effective as expected with high-risk patients.

Limitations of the study are noted, particularly the reluctance of patients to self-administer a promethazine suppository at home. The researchers clearly have an interest in conducting future research to determine if IPA is effective in combination with ondansetron in preventing PONV. They conclude that the findings of the current study show that IPA inhalation is as effective as promethazine in treating breakthrough PONV in patients who are at high risk for PONV and have received ondansetron; they further note that it works faster and is easier to administer than promethazine.

The results of this study add to the knowledge about IPA effectiveness by focusing on patients who are at high risk for PONV. It is a good example of the methods of experimental design.

http://go.jblearning.com/brown3e

References

Burns, N., & Grove, S. K. (2009). *Practice of nursing research: Conduct, critique, and utilization* (5th ed.). St. Louis, MO: Elsevier Saunders.

Kerlinger, F. N., & Lee, H. B. (2000). Foundations of behavioral research (4th ed.). Fort Worth, TX: Harcourt College.

Pellegrini, J., DeLoge, J., Bennett, J., & Kelly, J. (2009). Comparison of inhalation of isopropyl alcohol vs. promethazine in the treatment of postoperative nausea and vomiting (PONV) in patients identified as at high risk for developing PONV. *AANA Journal, 77*(4), 293–299.

Polit, D. F., & Beck, C. T. (2012). *Nursing research: Generating and assessing evidence for nursing practice* (9th ed.). Philadelphia, PA: Lippincott Williams & Wilkins.

Sackett, D. L., Straus, S. E., Richardson, W. S., Rosenberg, W., & Haynes, R. B. (2000). *Evidence-based medicine: How to practice and teach EBM*. Edinburgh, Scotland: Churchill Livingstone.

Shu, T-T. (2010). *Effects of duration of selected music as an intervention on postoperative pain in open-heart surgery patients during chair rest on the first postoperative day*. (Masters theses and doctoral dissertations, paper 321). Eastern Michigan University, Ypsilanti, MI. http://commons.emich.edu/theses/321

CHAPTER EIGHT

Cohort Research

Studying the cause-effect relationship between risk factors and health outcomes presents unique challenges. Random assignment of participants to a risk factor exposure that could result in disease or a poor health outcome ethically is not an option. Thus, cohort studies evolved as a way of studying risk factors associated with heredity, environment, behavior, a particular life experience, or a medical treatment. For instance, a cohort design could be used to compare the cognitive health of urban elderly persons who were live in senior versus nonsenior housing.

Cohort Studies

Design

In a cohort study, a sample is drawn from a larger population and classified into two distinct groups—those with the risk factor and those without it. The two groups, called cohorts, are followed over an appropriate length of time to determine how often the outcomes of interest occur in both groups. Cohort studies are like experiments in that they involve comparison of outcomes in contrasting groups of a specified population; however, they are unlike experiments in that the contrasting groups are not created by random assignment. Rather, the groups are defined based on whether or not they have had exposure to a particular risk factor. Most often, the cohorts are identified after exposure to the risk factor and before the outcomes of interest develop; they are then followed to determine the rate at which the outcome of interest occurs.

For instance one study screened patients admitted to four ICUs for risk factors known or thought to contribute to delirium (Van Rompaey et al., 2009). The risk factors included patient characteristics (age, alcohol intake, smoking), environmental conditions (e.g., no daylight visible), illness conditions (e.g., fever, tubes), and chronic illnesses. The researchers then followed the patients to determine who developed delirium and who did not. Among the findings were that the presence of an endotracheal tube or tracheostomy, sedation, the use of physical restraints, history of daily heavy use of alcohol, and no visitors had great influence on the development of delirium.

A 2 × 2 matrix, which is used to portray the results of a cohort study, is helpful in understanding the logic of cohort design (**Table 8–1**). The first division of the sample is into the exposed or not exposed group. Later, when the outcome is measured, everyone in the sample is classified into one of the four groups (a, b, c, or d), which becomes the basis for the analysis of the data.

Cohort studies often use information in health system databases to reconstruct the presence of a risk factor at a point in time or over time and the subsequent development of a particular outcome. A cohort study looked at adverse drug reactions among frail elderly persons after discharge from hospital (Hanlon et al., 2006). Data were collected from patients' healthcare records regarding various risk factors for adverse drug reactions, and patients were followed to determine those who experienced an adverse drug reaction. The main finding was that the number of medications the patient took and the use of the drug warfarin increased the risk of adverse drug events.

Confounding

The major concern in cohort studies is that the two groups could be different in some way other than the presence or absence of the risk factor, and that difference may produce different outcomes for the two groups. For instance, they may have different biophysical characteristics, lifestyles, or experiences. The difference could be something as easy to identify as an age difference or something as buried as different levels of nutrition during youth. If the difference is a determinant of the outcomes being studied and is unequally distributed in the two groups, it is called a **confounding variable**, or a confounder (Mamdani et al., 2005). Recognizing confounders in advance of doing a study allows researchers to collect data about them and run analyses to check on their influence on the outcome variables. Even when the analysis has ruled out suspected confounders, cohort studies

TABLE 8–1 Logic of a Cohort Study

		Adverse Outcome		
		Present	Absent	Totals
Exposed to	Yes	a	b	a + b
Risk Factor	No	c	d	c + d
Totals		a + c	b + d	

Exposed Cohort
a = exposed to risk factor and develop adverse outcome
b = exposed to risk factor but do not develop adverse outcome

Unexposed Cohort
c = not exposed to risk factor but develop adverse outcome
d = not exposed to risk factor and do not develop adverse outcome

are still vulnerable to unknown confounders. Thus, when reading cohort studies, you must think about whether a confounder other than those considered by the researcher might exist, because it could have had an independent effect on the outcomes, apart from the effect of the risk factor of interest. In the study you will read later in this chapter, you will learn about the techniques researchers can take to rule out confounding.

Other Limitations

Cohort studies that follow participants for long periods of time often suffer from high dropout rates. High dropout rates can bias the incidence of the outcome in either or both groups, thus confounding the results. Another limitation of cohort design is that it does not work well if the outcome being studied occurs rarely. A rare outcome would require following a very large number of people to detect a connection between the risk factor and the outcome. Therefore, when the outcome being studied is rare, researchers may use another design, case-control design.

Case-Control Studies

In a sense, a case-control study is the opposite of a cohort study. Remember: A cohort study starts by identifying cohorts of persons and then follows them forward to determine if they develop certain outcomes. In contrast, a case-control study starts by identifying persons with and without a particular outcome, for example, a disease, and then looks backward in their history to identify how the two groups were different in regard to suspected causes of the outcome. See **Figure 8–1**.

Generally, cohort studies are used to study exposures and outcomes that occur rather frequently and outcomes that develop or occur not too long after the risk factor or exposure, whereas case-control studies are used to study outcomes that are rare or take a long time to become evident (e.g., osteoporosis fracture, lung cancer). Case-control studies are even more prone to confounding by unknown factors than are cohort studies. They are highly prone to confounding because the study involves looking back in time and important data may not be available or may be forgotten or distorted by memory.

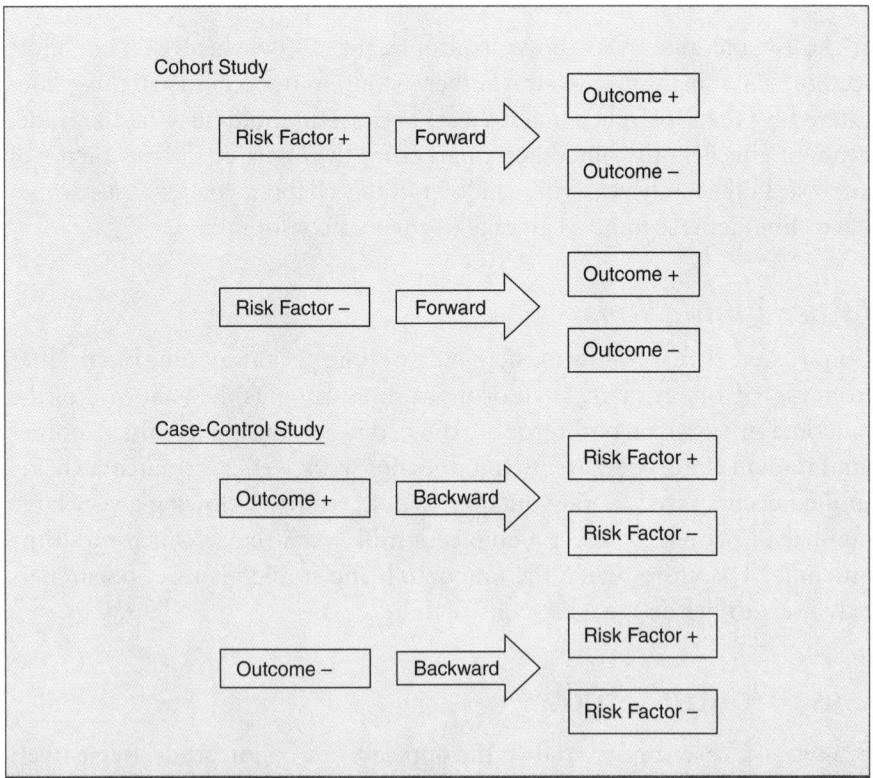

Figure 8-1 Cohort Study Versus Case-Controlled Study

A case-control study was conducted to determine the association between unplanned extubations in a pediatric intensive care unit and several patient, staffing, and care variables (Marcin, Rutan, Rapetti, Rahnsmayi, & Pretzlaff, 2005). During a 4-year period, 55 patients with unplanned extubations were identified. They were matched for age, intubation duration, and severity of illness with 165 control patients who did not experience unplanned extubation. Looking back at data from both groups' records of their time in ICU, they determined that patient agitation and nurse-to-patient assignment ratios of 1:2 were associated with unplanned extubations, whereas nurses' years of experience in pediatric intensive care nursing, patient restraints, and method of sedation delivery were not associated. Thus, by looking back after the event at possible risk factors, this case-control study identified 2 that put patients at risk.

Wrap-Up

Cohort studies provide a way of evaluating risk factors for health conditions or events; they do so by comparing groups with and without exposure to a preidentified risk factor or factors. Because random assignment is not used to form the comparison groups, cohort studies are prone to confounding, which threatens the validity of study conclusions about the relationship between the risk factor and the outcome of interest. However, cohort studies do provide control over follow-up and diagnosis of the outcome. An alternative design that is used to study risk factors when the outcome of interest is rare is the case-control study, but this design has even greater potential for confounding.

Exemplar

Reading Tips

The big phrase in the title of this article, *hemicallotasis technique*, is an orthopaedic surgical procedure performed to straighten knees deformed by arthritis. For our purposes, the exact nature of the surgery is not important except to note that metal pins are inserted into the bone and remain in place until the realigned bones fuse (see **Figure 8–2**). The pins go into the bone, but the ends remain outside the skin where they are attached to a rigid external frame, which is what provides the immobilization. The pin tract is a potential site for infection.

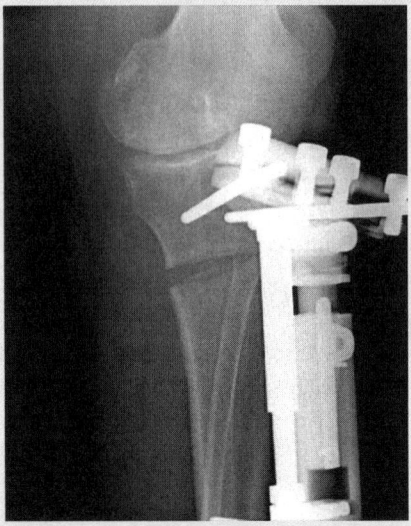

Figure 8-2 Radiograph of High Tibial Osteostomy

Source: W-Dahl, A., Toksvig-Larsen, S., & Roos, E. M. (2009). Association between knee alignment and knee pain in patients surgically treated for medial knee osteoarthritis by high tibial osteotomy. A one year follow-up study. *BMC Musculoskeletal Disorders 2009, 10,* 154. doi:10.1186/1471-2474-10-154.

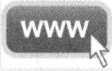

Cigarette Smoking Delays Bone Healing: A Prospective Study of 200 Patients Operated On by the Hemicallotasis Technique

ANNETTE W. DAHL AND SOREN TOKSVIG-LARSEN

ACTA ORTHOPAEDICA SCANDINAVICA (2008), *75*(3), 347–351.

DEPARTMENT OF ORTHOPEDIAS. UNIVERSITY HOSPITAL. LUND. SWEDEN

CORRESPONDENCE AWD: ANETTE.W-DAHL@ORT.LU.SE

SUBMITTED 03–04–26. ACCEPTED 03–10–14

Background: Cigarette smoking is known to impede bone healing. The hemicallotasis technique is based on an external fixation and delayed healing prolongs treatment and increases the risk of further complications.

Patients and methods: 200 patients, 34 smokers and 166 nonsmokers, operated on by the hemicallotasis technique in the proximal tibia for deformities of the knee (knee arthrosis in 186 patients) were consecutively studied. We recorded their preoperative smoking habits, postoperative complications and the duration of treatment with external fixation.

Results: Half of the smokers and one fifth of the nonsmokers developed complications. Their mean time in external fixation was 96 (SD 20) days. Smokers required an average of 16 days more in external fixation. Delayed healing and pseudoarthrosis were commoner in smokers than nonsmokers. The risk ratio for smokers to develop complications was 2.5, as compared to nonsmokers.

* * *

Tibia osteotomy by the hemicallotasis technique (HCO) is based on external fixation. Delayed healing and nonunion prolong the treatment and increase the risk of further complications.

Studies on rabbits have shown delayed bone healing and decreases in bone mineral density (BMD) and strength in the lengthened tibia caused by cigarette smoking (Ueng et al. 1997, 1999). Smoking was the single most important risk factor for the development of serious postoperative complications after elective arthroplasty of the hip and knee (Møller et al. 2003).

We studied whether smokers had longer healing times and more complications than nonsmokers who underwent HCO.

Methods

Patients

In a prospective study 200 consecutive patients (119 men), mean age 53 (18–75) years, were operated on by HCO for knee deformities (Tables 1–2).

The patients' smoking habits (smoker or nonsmoker) were noted preoperatively.

They were called nonsmoker if, at the preoperative examination, they stated that they had never smoked or had stopped smoking more than 6 months previously. Thirty-four (17%) were smokers and 166 (83%) nonsmokers. Seven patients underwent simultaneous bilateral surgery (1 smoker and 6 nonsmokers).

Hemicallotasis Osteotomy

Four conical pins were inserted, 2 hydroxyapatite-coated in the metaphyseal bone and 2 standard pins (Orthofix®, Bussolengo, Italy) in the diaphyseal bone. The Orthofix® T-garche was used. The patients were allowed free mobilization and full weight bearing after the operation.

Table 1 Patient Characteristics of the Study Group

	Nonsmokers n = 166	Smokers n = 34
Gender		
Men	102 (61)	17 (50)
Women	64 (39)	17 (50)
Age		
Mean	53	53
SD	10	6
< 50	47 (28)	9 (26)
50–59	77 (46)	22 (65)
60+	42 (25)	3 (9)
Preop HKA-angle in medial cases		
Mean	170°	170°
SD	5°	4°
≤ 189°	17 (11)	2 (3)
> 190°	5 (5)	3 (12)
BMI		
< 25	25 (16)	12 (35)
25–29	77 (48)	13 (38)
30+	58 (36)	9 (27)

Percentages within parentheses
Preop HKA-angle = Preoperative hip-knee-ankle-angle
BMI = Body mass index

Table 2 Indication for Surgery in 200 Patients Who Underwent HCO

	All n = 200	Nonsmokers/Smokers n = 166/34
Knee osteoarthrosis	186	153/32
Medial	163	134/29
Lateral	20	15/5
Pre[a]	2	2/0
Fracture sequelae	8	6/2
Knee deformity	4	4/0
Osteonecrosis	1	1/0
Sequelae of tibia osteotomy	1	1/0

[a]Arthroscopic osteoarthrosis with symptoms but no osteoarthrosis, according to radiographic Ahlback grade I.

The distraction started 7–10 days postoperatively. Eight weeks after surgery, the fixation was dynamised to stimulate healing of the bone. The first evaluation of bone healing was done 12 weeks postoperatively. If healing of the osteotomy was deemed satisfactory on both the radiographic and ultrasound examinations, the patient did a weight-bearing test—i.e., walked for a few hours or even some days without the instrument, but with the pins in situ. If no symptoms developed, the pins were removed in the outpatient clinic, but if the patient developed symptoms, the T-garche was applied again for 2–4 weeks.

Outcome

We recorded the duration of external fixation (from surgery until the external pins were removed) and the complications, such as delayed healing (> 16 weeks in external fixation), pseudoarthrosis, septic arthritis, deep venous thrombosis, nerves injury, and interrupted treatment (i.e., loose pins due to a pin site infection).

Statistics

The analysis of variance (ANOVA) test, *t*-test and Chi-square test were used for the statistical analysis, and the statistical significance was set at $p < 0.05$. A multiple logistic regression analysis (checked for potential confounder) was used to estimate the odds ratio (OR) of complications, delayed healing and pseudoarthrosis.

The study was approved by the Ethics Committee, Lund University, Sweden.

Results

More complications occurred among the smokers than the nonsmokers. Fifty-one patients had one or more complications (delayed healing, pseudoarthrosis, septic arthritis, deep venous thrombosis, nerves injury or interrupted treatment) (34/166 (Table 3) nonsmokers and 17/34 smokers, $p < 0.001$). 12/51 patients had 2 or more complications (7 nonsmokers and 5 smokers, $p = 0.02$). The risk ratio for the smokers who developed complications, as compared to the nonsmokers, was 2.5 (95% CI 1.5–3.9).

Delayed healing and pseudoarthrosis occurred more often among the smokers. The risk ratio for delayed healing was 2.7 (95% CI 1.5–4.7) in the smokers. Eight patients with delayed healing developed pseudoarthrosis. The risk ratio for smokers to develop pseudoarthrosis was 8.1 (95% CI 1.8–42.0) (Table 3). Six of the patients who developed pseudoarthrosis required additional surgery for healing (5 smokers and 1 nonsmoker) and 2 patients (nonsmokers) healed after low intensity ultrasound stimulation (Exogen®, Tuttlingen, Germany).

In the 3 patients who developed septic arthritis (2 nonsmokers and 1 smoker), the treatment was interrupted and in one patient (nonsmoker), the treatment was interrupted due to loose pins. The mean time in external fixation was 96 (SD 20)

Table 3 Complications in 200 Patients Operated On by HCO

			Relative Risk	
	Nonsmokers	Smokers	(RR)	(95% CI)[a]
Delayed healing[b]	25	14	2.7	(1.5–4.7)
Pseudoarthrosis	3	5	8.	(1.8–42)
Septic arthritis	2	1	2.4	(0.1–34)
Deep venous thrombosis	3	2	3.3	(0.4–23)
Nerve injury	1	0	0	(1.0–84)
Interrupted treatment	3	1	1.6	(0.1–17)

[a](95% CI) = 85% confidence interval.

[b]Includes 5 patients who developed pseudoarthrosis after removal of external fixation.

days in all patients. The mean time in external fixation for nonsmokers was 94 (SD 18) days and 110 (SD 25.2) days for smokers ($p < 0.001$). The smokers had 16 days ($p < 0.001$, 95% CI 7.0–25) longer mean time in external fixation than the nonsmokers. In patients with a frame time > 112 days, the smokers had a mean of 17 days more ($p = 0.004$, 95% CI 5.5–26) in external fixation than the nonsmokers (Table 4). Among the 7 patients who underwent bilateral HCO in one séance, 3 patients had complications—i.e., 2 had delayed healing, 1 smoker and 1 nonsmoker. And 1 (nonsmoker), with osteonecrosis after treatment for leukemia, developed pseudoarthrosis (rapid loss of correction) in one of the osteotomies.

The multivariate analysis, used to detect potential confounder, showed that cigarette smoking was the greatest preoperative risk factor for complications OR 5.1 ($p = 0.001$, 95% CI 2.2–12), delayed healing OR 4.0 ($p = 0.004$, 95% CI 1.7–9.5), and pseudoarthrosis OR 8.9 ($p = 0.02$, 95% CI 1.7–47.1) (Table 5).

Table 4 Frame Time > 112 days in Patients Operated On by HCO

	Nonsmokers	Smokers	P-value
Mean (days)	126	143	0.004
SD	13	16	
n	23	11	

Table 5 Relationship of Risk Factors to Complications, Delayed Healing and Pseudoarthrosis in Patients Operated On by HCO

	Complications Adjusted OR[a]	Delayed healing Adjusted OR[a]	Pseudoarthrosis Adjusted OR[a]
Gender			
Men[b]	1.0	1.0	1.0
Women	1.4 (0.7–2.9)	1.8 (0.8–4.1)	5.0 (0.8–31)
Age			
< 50[b]	1.0	1.0	1.0
50–59	0.9 (0.4–2.3)	1.0 (0.4–2.6)	0.5 (0.09–3.3)
60+	1.4 (0.5–3.9)	0.9 (0.3–3.0)	1.4 (0.2–12)
BMI			
< 25b	1.0	1.0	1.0
25–29	0.7 (0.3–1.8)	0.7 (0.3–2.1)	0.9 (0.1–6.0)
30+	1.2 (0.5–3.1)	1.1 (0.4–3.1)	0.5 (0.06–3.6)
Preop HKA-angle[c] medial/lateral			
> 171/< 189[b]	1.0	1.0	1.0
< 170/> 190	1.8 (0.9–3.7)	1.7 (0.8–3.8)	3.6 (0.6–21)
Smoking			
Nonsmokers[b]	1.0	1.0	1.0
Smokers	4.1 (1.8–3.7)	3.7 (1.5–8.9)	7.5 (1.4–41)

[a]Odds ratio (OR) adjusted simultaneously for all other risk factors listed and 95% confidence interval in parenthesis.[b]

Reference category.[c]

Hip-knee-ankle-angle preoperatively (varus or valgus).

Discussion

Smokers operated on by HCO for knee deformities needed a longer time in external fixation and had more complications, such as delayed healing and pseudoarthrosis than nonsmokers. Half of the smokers developed complications. The risk for the smokers developing complications was 2.5 times higher than in the nonsmokers.

A recent study by Møller et al. (2003) on patients operated on for arthroplasty of the hip and knee confirmed our findings—i.e., smoking is the greatest risk factor for developing postoperative complications.

The number of smokers (34 of 200 patients) in our material is similar to the percentage of smokers in the Swedish population, 19% (18% men and 20% women) (Mackay and Eriksen 2002).

The mean time in external fixation in patients operated on by HCO has ranged from 79 to 91 days in various studies (Magyar et al. 1998, Klinger et al. 2001, Gerdhem et al. 2002), as compared to our 96 days. These differences may be due to the time when the first examination for healing was done, the methods used to assess healing, the experience in evaluating the healing on radiographs and perhaps the use of ultrasound. The size of the correction and whether bilateral osteotomies were done in one séance could also account for a longer treatment time. We found no differences between unilateral and bilateral osteotomies or the preoperative HKA-angle, as regards the longer healing time.

Cigarette smoking has been shown to cause slower healing and pseudoarthrosis in tibial fractures, both after closed (Kyro et al. 1993) and surgical treatments (Adams et al. 2001). In closed and grade I open tibial shaft fractures, Schmitz et al. (1999ccc) found statistical differences in clinical and radiographic healing rates in smokers and nonsmokers in patients who underwent intramedullary or external fixation.

Cobb et al. (1994) reported that the relative risk of nonunion after ankle arthrodesis was 4 times higher in smokers. When patients had no known risk factors for nonunion, the risk of nonunion was 16 times higher in smokers.

Examination after a laminectomy and fusion showed more pseudoarthrosis among smokers than nonsmokers (Brown et al. 1986). After ulna-shortening osteotomy, the smokers had longer healing times and nonunion than the nonsmokers. The mean union rates were 7 months in smokers and 4 months in nonsmokers (Chen et al. 2001). Our study of patients who underwent HCO can be added to the list of treatments showing that smoking is an important risk factor for the development of complications in orthopaedic surgery.

In a preoperative smoking intervention study, cessation of smoking from 6–8 weeks preoperatively and 10 days postoperatively reduced the postoperative complications in patients undergoing hip and knee replacement. The smoking cessation group was compared to one with an at least 50% reduction in smoking. The patients who reduced their smoking did not differ from the smoking group in other respects (Møller et al. 2002). Patients undergoing arthroplasty of the hip and knee who smoked previously had a better short-term outcome than those who were smoking (Lavernia et al. 1999). Glassman et al. (2000) showed that the cessation of smoking after surgery helped to reverse the effects of cigarette smoking on the outcome of spinal fusion.

These studies indicate that smoking cessations both preoperatively and postoperatively decrease the risk for complications, whereas smoking reduction is not enough to decrease the risk.

The conclusions of the present study were that information about smoking cessations prior to surgery should be an important part of the preoperative information as well as cigarette smoking should be a factor to consider when selecting patients for callus distraction.

References

1. Adams C I, Keating J F, Court-Brown C M. Cigarette smoking and open tibial fractures. Injury 2001; 32 (1): 61–5.
2. Brown C W, Orme J T, Richardson H D. The rate of pseudoarthrosis (surgical nonunion) in patients who are smokers and patients who are nonsmokers: a comparison study. Spine 1986; 11 (9): 942–3.
3. Chen F, Osterman A L, Mahony K. Smoking and bony union after ulna-shortening osteotomy. Am J Orthop 2001; 30 (6): 486–9.
4. Cobb T K, Gabrielsen T A, Campbell D C, Wallrichs S L, Ilstrup D M. Cigarette smoking and nonunion after ankle arthrodesis. Foot Ankle Int 1994; 15 (2): 64–7.
5. Gerdhem P, Abdon P, Odenbring S. Hemicallotasis for medial gonarthrosis: a short-term follow-up of 21 patients. Arch Orthop Trauma Surg 2002; 12 (3): 134–8.
6. Glassman S D, Anagnost C S, Parker A, Burke D, Johnson J R, Dimar J R. The effect of cigarette smoking and smoking cessation on spinal fusion. Spine 2000; 25 (20): 2608–14.
7. Klinger H M, Lorenz F, Harer T. Open wedge tibial osteotomy by hemicallotasis for medial compartment osteoarthritis. Arch Orthop Trauma Surg 2001; 121 (5): 247–7.
8. Kyro A, Usenius J P, Aarnio M, Kunnamo I, Avikainen V. Are smokers a risk group for delayed healing of tibial shaft fractures? Ann Chir Gynaecol 1993; 82 (4): 254–62.
9. Lavernia C J, Sierra R J, Gomez-Marin O. Smoking and joint replacement: resource consumption and short-term outcome. Clin Orthop 1999; (367): 172–80.
10. Mackay J, Eriksen M. The Tobacco Atlas. Myriad Edition Limited. Brighton 2002.
11. Magyar G, Toksvig-Larsen S, Lindstrand A. Open wedge tibial osteotomy by callus distraction in gonarthrosis. Operative technique and early results in 36 patients. Acta Orthop Scand 1998; 69 (2): 147–51.
12. Møller A M, Villebro N, Pedersen T, Tonnesen H. Effect of preoperative smoking intervention on postoperative complications: a randomised clinical trial. Lancet 2002; 359 (9301): 114–7.
13. Møller A M, Pedersen T, Villebro N, Munksgaard A. Effect of smoking on early complications after elective orthopaedic surgery. J Bone Joint Surg Br 2003; 85 (2): 178–81.
14. Schmitz M A, Finnegan M, Natarajan R, Champine J. Effect of smoking on tibial shaft fracture healing. Clin Orthop 1999; (365): 184–200.

15. Ueng S W, Lee M Y, Li A F, Lin S S, Tai C L, Shih C H. Effect of intermittent cigarette smoke inhalation on tibial lengthening: experimental study on rabbits. J Trauma 1997; 42 (2): 231–8.
16. Ueng S W, Lin S S, Wang C R, Liu S J, Tai C L, Shih C H. Bone healing of tibial lengthening is delayed by cigarette smoking: study of bone mineral density and torsional strength on rabbits. J Trauma 1999; 46 (1): 110–5.

Profile & Commentary

STUDY PURPOSE

This study was conducted to determine if cigarette smokers and nonsmokers had the same rates of healing and complications after having an orthopedic surgical procedure called tibial hemicallotasis osteotomy.

In brief, then:

- Population: Persons having this orthopedic surgical procedure
- Risk cohorts: Smokers and nonsmokers—note the definition of smoker
- Outcome variables: Complications, delayed bone healing, infection, loose pins

DESIGN

The design of this study is a consecutive series, prospective cohort design. *Consecutive series* indicates that the sample was created by asking a series of patients who were having the surgical procedure to participate in the study. *Prospective* indicates that the participants were entered into the study and followed to determine how many developed complications after the surgery. In fact, this study design is the only way to compare complication rates in smokers and nonsmokers after surgery because random assignment to a smoking or not smoking group is not logistically possible.

Risk Factor of Interest

Prior research indicates that a history of recent smoking and current smoking slow, and in some cases prevent, bone healing after orthopedic surgeries. This is the first study examining the effects of smoking with this particular procedure. Note that the definition of who was considered a nonsmoker depended on the patient's report. Many cohort studies rely on patient reports regarding exposure to the risk factor, although some cohort studies use a very rigorously applied set of criteria to classify patients into one risk group or the other. I assume from the definition of nonsmoker that persons who were categorized as smokers preoperatively continued to smoke postoperatively—although this was not explicitly stated.

Sample

The target population was persons having a particular knee reconstruction procedure. The researchers obtained a sample of this population by studying 200 consecutive patients in one Swedish hospital. Enrolling consecutive patients is a reasonably unbiased way of obtaining a sample because it does not allow anyone on the research team to pick and choose who is in the study. In this study, consecutive enrollment of patients does not present any obvious concerns about the sample being different from persons who have the surgery at other times. The smokers cohort comprised 17% of the sample and the nonsmokers cohort made up the rest (83%).

Outcomes

Note how the outcomes were measured and the timing of the measurements. The outcome of time in external fixation was measured using an interval scale (days). Other outcomes (various complications) were measured as dichotomous outcomes; that is, the complication either occurred or did not occur. The overall complication rate (one or more complications) was measured as well as the rate of each of six complications.

In a cohort study, the first table often profiles the two cohorts as a first step in identifying potential confounders. Accordingly, Table 1 provides a profile of the smoker and nonsmoker groups with specifics about variables the researchers think could have an influence on the occurrence of complications. We note that there are differences between the composition of the two groups, particularly in terms of gender and proportion of persons over age 60. This raises a concern that perhaps these differences influenced the occurrence of complications and contributed to the differences found. At this point, the differences just send up a red flag and remind us to note whether the researchers deal with them during data analysis.

Dichotomous Outcomes In the text, the researchers tell us that 20% of nonsmokers (34/166) and 50% of smokers (17/34) had one or more complications; thus, the absolute difference in the complication rates of the two groups is 30% (50% minus 20%). Further, the *p*-value associated with this difference indicates that this is a real difference, not a chance difference ($p < .001$). To provide additional clinical perspective on the risk of one or more complications, the risk for smokers to develop complications was compared to the risk for nonsmokers. This was reported as relative risk (RR), which is the ratio between risk in the smoker group and risk in the nonsmoker group.[1] Because the risk of the smoker group was 50% and the risk of the nonsmoker group was 20%, the ratio was 50:20 = 2.5.

To understand the meaning of this RR, you need to know that an RR greater than 1.0 indicates the smoker group had a higher risk of the complication than did the nonsmoker group, whereas an RR of less than 1.0 would mean that the smoker group had a lower risk of complication than did the nonsmoker group. If the two groups had equal risk, the RR would be 1.0.

Thus, the RR = 2.5 for smokers having at least one complication means that the risk for smokers developing complications was 2.5 times higher than was the risk for nonsmokers.

Relative risk (RR) was also used in Table 3 to portray the risk of smokers in relation to nonsmokers for six poor outcomes. From this table, you can tell that being a smoker puts persons at much higher *relative risk* (8.1) of developing pseudoarthrosis and a lower level of *relative risk* of delayed healing (2.7). This means that the risk of smokers developing pseudoarthrosis was 8 times that of nonsmokers and their risk of developing delayed healing was 2.7 times that of nonsmokers. When interpreting RR, the operative word is *relative*—glossing over it can easily lead to misinterpretations of RR.

RR allows a comparison of smokers' relative risks for several outcomes. Comparing smokers' RRs for delayed healing (2.7) and pseudoarthrosis (8.1) tells us that being a smoker increases the risk of pseudoarthrosis more

---

[1] $\text{Risk} = \dfrac{\text{Number in the group who have the complication}}{\text{Total number in group}}$

$\text{Relative risk} = \dfrac{\text{Risk of smoker group}}{\text{Risk of nonsmoker group}}$

than it increases the risk of delayed healing (note the relative word *more*). When looking at smokers' RRs for delayed healing and pseudoarthrosis, *do not* make the mistake of interpreting it to mean that smokers are at a higher risk of pseudoarthrosis than they are of delayed healing. Because this can be confusing, I like to see the absolute rates and the RRs together, so I did my own fiddling with Table 3 (see **Table 8–2**). This display reminds me that the absolute risk rate of a complication in a group and its relative rate when compared to another group are quite different takes on the data.

One last point related to Table 3 concerns the far right column, *95% CI for Relative Risk*. To take just one line, *Delayed healing*, the sample had an RR of 2.7. This value is also the best single number for estimating what might occur in the larger population of persons having the HCO surgery. However, the 95% confidence interval provides additional information about what might occur in the population. It tells us that in the population the RR for delayed healing could be anywhere from 1.5 to 4.7. This is a moderate size interval; therefore it would be described as a *moderately precise estimate of treatment effect*. Generally, precise estimates of treatment effects (narrower confidence intervals) are preferable because they give clinicians a better sense of what difference they might see in real-world practice.

That explanation may have been difficult to grasp, and RRs can be misleading if you do not work with them frequently. My thinking regarding RR is this: If you do not regularly read reports with RR statistics, do not worry about understanding all the implications of RR beyond knowing that it is a way of comparing the risk of two groups for an outcome. Rather, focus on the absolute difference in the risk rates of the two groups for each outcome. They make sense in a very straightforward way and are less likely to lead you to wrong conclusions than RRs are. If your clinical field requires that

TABLE 8–2 Reformulation of Results to Clarify Risk

	Risk Nonsmokers	Risk Smokers	Absolute Difference	Relative Risk
Outcome	$n = 166$	$n = 34$	in Risk	
Delayed healing	25 (15%)	14 (41%)	26%	2.7
Pseudoarthrosis	3 (1.8%)	5 (14.6%)	12.8%	8.1

Source: Adapted from Dahl, A. W., & Toksvig-Larsen, S. (2004). Cigarette smoking delays bone healing: A prospective study of 200 patients operated on by the hemicallotasis technique. *Acta Orthopaedica Scandinavica, 75*(3), 347–351.

you read reports that use RR, then get a good source book and get a handle on just what RR means. As a starting point, I recommend a short but clear article by Sheldon (2000), "Statistics for Evidence-Based Nursing."

Interval Level Outcomes Switching to the analysis of days in external fixation, which is an interval level outcome, the mean days in external fixation for smokers and nonsmokers were compared. In the text of the Results section, we learn that smokers spent 16 more days than nonsmokers in external fixation (110 minus 94). From a clinical perspective, this difference in means is clinically significant because it represents on average two more weeks of being in the fixation device. From a statistical perspective, the *t*-test comparing the two means was statistically significant at the $p < .001$ level. This means that there is less than 1 chance in 1,000 that a difference as large as the one found could have occurred just by chance—thus a difference is likely to exist in the larger population as well as in this sample.

Note in the text that, although the mean *difference* of days in external fixation for the two groups was 16 days, the 95% confidence interval for the days in external fixation is 7.0–25.0; this means that in the target population smokers could spend as much as 25 days or as few as 7 days more in external fixation than nonsmokers do. Unfortunately, this CI is rather wide (in part because the sample size of the study was not large); a wide CI provides a less precise estimate of what might actually occur in the population than does a narrow one. Still, it is a better estimate of what might occur in the population than is the sample mean all by itself.

At this point, if you do not understand confidence intervals, you should go back to your statistical text because you are likely to encounter them when reading research reports and SRs. They are of practical, clinical value because they provide good estimates of the likely results that will be realized when applying the study's intervention in everyday practice.

Looking for Potential Confounders The researchers were aware that smoking was not the only risk factor for complications and that the smoking and nonsmoking groups could be different in ways other than just their smoking status. And we remember that Table 1 revealed some of those differences; for example, a greater percentage of women in the smoker group and a greater percentage of people over age 60 years in the nonsmoker group. To more definitively address the possibility that differences between smokers and nonsmokers on these other risk factors could have influenced the occurrence of complications, the researchers ran a multiple logistic regression analysis.

The results, shown in Table 5, were reported using a statistic called odds ratio. First, let us consider the concept of odds and how it compares to risk. Odds of a complication are similar to risk of a complication but slightly different. A risk is the likelihood (i.e., probability) of something occurring in relation to the number of times it could have occurred. You roll a die (just one) and are hoping to roll a five. There is one chance in six that you will get a five; thus, the risk of a five is one in six, which is 0.17 when converted to a decimal (1/6 = 0.166) and rounded up. In contrast, odds are the chances of something occurring in relation to the chances of it not occurring; thus, the odds of rolling a five are one to five (1/5) or 0.20. The numerator is the same in both calculations, but the denominator is different (compare the formula below[2] to the one given earlier for risk).

Like relative risk, an odds ratio is a ratio, specifically the odds of a particular outcome occurring in a comparison group (the numerator) relative to the odds of it occurring in the reference group (the denominator). It is interpreted like relative risk (RR). An odds ratio of 1 means the two groups have the same odds of experiencing the particular outcome.

Odds ratios are appearing with increased frequency in the nursing literature, so it is worth an effort to understand them. For a further explanation of odds ratios, I again refer you to Sheldon (2000).

An odds ratio (OR) is used instead of RR in some analyses for technical reasons. As a clinical reader, you are not expected to know when one or the other should be used. The researcher and the peer review team are responsible for getting this right. One other point is that an adjusted OR is an OR that takes into account the other variables in the analysis; the adjustment essentially holds the other variables constant while calculating the OR of each variable.

Getting back to the study results, in Table 5 we notice that the smokers were the only subgroup having an odds ratio (adjusted OR) significantly larger than 1.0; their confidence intervals were the only ones that did not include 1.0. Therefore, being a smoker is the only risk factor that determined whether each of the complications occurred. This analysis in essence ruled out the other risk factors as confounders, leaving smoking as the best explanation for why complications occurred at different rates in the smoker and nonsmoker groups.

---

[2] $$\text{Odds} = \frac{\text{Number in group with complication}}{\text{Number in group without complication}}$$

$$\text{Odds ratio} = \frac{\text{Odds of complication in smokers}}{\text{Odds of complications in nonsmokers}}$$

Potential confounding influences could have been controlled by inclusion criteria that allowed into the study only persons who do not have a particular characteristic. So, in this study, the researchers could have excluded people over age 60 if they thought that the smoking group might be older and that age would have a great influence on complications after surgery. This would have had the effect of reducing the number of people eligible for the study and would have produced findings that were less generalizable. Moreover, the results bear out that it was not necessary to exclude this group because the risk factor of age over 60 did not predict any of the three complications (all three 95% CIs include 1.0).

Discussion

Importantly, the researchers placed their findings in the context of other work that has been done on the subject and concluded that the findings of this study add to the list of studies showing that smoking is a risk factor for postoperative complications after orthopedic surgery.

http://go.jblearning.com/brown3e

References

Dahl, A. W., & Toksvig-Larsen, S. (2004). Cigarette smoking delays bone healing: A prospective study of 200 patients operated on by the hemicallotasis technique. *Acta Orthopaedica Scandinavica, 75*(3), 347–351.

Hanlon, J. T., Pieper, C. F., Hajjar, E. R., Sloane, R. J., Linblad, C. I., Ruby, C. M., & Schmader, K. E. (2006). Incidence and predictors of all preventable adverse drug reactions in frail elderly persons after hospital stay. *Journals of Gerontology. Series A, Biological Sciences and Medical Sciences, 61*(5), 511–515.

Mamdani, M., Skyora, K., Li, P., Normand, S. L., Streiner, D. L., Austin, P. C., . . . Anderson, G. M. (2005). Reader's guide to critical appraisal of cohort studies: 2. Assessing potential for confounding. *British Medical Journal, 330*, 960–962.

Marcin, J. P., Rutan, E., Rapetti, P. M., Rahnsmayi, R., & Pretzlaff, R. K. (2005). Nurse staffing and unplanned extubation in the pediatric intensive care unit. *Pediatric Critical Care Medicine, 6*(3), 254–257.

Sheldon, T. (2000). Statistics for evidence-based nursing. *Evidence-Based Nursing, 3*, 4–6.

Van Rompaey, B., Elseviers, M. M., Schuurmans, M. J., Shortridge-Baggett, L. M., Truijen, S., & Bossaert, L. (2009). Risk factors for delirium in intensive care patients: A prospective cohort study. *Critical Care Forum, 13*, R77. Retrieved from http://ccforum.com/content/13/3/R77

CHAPTER NINE

Systematic Reviews

With an Emphasis on Integrative Research Reviews

Once several, or many, studies have been conducted on an issue, clinicians or researchers will feel the need to pull together the findings of the various studies into one document so as to see the bigger picture. This pulling together is called a systematic review. It has to be done carefully so as to not introduce bias into the conclusions. For this reason, the methods for conducting systematic reviews have been explicitly set forth by the healthcare disciplines, most notably by the Joanna Briggs Institute (2011), the international Cochrane Collaboration (Higgins & Green, 2011), and the Institute of Medicine (2011) in the United States. When done well, a systematic review helps clinicians and researchers identify what is known with certainty, what is tentatively known, and what the gaps in knowledge are regarding an issue. Not infrequently, systematic reviews serve as a link between individual studies and clinical decision making and between individual studies and clinical practice guidelines (Eden et al., 2008).

Sometimes a well-conducted systematic review calls into question a widely used clinical practice method. For instance, a systematic review of studies examining the effectiveness of rapid response teams (RRTs) found that implementation of an RRT does not always produce the expected benefits (Chan et al., 2010). In that review and meta-analysis of 18 studies involving 1.3 million hospital admissions, implementation of RRTs was associated with a 34% reduction in cardiopulmonary arrests outside intensive care units but was not associated with lower hospital mortality rates. These findings have challenged hospital staffs to consider whether the time, effort, and money invested in RRTs are the best expenditure of precious resources.

Types of Systematic Reviews

The overarching goal of systematic reviews (SRs) is to reach conclusions regarding specific issues by compiling and analyzing findings from several (or many) studies. There are three ways of accomplishing this: **integrative research reviews**, **meta-analysis**, and **metasynthesis**. Integrative research reviews (IRRs)[1] are narrative summaries of past research in which the reviewer extracts findings from original studies, creates findings tables, and uses analytical reasoning to produce conclusions about the findings of a body of research. The meta-analysis method of summarizing research findings uses statistical techniques to combine the results of studies from several or many studies. With intervention studies, this statistical combining can often reveal effectiveness that was not detectable in the individual studies. A metasynthesis combines results or findings from several or many qualitative studies. For example, a metasynthesis was of done of 13 qualitative studies regarding how illness disrupts a woman's ability to mother her child/children; 5 themes were identified (Valido, Wilkes, Carter, & Jackson, 2010).

SYSTEMATIC REVIEWS

- **Integrative research reviews**
- **Meta-analysis**
- **Metasynthesis**

Although all three types of SRs produce important knowledge for practice, IRRs are more commonly found in clinical nursing journals. Thus, they will be the focus of this chapter and again later in the text. Before heading into a description of IRRs, I point out that all three types of systematic

[1]IRRs are also called state-of-the-science summaries, narrative reviews, and qualitative systematic reviews (to differentiate them from quantitative research reviews, that is, meta-analyses).

reviews are different from literature reviews in several ways (see also **Table 9–1**), including:

- Prescribed criteria regarding how an SR should be done have been established. Additionally, SR reports include detailed descriptions about each step in the production process. Adherence to a prescribed process and detailed reporting about how the process played out reduce the likelihood of biased conclusions. In contrast, no production process is prescribed for literature reviews; rather they are done according to the reviewers' predilections. And there is no expectation that the production process be described. The lack of a prescribed process for literature reviews and the lack of detailed reporting about how they are done increase the likelihood that they are prone to bias.
- Systematic reviews incorporate only research reports and sometimes data from large **databases**. Literature reviews typically include a wide variety of types of articles including essays, anecdotal accounts, and opinion.
- Systematic reviews are based on a wide and diligent search for studies, whereas literature reviews can be, and often are, selective in what they report.
- Systematic reviews use a **quality filter** either to exclude poor quality studies or to categorize the quality of studies included.

TABLE 9–1 Differences Between Systematic Reviews and Literature Reviews

Feature	Systematic Review (SR)	Literature Review
Purpose	Thorough examination of a specific issue	Highlights of an issue; varying degrees of thoroughness
Production process	Standards exist and the process used is described in report	No standards; process not described
Search	As exhaustive as possible	Often limited
Inclusion	Original study reports, previous SRs, information from large databases	Original study reports, theoretical literature, essays, opinion articles
Selection	Should use a quality appraisal filter	Quality filter not used
Report	Inclusive of all qualifying studies	Often selective based on purpose (cherry picking)

The IRR Production Process

The steps taken to produce an SR are as follows:

Formulate the topic or question of interest.

↓

Systematically search for studies and screen for relevance.

↓

Appraise the studies to select only those that are relevant and not biased.

↓

Extract information, analyze it, and synthesize the findings of the studies as a body of evidence.

↓

Produce a report.

These steps are in accordance with the more detailed process and standards set by the Joanna Briggs Institute (2011) and by the Institute of Medicine (2011). The steps have been set forth in detail to control error and bias, which can enter at any point along the way.

Formulate the Topic

Panels or individuals with expertise in the issue of interest conduct integrative research reviews. The word *conduct* is used because doing an IRR is a demanding and rigorous undertaking. A review panel has greater potential to conduct an IRR that is free of error and bias than does an individual because the panel members act as checks and balances to each other's work and uncover unconscious bias.

Scope The review panel starts by identifying a topic, issue, or problem it believes is in need of summarization. Sometimes, the topic is broad; other times the issue is quite narrow. A broad topic addresses several aspects of an issue, whereas a narrow topic focuses on one particular aspect; this is the IRR's scope. A review of studies about preventing falls in the elderly would be broader than a review about preventing falls in the home-dwelling elderly would be. A review titled "Environmental alterations to prevent falls in home-dwelling elders" would be even narrower.

Broad and narrow scope is not a good–bad issue; rather, broad topics require retrieving and appraising a greater number of studies than do narrow topics. A review about preventing falls in home-dwelling elders would have to include studies regarding the functional status of patients (e.g., balance and gait), the role of medications, orthostatic hypotension, environmental issues, and more. In contrast, an IRR about environmental alterations to prevent falls in the home could focus on a smaller subset of studies having to do with floor surfaces, grab bars, lighting, steps, etc. Similarly, a review of smoking cessation interventions would be quite broad, but by specifying a population, such as adolescents, the review becomes considerably narrower. The broader the issue or topic, the more resources required to conduct the review, the more difficult the summary is to produce, and the longer the report.

Early on, reviewers consider the types of studies they will include in the IRR and how far back they will go in the search for studies. Sometimes changing technology or patterns of care signify that it does not make sense to go back beyond a certain date.

Types of Studies Reviewers can decide to include studies using the full range of designs or just those with certain design characteristics. For instance, a physician group interested in reviewing interventions for urinary incontinence in nursing home residents included only randomized trials (Fink, Taylor, Tacklind, Rutks, & Wilt, 2008). In contrast, a nurse reviewer interested in women's experiences of cardiac pain included only qualitative studies because she was interested in understanding the women's perspective (O'Keefe-McCarthy, 2008). The difference in the types of studies included in the two reviews was determined by the clinical issue of interest.

In the recent past, when conducting an SR about the effectiveness of a clinical treatment, the standard in medicine was to include only randomized studies, i.e., experimental studies. Increasingly, however, researchers conducting systematic reviews about treatment effectiveness are recognizing the contribution of findings from qualitative and observational/nonexperimental studies. The following statement is from the Cochrane Consumer Network (2012):

> Systematic reviews are based on clinical studies that carefully select their participants. As a result, more complex combinations of clinical problems and the social aspects of health care are not considered. The Cochrane Collaboration is working on how qualitative studies can be used to inform and add to the information obtained from the randomised controlled studies that currently inform Cochrane reviews—where the outcomes are often measured in numerical terms (and so are termed quantitative studies). (p.1)

So qualitative research is gaining respect for its unique contribution to intervention knowledge. Qualitative studies are seen as providing information about:

1. Patients' perceptions about the treatment.
2. Problems patients have following a particular regimen.
3. The extent to which patients consistently integrate treatment recommendations into their daily lives.
4. Quality of life outcomes associated with treatments

Clearly, these are important considerations when evaluating the evidence in support of a treatment. They shed light on its actual use, burden to the patient, and adherence aspects of effectiveness, all of which complement information about the treatment's effect on physiological and other clinical outcomes. In fact, real patient-world effectiveness of a treatment or intervention is most likely a combination of direct physiological or psychological effectiveness and patient response and use factors.

Similarly, nonrandomized studies, i.e., cohort studies, case-controlled studies, and controlled before-and-after studies, provide evidence of benefit or harm of interventions, particularly long-term and rare outcomes, which are rarely studied in randomized trials. Risk of bias in nonrandomized studies can be assessed in a similar manner to that used for randomized trials, although more attention must be paid to the possibility of selection bias (Higgins & Green, 2011, Section 13.1.2).

Early on, review panels decide how they will handle studies that are of dubious methodological quality. Some panels will include them but note their poor or modest quality, whereas other panels will eliminate them altogether. Still others will analyze the results of low-quality and high-quality studies together and then separately to determine if study quality affects the conclusions.

Search for Studies and Screen for Relevance

When the topic and scope have been clearly specified, the search for studies begins. Most review panels include a health science librarian who has expertise in locating research reports. The most common search-starting place is the computerized databases of the published healthcare literature (CINAHL, MEDLINE, and others). Reviewers typically search several healthcare databases using a variety of search terms, combinations of search terms, and search options.

Usually, the panel's initial goal is to identify all potential studies on the issue; however, database indexing and retrieval may fail to identify some eligible studies, which can be a source of bias. Moreover, databases include only published studies, and some studies may have been done but were never published. Thus, retrieval of eligible studies from databases is only a starting point. The panel often go on to peruse reference lists, check research registries and conference presentations, contact colleagues, and even run searches using Web search engines.

At this point, hundreds of citations may be under consideration. Careful reading of abstracts can reduce the number considerably by eliminating those that are not research reports or do not actually address the topic. Then, all potentially relevant research reports are retrieved. Using a prespecified set of inclusion criteria, two or more persons decide which studies are relevant.

Appraise

All of the relevant studies should be carefully appraised for quality; the goal of this appraisal is to eliminate studies that are biased or not credible because of the methods used. The number of studies that survive relevance screening and quality appraisal may be much smaller than the number initially identified during the search phase. It is not uncommon to have hundreds of citations identified by the search, but end up with 30, or even 8 studies, in the final review.

The panel will then sort the final body of articles into stacks by key questions or subtopics, such as those using similar forms of the intervention or those evaluating a particular clinical outcome. For instance, in a study of parenting in the neonatal intensive care unit (Cleveland, 2008), studies were grouped by whether they examined (1) the learning needs of parents or (2) the support needed by parents.

Extract, Analyze, and Synthesize

Panel members read each report and carefully extract basic information about design, sample, variables studied, and results. They then enter the information into evidence tables (see **Table 9–2**) and create lists to help

TABLE 9–2 Example of a Findings Table from an IRR Comparing Exercise Programs

Study	N Randomized/ Followed-up*	Participants Inclusion Criteria and Mean Age	Interventions	Primarily Aimed at†	Follow-up‡	Outcome measures§	Results‖
Binder, 2002, USA	IG: 69/66 CG: 50/49	Two out of three criteria: Score between 18–32 on Modified PPT, peak oxygen uptake between 10–18 mL/kg/min, self-reported difficulty in max. 2 ADLs or 1 IADL (Mean age: 83)	*IG:* 9-month program provided by physiology exercise technicians consisting of three phases of each 36 sessions. Phase 1: Group format: 22 exercises on flexibility, balance, coordination, speed of reaction and strength. Phase 2: Progressive resistance training combined with shortened version of phase 1 exercises. Phase 3: Endurance training combined with shortened version of phase 1 and phase 2 exercises.	Reduce or delay frailty	3, 6, and 9 months	Self-reported use of assistance or assistive technology (OARS ADL and IADL scale)	No differences between groups (data not presented).
						Self-reported difficulty with ADL and IADL (Physical Function subscale of FSQ)	Difference (SS) in favor of IG.
			CG: 9-month home exercise program including 9 of the 22 exercises from phase 1. Participants were asked to perform exercises 2–3 times a week and attended a monthly class.			Modified PPT items Knee extension/ flexion strength VO_2-peak Balance Body weight	Differences (SS) in favor of IG for modified PPT score knee strength, VO_2-peak and balance. No SS difference for body weight (data not shown).

TABLE 9–2 Example of a Findings Table from an IRR Comparing Exercise Programs *(continued)*

Study	N Randomized/ Followed-up*	Participants Inclusion Criteria and Mean Age	Interventions	Primarily aimed at†	Follow-up‡	Outcome measures§	Resultsf
Boshuizen, 2005, Netherlands	IG: High guidance (HG) 24/16 IG: Medium guidance (MG) 26/16 CG: 22/17	Experiencing difficulty in rising from chair and maximum knee extensor torque < 87.5 N-m (Mean age: ~79)	*IG:* High-guidance: 10-wk exercise program, each week two group sessions (60 min) by PT and one unsupervised home session. Focus on exercises with a variation in concentric, isometric, and eccentric knee-extensor activity. *IG:* Medium-guidance: Same program, though each week one supervised session and two unsupervised home sessions. *CG:* No training or other encouragement	Increasing strength knee extensors	10–12 weeks	Self-reported performance in activities of daily living (GARS) Knee extensor strength Walking function Balance Box stepping Timed Up and GO	No differences between groups. Difference (SS) in knee strength and walking function for HG group compared to CG. Differences (NS) between HG and MG for walking function in favor of HG.

(continues)

TABLE 9–2 Example of a Findings Table from an IRR Comparing Exercise Programs *(continued)*

Study	N Randomized/ Followed-up*	Participants Inclusion Criteria and Mean Age	Interventions	Primarily aimed at†	Follow-up‡	Outcome measures§	Results‖
Chandler, 1998, USA	IG: 50/44 CG: 50/43	Inability to descend stairs step over step without holding the railing (Mean age: ~78)	*IG:* 10-wk exercise program, each week three individual in-home sessions by PT. Focus: Progressive resistive lower extremity exercises with Thera-Band. *CG:* No training or any encouragement.	Increasing lower extremity strength	10 weeks	Self-reported limitations in physical activities (MOS-36 physical functioning subscale) Lower extremity strength Physical performance	No significant differences between groups (data not presented). Greater lower extremity (SS) strength gain in favor of IG (data on physical performance not presented).

Source: Adapted from Daniels, R., van Rossum, E., de Witte, L., Kempen, G. I., & van den Heuvel, W. (2008). Interventions to prevent disability in frail community-dwelling elderly: A systematic review. *BMC Health Services Research, 8,* 278. Retrieved from http://www.biomedcentral.com/content/pdf/1472-6963-8-278.pdf

*Randomized relates to the number of participants randomized to intervention guidance (IG) and control group (CG). Followed-up relates to the numbers of participants taken into data analysis.

† Outcome that the authors primarily aimed to improve by conducting the intervention.

‡ Follow-up measurement in weeks or months after randomization.

§ Measured disability concept and instrument, followed by outcome measures for frailty components.

‖ SS = Statistically significant difference if $p < .05$; NS = Not statistically significant.

identify differences, commonalities, and patterns across the studies. Different research questions, ways of measuring a variable, or timing of the outcome measurement are noted. Similarities and differences in results and findings are identified and reasons for the differences explored.

The goal of analysis is to reach conclusions that represent the findings of the individual studies as a body of findings, which is different from looking at each one in isolation from the others. This combining of findings from many studies in the form of conclusions is often referred to as *synthesis* because new knowledge claims are produced—claims that go beyond what any single study produced. The term *synthesis* makes the process of bringing research findings together sound quite exacting—which is not quite the reality. In the conduct of all three forms of SRs, even when the reviewers are conscientious, interpretation is inherent in the process; assumptions, decisions about inclusion and exclusion, and faulty reasoning can affect the conclusions—and even produce misleading ones. However, these sources of bias can be minimized by following the recognized ways of conducting IRRs.

Report

IRR reports open by stating the issue they examine and why the reviewers think it is important. You should note if the review focused on a certain population or setting, and whether it is focused on one or several outcomes. For instance, a review about the effectiveness of relaxation techniques could focus just on the outcome of pain, or it could also include studies that examined relaxation techniques for anxiety, onset of panic attacks, or smoking cessation.

Next, the process that was used to search for study reports is described in detail, including databases searched, key terms used, and any inclusion or exclusion criteria used. The process used to extract information from the reports and the methods used to evaluate the quality of the studies are also described.

Typically, tables display much-abbreviated profiles of the studies and the findings. Table 9–2 is part of an evidence table from a review of interventions to prevent disability in frail community-dwelling elderly (Daniels, van Rossum, de Witte, Kempen, & van den Heuvel, 2008). Note how this table provides a quick overview of the methods and the results of the studies.

In the text, findings that are consistent, conflicting, and equivocal, as well as gaps in the research base, are reported, and bottom-line conclusions are set forth. Finally, the panel or authors indicate whether and how their conclusions square with any prior work that has been done on the topic, summarize the limitations of the body of research, and offer opinions regarding the clinical implications of the conclusions.

Use of IRRs

IRRs are being published in clinical journals with increasing frequency, which is very helpful to clinician teams designing nursing protocols. They are helpful because they distill the findings of several, or many, studies in a few pages. Locating a well-conducted, recent IRR saves a clinical project team all the work of identifying, retrieving, appraising, analyzing, and summarizing the research findings pertaining to the protocol they are designing.

At the same time, users of IRRs need to keep in mind that the conclusions are interpretations of findings, and as such they are prone to unidentified assumptions, oversight, and unconscious bias. Two review groups examining the same body of research findings could arrive at different conclusions. From the search of studies to the appraisal of the quality of the individual studies and on through the conclusions, there are numerous points at which the opinion of two review groups could differ. One group may discount the findings of a study that another group thinks is important. One group may focus on one outcome, while another group thinks another outcome is more important. Often the conclusions are similar or complementary but sometimes they are contradictory.

Healthcare organizations around the world produce and index systematic reviews. In Chapter 12, you will learn how to search for them and in Chapter 15, you will learn how to appraise the quality of an IRR.

Exemplar

Reading Tips

It may help to tell you in advance that in the Results and the Discussion sections of this IRR article, the references provided in the text most often refer to background information provided by studies that were not included in this IR. They were not included in the review itself because they did not directly address the issue of interest, yet they relate to the findings of this IR.

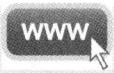

Patients' reports of the factors influencing medication adherence in bipolar disorder—An integrative review of the literature

MARIE CROWE*, LYNERE WILSON, MAREE INDER

DEPARTMENT OF PSYCHOLOGICAL MEDICINE, UNIVERSITY OF OTAGO, PO BOX 4345, CHRISTCHURCH, NEW ZEALAND

ARTICLE INFO

Article history:

Received 22 September 2010
Received in revised form 24 January 2011
Accepted 11 March 2011

Keywords:

Bipolar disorder, depression, medication adherence, mania, nursing, review

ABSTRACT

Background: As with other long-term conditions patients with bipolar disorder are rarely totally adherent or non-adherent. Rates of non-adherence have not changed since the first introduction of psychotropic medications in the 1950s despite vast numbers of new compounds being marketed. Non-adherence with medication in bipolar disorder is associated with affective relapse and consequently poor quality of life. The reasons that patients are non-adherent with medication are not well understood by clinicians who often assume it is related to the illness itself.

© 2011 Elsevier Ltd. All rights reserved.

*Corresponding author. Tel.: +64 3 3720400; fax: +64 3 3720407.
E-mail address: Marie.crowe@otago.ac.nz (M. Crowe).

0020-7489/$ – see front matter (2011 Elsevier Ltd. All rights reserved. doi:10.1016/j.ijnurstu.2011.03.008

Objectives: To identify patients' perceptions of medication adherence in bipolar disorder.

Design: An integrated review of the literature published between 1999 and 2010.

Data sources: Ovid (Medline, CINAHL, Embase, PsycINFO) and manual searching.

Review methods: An integrative review of the literature was conducted which included: (a) problem formation, (b) literature search and initial screening, (c) gathering data from studies, (d) evaluating study quality, (e) data analysis and integration, (f) data interpretation, and (g) presentation of the findings.

Results: Thirteen articles met criteria for inclusion in the review. These articles identified how patients reported their perceptions on medication and were integrated into four categories: illness factors, personal attitudes and beliefs, medication factors and environmental factors.

Conclusions: These findings suggest a need to address adherence from the full range of influencing factors (patient, illness, medication and environmental). Clinicians need to utilise a collaborative approach to working together with patients in order to identify the meaning that patients attribute to the symptoms, diagnosis, prognosis and medication. Understanding patients' perceptions and accepting these may facilitate greater medication adherence and the consequent improved clinical outcomes for patients with bipolar disorder.

What is already known about the topic?

- Medication adherence is a significant issue across many long-term conditions.
- Relapse in bipolar disorder is associated with medication non adherence.

What this paper adds

- This review identifies what studies have identified about patients' perceptions of medication non adherence.
- This review identifies that patient perspectives on medication adherence are related to patient factors, illness factors, medication factors and environmental factors.
- Increasing medication adherence in the context of a strong treatment alliance may be important in reducing relapses and recurrences, minimising the negative impacts on individuals' lives and improving their well-being.

1. Introduction

Medication adherence is an issue that impacts across many long-term conditions. The World Health Organization (2003) has reported that 50% of patients from developed countries with chronic disease do not use their medications as recommended. Adherence has been described as the extent to which the patient's behaviour matches agreed recommendations from the prescriber (Horne, 2006). The term 'adherence' has generally superseded 'compliance' and its patriarchal connotations, and emphasises the patient's role in deciding to adhere to the doctor's recommendations and removes a sense of blame if the patient chooses not to follow those recommendations. It emphasises the need for agreement between patient and prescriber.

Non-adherence is not significantly related to the type or severity of disease, quality of information provided to the patient or socio-demographic variables (Horne, 2006). It takes a number of forms but is generally defined as taking medications differently from the prescriber's recommendations—reducing dosages and frequency, using symptomatically rather than as a prophylactic, temporary cessation and full cessation. It occurs in the context of the patient's determination of their needs without consultation with the prescriber. As Horne (2006) has noted most people do not blindly follow treatment recommendations, even when they are made by trusted clinicians. Instead, they tend to evaluate whether the advice makes common sense in the light of their personal understanding and beliefs about the illness. A significant proportion of individuals have strong negative beliefs about prescribed medicines: that they are harmful, chemical (i.e., unnatural), and better avoided, and that doctors are far too willing to prescribe medications (Horne et al., 1999).

As with other long-term conditions patients with bipolar disorder are rarely totally adherent or non-adherent but use their medication somewhere in between (Scott and Pope, 2002). Traditionally non-adherence with medications for mental disorders has been blamed on 'lack of insight' (El-Mallakh, 2007; Yen et al., 2005) or 'denial' (Keck et al., 1997; Pollack, 1995) as a symptom of the disorder, but this suggests a limited explanation of the factors that influence adherence both generally and those specifically associated with the disorder and the medications recommended for its treatment. Because medication adherence has been associated with recurrence of episodes, particularly mania (Miklowitz, 2008), it is important to gain a better understanding of the factors that influence how patients with bipolar disorder decide to take medications.

2. Background

Bipolar disorder is characterised by chronic and recurrent marked mood instability. Studies have identified that the longitudinal course of both Bipolar I and Bipolar II disorders was chronic and primarily depressive (Judd et al., 2002). According to the Diagnostic and Statistical Manual-IV (American Psychiatric Association, 2000) Bipolar I disorder is characterised by episodes mania (extreme mood elevation), mixed moods (usually agitated dysphoria) and major depression. Bipolar II disorder is characterised by major depressive episodes and at least one episode of hypomania (mood elevation). Generally medication is effective in the treatment of acute episodes but there is increasing evidence that while a large majority of patients recover from these episodes of mania and/or depression, many do not achieve a functional recovery (Bauer et al., 2001; Judd et al., 2002; Keck, 2006). According to clinical guidelines after the resolution of an acute illness episode, long-term prophylaxis is required to prevent recurrence (Royal Australian and New Zealand College of Psychiatrists Clinical Practice Guidelines Team for Bipolar Disorder, 2004). However rates of relapse in bipolar disorder (even when taking prophylaxis) are as high as 40% in the first year, 60% in the second year and 73% over five years or more (Gitlin et al., 1995). Johnson and McFarland (1998) found that the median duration of continuous use of lithium after it was first prescribed was only 76 days. Precise evaluation and assessment of treatment adherence is difficult in patients with bipolar disorder (Sajatovic et al., 2004). The most commonly used measures of adherence are self-report and plasma levels. Scott (2000) found that self-report measures correlated highly with plasma levels.

Scott (2002) has noted that between 30% and 50% of individuals prescribed a prophylactic mood stabiliser stopped taking medication against medical advice at least once over the course of a year. These rates of non-adherence have not changed since the first introduction of psycho-tropic medications in the 1950s despite vast numbers of new compounds being marketed (Tacchi and Scott, 2005). Pope and Scott (2003) found that clinicians misunderstood the reasons patients were not adherent with medication and had inaccurately identified that patients missed highs or felt well as the reasons for non-adherence.

There is increasing evidence that psycho-pharmacological-only interventions are not as effective as first promoted for the management of bipolar disorder primarily because of high rates of non-adherence (Crowe et al., 2010). Angst and Sellaro (2000) found in a review of two centuries of literature on bipolar disorder that the findings of modern follow-up studies are closely compatible with those of studies conducted before the introduction of modern antidepressant and mood-stabilizing treatments. Many mental health services provide medication as the only treatment option and many do not address the issues that underpin treatment non-adherence.

Non-adherence in bipolar disorder is associated with higher rates of relapse, hospital admissions and suicide which suggests that there is clearly a need for a better understanding of the reasons behind it (Clatworthy et al., 2007). Perlis et al. (2006) have identified that even patients receiving optimal medication are likely to have recurrences, have trouble holding jobs, maintaining relationships and getting along with significant others. It was an interest in trying to identify the effective treatment options for people with bipolar disorder that initiated this review of factors that influence adherence to medication.

3. Method

An integrative review of the literature was conducted utilising the general framework for research synthesis described by Cooper (2010) which describes seven stages in research synthesis methodology, including: (a) problem formation (MC, MI, LW), (b) literature search (MC and research librarian) and initial screening (MC & MI independently), (c) gathering data from studies (MC, MI), (d) evaluating study quality (MC, MI, LW independently), (e) data analysis and integration (MC), (f) data interpretation (MC, MI LW), and (g) presentation of the findings (MC).

3.1. Problem

What factors do people with bipolar disorder identify as contributing to medication non-adherence?

3.2. Search strategy

Databases searched included: Ovid (Medline, Embase, CINAHL and PsycINFO) and manual searching from the reference lists from articles identified by electronic search. The key words were identified in consultation with a research librarian using The Medical Subject Headings vocabulary: bipolar disorder; medication adherence; drug therapy; client attitude; patient attitude; health knowledge, attitudes, practice; concordance.

3.3. Criteria for considering studies

The following inclusion criteria were determined as they captured the focus of the research question and reflected both clinical and research requirements i.e., clinical guidelines for the treatment of bipolar disorder identify the need for medication yet research has identified that many people with bipolar disorder are non-adherent with medications.

1. Studies examining factors associated with non-adherence for people with bipolar disorder.
2. Studies utilising quantitative measures and qualitative exploration.
3. The focus of studies was patients' perceptions of their medication adherence.
4. Reported outcome data using any measurement instrument.
5. Published between 1999 and 2010. These parameters were chosen because an initial search identified few if any articles exploring the patient's perspective prior to 1999. Only two articles found prior to this time met inclusion criteria but were did not seek patient's perception but focused on clinical attributes.

3.4. Exclusion criteria

Studies were excluded if more than one diagnosis was the focus and the results did not separate bipolar disorder from other diagnoses.

Table 1 Key search terms and results. Database: Ovid (Includes Medline, Cinahl, EmBase and PsychInfo) Manual Searching (from Reference Lists).

Search #	Search terms	Results
1	Bipolar disorder/or bipolar.mp	15,269
2	Medication adherence.mp. or medication adherence/	3446
3	1 and 2	100
4	Drug therapy. mp or drug therapy/	89,824
5	Client attitude. mp	1
6	Health knowledge, attitudes, practice/or patient attitude. mp.	45,264
7	1 and 4 and 6	1
8	1 and 2 and 6	3
9	Concordance. mp	12,237
10	1 and 4 and 9	0
8	Manual searching	8

3.5. Assessment of relevance for inclusion in the review

The abstracts of all studies identified by the search strategies were examined. Articles were screened by two investigators working independently. Those that identified patient perspectives as their foci were selected for more detailed examination. The full-text versions of these studies were then obtained.

3.6. Study quality assessment

The quality of the identified trials was assessed using the following criteria that were adapted from previously published systematic reviews (Bee et al., 2008; Curran and Brooker, 2007) and enabled us to assess methods of research design, sampling and conclusions:

- Identified aims are congruent with methodology and measurements.
- Sufficient details of sampling procedure reported along with demographic characteristics.
- Methods for collecting data described.
- Validated measures and/or method for obtaining qualitative data.
- Sufficient detail of the process of analysis is provided to follow method.
- Results presented systematically.
- Conclusions reflect the results from the study.

All three investigators completed the quality evaluation independently and met to discuss results and obtain consensus on those studies excluded or included. A total of 100 articles were identified by key search terms (see Table 1) but most of these failed to meet all inclusion criteria (see Table 2 for flow diagram of process).

4. Results

A total of 13 studies were included in the review with a total of 1897 participants with bipolar disorder. Because of the low number of published studies all were included if they measured patients' perceptions of medication adherence. All studies included met the minimum quality requirements outlined above. The number of participants in each study ranged from 10 to 435 with most studies conducted in the United States or England. The studies were predominantly quantitative in design although there were two qualitative studies included and one that was mixed methods. Some were designed as stand-alone studies and some were adjunctive to other studies of bipolar disorder. The combination of both quantitative and qualitative methods and the variety of measures used meant a meta-analysis was not possible. The majority of the studies were conducted with patients in out-patient settings but one study was conducted with members of a bipolar support network.

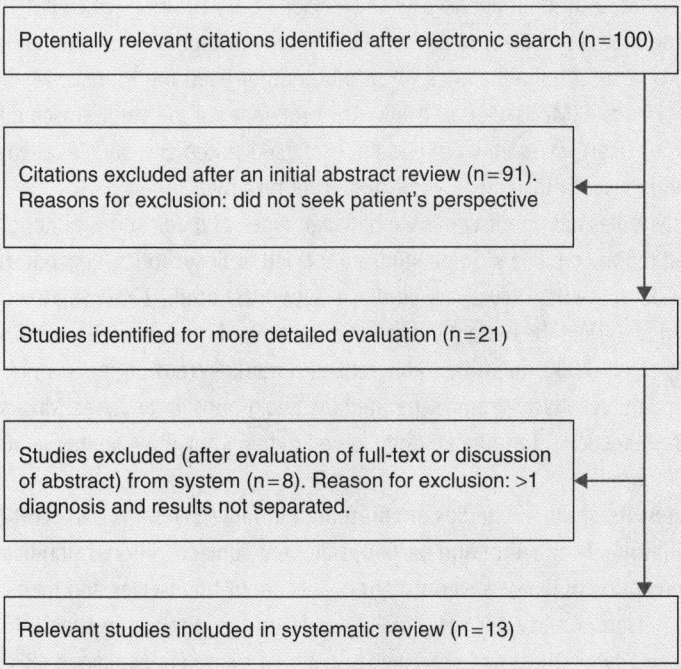

Table 2 Flow Diagram of Process

The studies used a variety of measures that included a measure of adherence e.g., the Medication Adherence Rating Scale (MARS) (Thompson et al., 2000) and other measures that reflected the primary outcome of the study e.g., Health Care Climate Questionnaire (Ludman et al., 2002); Beliefs About Medication Questionnaire (Horne et al., 1999); Attitudes to Mood Stabilizers Questionnaire (Harvey, 1991). One study collected qualitative data using the Subjective Experience of Medication Interview (Jenkins et al., 2005) that explored what patients thought the medication was doing, worries or concerns about medications and what they want their medications to do for them. These measures are primarily quantitative in design and yielded descriptive statistical analysis. The qualitative study and the qualitative component of mixed methods studies utilised thematic and content analyses.

The studies were not consistent in the choice of measure of adherence. Three studies used the Medication Adherence Rating Scale Thompson et al. (2000)—Bowskill et al. (2007), Clatworthy et al. (2007) and Rosa et al. (2007). This has series of questions that can score between five and 25 with <21 considered low adherence. Two studies (Adams and Scott, 2000; Sajatovic et al., 2009a,b) used the modified Tablet Routine Questionnaire (Peet and Harvey, 1991) which calculates nonadherence as missing >30% of medication. One study (Adams and Scott, 2000) used the Ratings of Medication Influences Scale (Weiden et al., 1994) in which patients are asked to place themselves in one of six categories ranging from total adherence (100%) and total nonadherence (0%) and another used the Morisky Medication Adherence Scale (Morisky et al., 1986). The remainder of the studies used different versions of Likert scales in which patients endorsed statements such as always take medication, usually take medication, and never take medication.

Most studies did not discriminate between types of medications although most included mood stabilisers. Some studies included antipsychotics, benzodiazepines and antidepressants. Only a few studies (Clatworthy et al., 2007; Sajatovic et al., 2009a,b) identified the patient's mood state at time of measurement. Some studies (Darling et al., 2008) identified adherent and nonadherent patients a priori and compared the results and some separated the two groups for analyses. Most studies were cross-sectional but one study followed patients for three years (Sajatovic et al., 2009a,b).

The results of the 13 studies are presented in Table 3. Adams and Scott (2000) found that highly adherent and partially adherent subjects differed significantly in their perception of illness severity, their beliefs about themselves and their control over the disorder and their concerns about future hospitalizations; and that perceived severity of illness and perceived benefits of treatment explained 43% of the variance in adherence and non-adherence.

Table 3 Summary of Papers Reviewed

Authors	Focus	*N*	Measures	Results	Conclusions
Adams and Scott (2000)	The relationship between patients' health beliefs and medication adherence.	39	Ratings of Medication Influences Scale Lithium Side Effects Questionnaire Dysfunctional Attitudes Scale Multi-dimensional Health Locus of Control Scale	Highly adherent and partially adherent subjects differed significantly in their perception of illness severity, their beliefs about themselves and their control over the disorder and their concerns about future hospitalizations. Perceived severity of illness and perceived benefits of treatment explained 43% of the variance.	Including questions related to severity of illness and fear of hospitalization combined with direct clinical inquiry about difficulties with adherence could help detect non-adherence.
Bowskill et al. (2007)	Satisfaction with information about medication	223	Satisfaction with Information about Medicines Scale	58% dissatisfied with information about how medicines acted 65% dissatisfied with information about side effects	Perceived satisfaction with information about medication is associated with low adherence

(continues)

Table 3 Summary of Papers Reviewed *(continued)*

Authors	Focus	*N*	Measures	Results	Conclusions
Clatworthy et al. (2009)	Patients attitudes to adherence	223	Beliefs About Medication Questionnaire Medication Adherence Report Scale	Low adherence reported by 30% and was predicted by greater doubts about personal need for treatment and stronger concerns about potential negative effects.	Interventions to facilitate adherence should elicit and address patients' beliefs about medication.
Clatworthy et al. (2007)	Patients' beliefs about bipolar disorder and its treatment associated with non-adherence	16	Qualitative interviews	81% reported some form of medication non-adherence. This was associated with patients' concerns about the medication side effects, beliefs that use could have adverse effects in future, doubts about personal need for medication.	Interventions to facilitate adherence should elicit patients' beliefs about their diagnosis and the nature of bipolar disorder and their concerns about medications.

Table 3 Summary of Papers Reviewed *(continued)*

Authors	Focus	*N*	Measures	Results	Conclusions
Darling et al. (2008)	Association of life contentment (family and health stress, level of coping and internal health locus of control) with medication adherence	100	Family Inventory of Life Events and Changes Family Health Status Inventory Family Crisis-oriented Personal Evaluation Scale Health Locus of Control Generalised Contentment Scale Adherence	Family stress, family coping, health stress, internal locus of control and general contentment scores were associated with adherence. The ability to address family stress associated with having bipolar disorder mediated the relationship between medication adherence and general contentment	Interventions need to focus on assessing the multiple factors associated with medication adherence and develop approaches that are individualised to the persons' unique needs.
Jonsdottir et al. (2009)	Patients' beliefs about medication and relation ship to medication adherence.	114	Beliefs About Medication Questionnaire Self-reported adherence Serum levels	Beliefs about necessity and the concerns about taking medication are related to adherence. Negative attitudes to medication were common. Service related factors and experience of psychiatric services influence these beliefs	Eliciting patients' beliefs about the necessity for taking medication and their concerns about taking medication need to be addressed to improve adherence.

(continues)

Table 3 Summary of Papers Reviewed *(continued)*

Authors	Focus	*N*	Measures	Results	Conclusions
Pope and Scott (2003)	Reasons patients give for stopping lithium	61	Reasons for Stopping Medication Questionnaire	Patients identified 'bothered by the idea that moods were controlled by medication', 'bothered by the idea of a chronic illness' and 'felt depressed' as the main reasons for stopping lithium.	Patients' reasons for stopping lithium appear to be influenced by concerns about what having an affective disorder and taking medication says about them. Clinicians are not fully aware of these reasons.
Rosa et al. (2007)	Degree of non-adherence to lithium, reasons for non-adherence and its consequences and attitudes towards long-term treatment.	106	Lithium Attitudes Questionnaire Medication Adherence Rating Scale Side Effects Questionnaire Lithium Knowledge Test Lithium plasma levels	85.6% of participants were adherent to lithium. There was a negative relationship between plasma levels and the LAQ, and a positive relationship between LKT and MARS and plasma levels.	Knowledge levels are related to treatment adherence, patients' attitudes, lower adherence, opposition to prophylaxis, fear of side effects, denial of therapeutic effectiveness and severity. The higher the knowledge level, the higher the adherence and the lower the toxicity risks.

Table 3 Summary of Papers Reviewed *(continued)*

Authors	Focus	*N*	Measures	Results	Conclusions
Sajatovic et al. (2008)	The association between baseline variables and average treatment adherence over a three year period.	306	Medication Adherence Rating Scale Structured Clinical Inter view for DSM-IV Global Assessment Scale SF-36 Working Alliance Inventory	Non-adherence associated with lower-intensity bipolar medication treatment, more barriers to care and more previous suicide attempts.	Consideration of non-adherence as a function not just of patient factors but also system factors will enhance understanding of non-adherence and ability to intervene more quickly.
Sajatovic et al. (2009b)	The relationship between demographic and clinical variables, illness severity and subjective illness and treatment attitudes; and medication adherence.	140	Tablets Routine Questionnaire Brief Psychiatric Rating Scale Attitudes to Mood Stabilizers Questionnaire Rating of Medication Influences Multidimensional Locus of Control	Adherent individuals did not differ from non-adherent ones on clinical variables (apart from substance abuse comorbidity). Non-adherent individuals had reduced insight into illness, more negative attitudes towards medications, and fewer reasons for adherence. The strongest attitudinal predictors for non-adherence were difficulties with medication routines and negative attitudes to drugs in general.	A patient-centred collaborative model of care that addresses negative attitudes towards medications and difficulty coping with medication routines may be the best way to address adherence issues

(continues)

Table 3 Summary of Papers Reviewed *(continued)*

Authors	Focus	*N*	Measures	Results	Conclusions
Sajatovic et al. (2009a)	Perceived treatment effects, concerns and expectations	90	Subjective experience of medication interview Insight and Treatment Attitudes Questionnaire	42% medication more stabilizing 19% decrease depression 10% mood improvement 10% improved sleep 39% no concerns 29% adverse effects	Concerns relate to long-term adverse effects and discrepancy between actual effects and hoped for outcomes
Scott (2002)	The utility of the Health Belief Models in explaining adherence	98	Ratings of Medication Influences Scale Lithium Side effects Questionnaire Self-reported adherence Tablets Routine Questionnaire	Self-report compares favourably with serum levels. Subjects' beliefs about themselves and their control over the disorder were more important than side-effects in predicting medication adherence	Exploring health beliefs may improve detection of patients at-risk of non-adherence.
Zeber et al. (2008)	Relationship between perceptions of the therapeutic environment and medication adherence	435		Positive therapeutic alliance was associated with better adherence. Notably those encouraged to maintain regular contact and those who had progress reviewed regularly were more likely to be adherent.	Recognising how individuals view their treatment will enable to better target clinical relationships towards medication adherence, quality of life and outcomes. Need to strengthen therapeutic relationships

Similar findings were identified by (Clatworthy et al., 2007; Sajatovic et al., 2008, 2009a,b). Only one study identified the importance of knowledge (Rosa et al., 2007). Two studies (Sajatovic et al., 2009a,b; Zeber et al., 2008) identified that access to treatment and the way in which treatment was delivered also influenced adherence. An integration of the findings of these studies suggests that the factors affecting adherence could be grouped into illness factors (Clatworthy et al., 2007; Sajatovic et al., 2008, 2009a,b), personal attitudes and beliefs (Adams and Scott, 2000; Clatworthy et al., 2009; Pope and Scott, 2003; Scott, 2002); medication related factors (Bowskill et al., 2007; Jonsdottir et al., 2009; Rosa et al., 2007) and environmental (relationship) factors (Darling et al., 2008; Zeber et al., 2008).

Illness factors included perceptions of illness severity and acceptance of their illness as well as the clinical features of substance abuse co-morbidity and a history of past suicide attempts. Personal attitudes and beliefs reflected individual's beliefs about themselves and their control over the disorder and adjusting to having a chronic disorder. Issues around medication included perceived benefits of medication, concerns about negative side effects, dissatisfaction with information about medications, doubts about the need for medication, concerns about future adverse effects and generally feeling negative about medication. Environmental issues affecting adherence reflected family stress and family coping, experiencing barriers to care, having less intense follow-up and the degree of therapeutic relationship.

5. Discussion

5.1. Limitations

This review is primarily limited by the small number of studies exploring medication adherence from the patient's perspective. Because of this we had fairly broad inclusion criteria. There is a significant body of studies that have examined adherence in relation to clinical characteristics of patients which were excluded because we were particularly interested in the patient's perceptions. The foci of the studies were not homogeneous and included attitudes, beliefs, satisfaction, associations with clinical characteristics, reasoning and perceptions. The range of foci and measures precluded any aggregation of results. Measurement of adherence included a number of validated measures and unvalidated Likert scales.

5.2. Reasons for nonadherence

The studies included in the review confirmed that medication non-adherence is a significant issue in bipolar disorder however measurement of adherence was not consistent. Patients' perceptions of the reasons for medication non-adherence could be categorised as: perception of illness severity, beliefs about themselves and their control over the disorder (impact of the disorder), and their perception of treatment.

Patients' adherence is more likely if the patient perceives that the advice to take the medication makes 'common-sense' in light of their experience of the illness and their personal beliefs about the cause of the illness (Leventhal et al., 1992). Broadbent et al. (2006) have identified that perception of illness has five dimensions: the label the person uses to describe the illness; the expected outcomes of the disease; personal beliefs about the cause of the disease; how long the person believes the illness will last; and the extent to which the patient believes they can recover from or control the illness. In bipolar disorder patients' perceptions of illness could be influenced by the fluctuating mood states common to the disorder. Anandit et al. (2009) have found that patients with bipolar disorder had beliefs that contradicted the biomedical model and that they seemed to simultaneously hold multiple and apparently contradictory causal and treatment models. Inder et al. (2010) has identified that ambivalence about the diagnosis and the need for treatment is common for people with bipolar disorder and is influenced by mood state. Many patients are unwilling to accept the disorder as chronic which may be because periods of unwellness are counterpoised against periods of wellness when patients begin to question both severity and chronicity.

5.3. Impact of the disorder

Beliefs about themselves and their ability to control bipolar disorder may also fluctuate according to mood state. The impact of depressive, manic and mixed mood symptoms can alter how the person perceives themselves. Inder et al. (2008) identified that the person's mood state was a central defining factor which led to the development of a sometimes inconsistent and at times contradictory sense of self. They found that some people with bipolar disorder had difficulty distinguishing their sense of self from the illness and that this could result in a lack of internalised personal sameness.

Shoemaker and de Oliveira (2008) have identified that the unremitting nature of chronic medication use often leads the individual to question the need for medication and subsequently seek to exert some control over their treatment experience by altering the way they take medication. This was supported by Berk et al. (2004) who identified that on average nearly half of the patients seen by a clinician for pharmacological treatment will not be fully compliant with prescribed medication.

5.4. Perception of treatment

Patient's perceptions of treatment relates to both the accessibility of services and the quality of the relationship that patients have with their clinician. Bhugra and Flick (2005) have suggested that only about 50% of patients receive appropriate treatment for bipolar disorder because of systemic barriers to patients gaining access to appropriate care. They suggest the current treatment environment relies too heavily on a crisis response rather than comprehensive, on-going, long-term illness management. Once accurate diagnosis is obtained patients need to be able to access care rapidly prior to the emergence of a full episode in order to have the best treatment outcome. The other crucial aspect of the patient's perception of treatment highlighted in the review is the quality of the therapeutic relationship. As Strauss and Johnson (2006) have identified a strong treatment alliance encourages greater acceptance of bipolar disorder and psychopharmacological interventions and thus contributes to improved medication adherence and clinical outcomes. One large study (Sajatovic et al., 2008) found that non-adherence was more likely to occur if follow-up was less intensive and if there were more barriers to receiving care. The relationship that patients had with their health service was also found to be significant in another large study (Zeber et al., 2008) which found that better adherence was associated with a more positive therapeutic alliance and more regular follow-up.

In a systematic review of interventions to improve medication adherence in bipolar disorder Sajatovic et al. (2004) found that psycho educational interventions that focus specifically on bipolar illness appear effective in improving outcomes and treatment adherence, although improved adherence does not necessarily correlate with improved symptoms. They suggest that effective therapies occur in the context of long-term management of illness that incorporates a good understanding of medications and their risks and benefits as well as education about illness awareness and illness self-management. A range of disorder-specific psychosocial therapies has evidence to support their implementation in routine in clinical practice (Crowe et al., 2010). This review suggested that all these therapies could be implemented in mental health nursing practice but that perhaps the manualised group psychoeducation (Colom and Vieta, 2006) could be the most easily integrated into practice. Because of the way in which patients perceive medication adherence stand-alone education sessions are likely to be of little value. Any effective intervention needs to longitudinal in design and encompassing strategies for self management of bipolar disorder.

5.5. Implications for nursing

Nursing interventions focused on improving medication non-adherence are complex and not always successful. Wijnveld and Crowe (2010) have identified that mental health nurses often feel conflicted about the need to maintain a therapeutic relationship and the clinical expectations that they ensure patients take their medication. The nurses in that study felt they were expected to do the job for doctors (rather than the patients) and approached this by stopping and listening to the patient or taking control when patients refused their medications. Overall they described their role in medication adherence as walking a fine line between keeping the relationship therapeutic and taking control.

A Cochrane review of interventions to manage medication non-adherence (Haynes et al., 2005) identified that only about 40% of the interventions studied to improve adherence demonstrated any significant improvement and even the most effective interventions did not lead to large improvements in adherence and treatment outcomes. For long-term treatments, such as those for bipolar disorder, no simple intervention, and only some complex ones, led to improvements in health outcomes. They included combinations of more convenient care, information, counselling, reminders, self-monitoring, reinforcement, family therapy, psychological therapy, mailed communications, crisis intervention, manual telephone follow-up, and other forms of additional supervision or attention. Even with the most effective methods for long-term treatments, improvements in drug use or health were not large.

A recent study has indicated the need for nurses to maintain a person-centred approach in relation to medication (Bolster and Manias, 2010). One such model that has promise at a theoretical level for bipolar disorder, but has yet to be studied systematically, is the dialogic risk communication framework described by Collins and Street (2009) This model proposes five steps: defining the nature of risk; clarifying the goal of communication; describing risk perspectives; managing difference and prioritising risk perspectives; and making a decision. Defining the nature of risk involves exploring medication use from both the nurse's and patient's perspective. The patient may have concerns about the risk to their lifestyle or well-being while the nurse may be concerned about relapse prevention. These concerns need to be explored and openly discussed. Clarifying the goal of communication involves making it explicit that the discussion is about coming to a shared decision and not one of advice-giving regarding the need to take medication. The nurse needs to explain that the goal is to incorporate both scientific evidence and personal feelings about the risks of taking long-term medication. Describing risk perspectives involves both patient and nurse sharing their perspectives on the nature. Managing the difference and prioritising risk perspectives involves the nurse and patient clarifying the values of the risks associated with the proposed treatments. If clinical evidence indicates that medication has both risks and benefits or there is differing evidence on the nature of the risk, then patients' values become more salient for determining the acceptability of risks. Making a decision involves both parties understanding which risks are acceptable, then they can justify specific treatment decisions. With a closer shared understanding, the patient is better equipped to make a quality decision because both the clinical evidence and their own perspective have been incorporated into the information sharing (Collins and Street, 2009).

Another more controversial approach may be to advocate for the symptomatic treatment of bipolar disorder symptoms for patients who do not respond to prophylactic treatment. Clinical experience suggests patients may be more likely to take medication for symptom relief when they understand how to use medication in this way, but there have been no studies to support this approach. The information that patients receive needs to be accurate and should not oversell the potential benefits of medication. Garnham et al. (2007) reviewed the charts of 120 patients with bipolar disorder and found that the rates of response to individual mood stabilizers were lithium 30%, valproate 13%, lamotrogine 11% and olanzapine 25%. Less than one third of patients had achieved remission from symptoms by taking the medication as prescribed. Factors not identified by patients themselves but identified in other studies include patient factors such as younger age, single status, male gender and low educational level (Colom and Vieta, 2002; Sajatovic et al., 2007); duration of being prescribed a mood stabilizer (Scott and Pope, 2002); polypharmacy (Patel and Anthony, 2007); and comorbid disorders such as personality disorders and substance use disorders (Colom et al., 2000).

6. Conclusion

The review has highlighted a limited number of studies investigating patients' perceptions of medication and adherence in bipolar disorder. These findings suggest a need for mental health nurses to address adherence from the full range of influencing factors (patient, illness, medication and environmental). Such a framework has been suggested by Goodwin and Jamison (2007) who identified four interacting domains—medication-related, patient-related, environmental and clinician-related factors.

Increasing medication adherence in the context of a strong treatment alliance may be important in reducing relapses and recurrences, minimising the negative impacts on individuals' lives and to increase their well-being. Patients with bipolar disorder need to be given full and accurate information about the medication they are receiving and what they can realistically expect from its actions and side-effects. An authoritarian or judgmental approach that involves telling the patient about the medication and why they need to take it is likely to be counter-productive. A more therapeutic and clinically effective approach would involve eliciting and validating the patient's perceptions of medications in general and psychotropic medications in particular and contributing information based on evidence of efficacy. Mental health nurses need to utilise a collaborative approach to working together with patients in order to identify the meaning that patients attribute to the symptoms, diagnosis, prognosis and medication. This may facilitate greater medication adherence and the consequent improved clinical outcomes for patients with bipolar disorder.

Conflict of interest

No conflicts of interest.

Funding

Not funded.

Ethical approval

Not declared.

References

1. Adams, J., Scott, J., 2000. Predicting medication adherence in severe mental disorders. Acta Scandanavica Psychiatrica 101, 119–124.
2. American Psychiatric Association, 2000. Diagnostic and statistical manual IV-TR. American Psychiatric Association, Washington.
3. Anandit, J.M., Beulah, S., Jacob, K., 2009. Perceptions of illness in self and others among patients with bipolar disorder. International Journal of Social Psychiatry 55, 462–470.
4. Angst, J., Sellaro, R., 2000. Historical perspectives and natural history of bipolar disorder. Biological Psychiatry 48 (6), 445–457.
5. Bauer, M.S., Kirk, G.F., Gavin, C., Williford, W.O., 2001. Determinants of functional outcome and healthcare costs in bipolar disorder: a high-intensity follow-up study. Journal of Affective Disorders 65 (3), 231–241.
6. Bee, P.E., Playle, J., Lovell, K., Barnes, P., Gray, R., Keeley, P., 2008. Service user views and expectations of UK-registered mental health nurses: a systematic review of empirical research. International Journal of Nursing Studies 45, 442–457.
7. Berk, M., Berk, L., Castle, D., 2004. A collaborative approach tot he treatment alliance in bipolar disorder. Bipolar Disorders 6, 504–518.
8. Bhugra, D., Flick, G.R., 2005. Pathways to care for patients with bipolar disorder. Bipolar Disorders 7 (3), 236–245.
9. Bolster, D., Manias, E., 2010. Person-centred interactions between nurses and patients during medication activities in an acute hospital setting. International Journal of Nursing Studies 46, 154–165.
10. Bowskill, R., Clatworthy, J., Parham, R., Rank, T., Horne, R., 2007. Patients' perceptions of information received about medication prescribed for bipolar disorder: implications for informed choice. Journal of Affective Disorders 100, 253–257.
11. Broadbent, E., Petrie, K.J., Main, J., Weinman, J., 2006. The brief illness perception questionnaire. Journal of Psychosomatic Research 60 (6), 631–637.
12. Clatworthy, J., Bowskill, R., Parham, R., Rank, T., Scott, J., Horne, R., 2009. Understanding medication non-adherence in bipolar disorders using a Necessity-Concerns Framework. Journal of Affective Disorders 116, 51–55.
13. Clatworthy, J., Bowskill, R., Rank, T., Parham, R., Horne, R., 2007. Adherence to medication in bipolar disorder: a qualitative study exploring the role of patients' beliefs about the condition and its treatment. Bipolar Disorders 9, 656–664.

14. Collins, D., Street, R., 2009. A dialogic conversation about risk: coordinating perceptions and achieving quality decisions in cancer care. Social Science & Medicine 68, 1506–1512.
15. Colom, F., Vieta, E., 2006. Psychoeducation manual for bipolar disorder. Cambridge University Press, London.
16. Colom, F., Vieta, E., 2002. Treatment adherence in bipolar patients. Clinical Approach to Bipolar Disorder 1, 49–56.
17. Colom, F., Vieta, E., Martinez-Aran, A., Reinares, M., Benabarre, A., Gasto, C., 2000. Clinical factors associated with treatment non-compliance. Journal of Clinical Psychiatry 61, 549–555.
18. Cooper, H.M., 2010. Research synthesis and meta-analysis: a step-by-step approach. Sage, Thousand Oaks, CA.
19. Crowe, M., Whitehead, L., Wilson, L., Carlyle, D., O'Brien, A.J., Inder, M., Joyce, P., 2010. Disorder-specific psychosocial interventions for bipolar disorder—a systematic review of the evidence for mental health nursing practice. International Journal of Nursing Studies 47 (7), 896–908.
20. Curran, J., Brooker, C., 2007. Systematic review of interventions delivered by UK mental health nurses. International Journal of Nursing Studies 44, 479–511.
21. Darling, C., Olmstead, S., Lund, V., Fairclough, J., 2008. Bipolar disorder: medication adherence and life contentment. Archives of Psychiatric Nursing 22, 113–126.
22. El-Mallakh, R., 2007. Medication adherence and the use of long-acting antipsychotics in bipolar disorder. Journal of Psychiatric Practice 13, 79–85.
23. Garnham, J., Munro, A., Slaney, C., MacDougall, M., Passmore, M., Duffy, A., O'Donovan, C., Teehan, A., Alda, M., 2007. Prophylactic treatment response in bipolar disorder: results of a naturalistic observation study. Journal of Affective Disorders 104, 185–190.
24. Gitlin, M., Swendsen, J., Heller, T.L., Hammen, C., 1995. Relapse and impairment in bipolar disorder. American Journal of Psychiatry 152, 1635–1640.
25. Goodwin, F.K., Jamison, K.R., 2007. Manic-depressive illness – bipolar disorders and recurrent depression. Oxford University Press, New York.
26. Harvey, N., 1991. The development and descriptive use of the lithium attitudes questionnaire. Journal of Affective Disorders 22, 211–219.
27. Haynes, R., Yao, X., Oliver, T., et al., 2005. Interventions to enhance medication adherence. Cochrane Database Systematic Review 1, 1–29.
28. Horne, R., 2006. Compliance, adherence and concordance: implications for asthma treatment. Chest 130, 56s–72s.
29. Horne, R., Weinman, J., Hankins, M., 1999. The beliefs about medicines questionnaire: the development and evaluation of a new method for assessing the cognitive representation of medication. Psychology and Health 14, 1–24.
30. Inder, M., Crowe, M., Joyce, P., Moor, S., Luty, S., Carter, J., 2010. "I really don't know whether it is still there": ambivalent acceptance of a diagnosis of bipolar disorder. Psychiatric Quarterly 81, 157–165.
31. Inder, M.L., Crowe, M.T., Moor, S., Luty, S.E., Carter, J.D., Joyce, P.R., 2008. "I actually don't know who I am": the impact of bipolar disorder on the development of self. Psychiatry: Interpersonal and Biological Processes 71 (2), 123–133.

32. Jenkins, J.H., Strauss, M.E., Carpenter, E.A., Miller, D., Floersch, J., Sajatovic, M., 2005. Subjective experience of recovery from schizophrenia-related disorders and atypical antipsychotics. International Journal of Social Psychiatry 51 (3), 211–227.
33. Johnson, R., McFarland, B., 1998. Lithium use and its discontinuation in a health maintenance organisation. American Journal of Psychiatry 153, 993–1000.
34. Jonsdottir, H., Friis, S., Horne, R., Pettersen, K., Rekvam, A., Andreassen, O., 2009. Beliefs about medications: measurement and relationship to adherence in patients with severe mental disorders. Acta Psychiatrica Scandinavica 119, 78–84.
35. Judd, L.L., Akiskal, H.S., Schettler, P.J., Endicott, J., Maser, J., Solomon, D.A., Leon, A.C., Rice, J.A., Keller, M.B., 2002. The long-term natural history of the weekly symptomatic status of bipolar I disorder. Archives of General Psychiatry 59 (6), 530–537.
36. Keck, P., McElroy, S., Strakowski, S.M., Bourne, M., West, S.A., 1997. Compliance with maintenance treatment in bipolar disorder. Psycho-pharmacology Bulletin 33, 87–91.
37. Keck, P.E., 2006. Long-term management strategies to achieve optimal function in patients with bipolar disorder. Journal of Clinical Psychiatry 67 (12), e17.
38. Leventhal, H., Diefenbach, M., Leventhal, E.A., 1992. Illness cognition: using common sense to understand treatment adherence and affect cognition interactions. Cognitive Therapy & Research 16, 143–163.
39. Ludman, E.J., Simon, G.E., Rutter, C.M., Bauer, M.S., Unutzer, J., 2002. A measure for assessing patient perception of provider support for self-management of bipolar disorder. Bipolar Disorders 4 (4), 249–253.
40. Miklowitz, D.J., 2008. Adjunctive psychotherapy for bipolar disorder: state of the evidence. American Journal of Psychiatry 165 (11), 1408–1419.
41. Morisky, D., Green, L., Levine, D., 1986. Concurrent and predictive validity of a self-reported measure of medication adherence. Medical Care 24, 67–74.
42. Patel, M., Anthony, D., 2007. Medication adherence: predictive factors and enhancement strategies. Psychiatry 6, 357–361.
43. Peet, M., Harvey, N., 1991. Lithium maintenance. 1. A standard education programme for patients. British Journal of Psychiatry 158, 197–200.
44. Perlis, R.H., Ostacher, M.J., Patel, J.K., Marangell, L.B., Zhang, H., Wisniewski, S.R., Ketter, T.A., Miklowitz, D.J., Otto, M.W., Gyulai, L., Reilly-Harrington, N.A., Nierenberg, A.A., Sachs, G.S., Thase, M.E., 2006. Predictors of recurrence in bipolar disorder: primary outcomes from the Systematic Treatment Enhancement Program for Bipolar Disorder (STEP-BD). American Journal of Psychiatry 163 (2), 217–224.
45. Pollack, L., 1995. Striving for stability with bipolar disorder despite barriers. Archives of Psychiatric Nursing 9, 122–129.
46. Pope, M., Scott, J., 2003. Do clinicians understand why individuals stop taking lithium? Journal of Affective Disorders 74, 287–291.
47. Rosa, A., Marco, M., Fachel, J., Kapczonski, F., Stein, A., Barros, H., 2007. Correlation between drug treatment knowledge and lithium treatment attitudes and knowledge by bipolar patients. Progress in Neuro-Pschopharmacology and Biological Psychiatry 31, 217–224.
48. Royal Australian and New Zealand College of Psychiatrists Clinical Practice Guidelines Team for Bipolar Disorder, 2004. Australian and New Zealand clinical practice guide-

lines for the treatment of bipolar disorder. Australian and New Zealand Journal of Psychiatry 38, 280–305.

49. Sajatovic, M., Biswas, K., Kilbourne, A., Fenn, H., Williford, W., Bauer, M., 2008. Factors associated with prospective long-term treatment adherence among individuals with bipolar disorder. Psychiatric Services 59, 753–759.
50. Sajatovic, M., Davies, M., Hrouda, D., 2004. Enhancement of treatment among patients with bipolar disorder. Psychiatric Services 55, 264–269.
51. Sajatovic, M., Ignacio, R., West, J., Cassidy, K., Safavi, R., Kilbourne, A., Blow, F., 2009a. Predictors of nonadherence among individuals with bipolar disorder receiving treatment in a community mental health clinic. Comprehensive Psychiatry 50, 100–107.
52. Sajatovic, M., Jenkins, J., Cassidy, K., Muzina, D., 2009b. Medication treatment perceptions, concerns and expectations among depressed individuals with Type I Bipolar Disorder. Journal of Affective Disorders 115, 360–366.
53. Sajatovic, M., Valenstein, M., Blow, F., Ganoczy, D., Ignacio, R., 2007. Treatment adherence with lithium and anticonvulsant medications among patients with bipolar disorder. Psychiatric Services 58, 855–863.
54. Scott, J., 2000. Predicting medication adherence in bipolar disorder. Acta Neuropsychiatrica 12, 128–130.
55. Scott, J., 2002. Using health belief models to understand the efficacy–effectiveness gap for mood stabilizer treatments. Neuropsychobiology 46 (Suppl. 1), 13–15.
56. Scott, J., Pope, M., 2002. Nonadherence with mood stabilizers: prevalence and predictor. Journal of Clinical Psychiatry 63, 384–390.
57. Shoemaker, S., de Oliveira, D., 2008. Understanding the meaning of medications for patients: the medication experience. Pharmacy World and Science 30, 86–91.
58. Strauss, J., Johnson, S., 2006. Role of treatment alliance in the clinical management of bipolar disorder: stronger alliances prospectively predict fewer manic symptoms. Psychiatry Research 145, 215–223.
59. Tacchi, M., Scott, J., 2005. Improving medication adherence in schizophrenia and bipolar disorders. John Wiley & Sons, Chichester.
60. Thompson, K., Kulkharni, J., Sergejew, A., 2000. Reliability and validity of a new medication adherence rating scale (MARS) for the psychoses. Schizophrenia Research 42, 241–247.
61. Weiden, P., Rapkin, B., Mott, T., Zygmunt, A., Goldman, D., Horvitz-Lennon, M., Frances, A.J., 1994. Rating of medication influences (ROMI) scale in schizophrenia. Schizophrenia Bulletin 20, 297–310.
62. Wijnveld, A.M., Crowe, M., 2010. Walking a fine line: managing the tensions associated with medication non-adherence in an acute inpatient psychiatric setting. Journal of Clinical Nursing 19 (9–10), 1378–1386.
63. Yen, C.F., Chen, C.S., Ko, C.H., Yeh, M.L., Yang, S.J., Yen, J.Y., Huang, C.F., Wu, C.C., 2005. Relationships between insight and medication adherence in outpatients with schizophrenia and bipolar disorder: prospective study. Psychiatry & Clinical Neurosciences 59, 403–409.
64. Zeber, J., Copeland, L., Good, C., Fine, M., Bauer, M., Kilbourne, A., 2008. Therapeutic alliance perceptions and medication adherence in patients with bipolar disorder. Journal of Affective Disorders 107, 53–62.

Profile & Commentary

PURPOSE

The reviewers start by acknowledging that the factors influencing whether persons take medications as prescribed are not well understood. This is particularly true of persons with bipolar disorder, which is characterized by considerable mood instability. The authors establish that both relapse rates and medication nonadherence are high in this population. However, the extent to which medication nonadherence contributes to relapse of symptoms is not specified or supported by research evidence—although it is presumed to be the case. The reviewers sought to better understand the factors that contribute to medication nonadherence from the perspective of persons with bipolar disorder. Focusing on the perspective of persons with the disorder narrowed the scope of the IRR considerably. This is not bad; in fact it could uncover issues that would be glossed over if all studies about medication nonadherence in persons with bipolar disorder were examined. It does, however, reduce the number of studies qualifying for review.

METHODOLOGY

A widely used method for conducting a research review was followed and described in considerable detail in Section 3. The search strategy is described as are inclusion and exclusion criteria. Notice how the number of studies identified by the search (108) was reduced by reading the abstracts to 21. Then review of the full reports reduced the number to 13; all met the quality assessment described in Section 3.6.

I must admit to wondering why the flow diagram only accounts for the 100 studies identified by electronic database search and doesn't account for the 8 identified by manual searching; also the sum of studies excluded after initial abstract review and those identified for more detailed evaluation is 112, not 108 as I would expect. So, as per my usual practice when I have such questions, I contacted the corresponding author, and she acknowledged a typographical error. In the end, it is not a critical issue as the flow diagram does indicate how the researchers went from their initial identification of potentially relevant citations to the 13 studies included in the review, and the text describes in detail how this was done.

Examine Table 3 and notice how diverse the studies are in terms of the issues and the measures used to quantify the variables (columns 2 and 3). The study design per se is not in the table, but the text informs us that most used quantitative designs; two collected qualitative data, one of which used a mixed design. The purely qualitative study was Clatworthy et al. (2007) and the mixed design study was Sajatovic et al. (2009a). I identified them because their information in the Measures column lists interview as the method of data acquisition.

The considerable variety of foci (attitudes, beliefs, perception, reasoning, life contentment) made it difficult to identify trends or patterns and reach conclusions based on the findings of several studies. However, in looking across the studies, the reviewers grouped the factors that affected adherence into the following four categories: (1) illness factors, (2) personal attitudes and beliefs, (3) medication-related factors, and (4) environmental factors. They give specific examples of each. This four-category framework was set forth in an earlier qualitative study but served well in organizing the findings of this IRR. Of note is that two studies in this IR (Zeber et al., 2008; Sajatovic et al., 2008) suggest that the quality of relationship that patients have with their provider may have an influence on medication adherence.

In looking at the results and discussion sections, it is striking how many studies found that persons thought they did not need the medication or did not like the idea of taking a mood medication long term. Their actual experiences of side effects or the daily logistics of taking a medication were mentioned as influencing factors in several studies but were not as consistently found as the influence of their self-perception and the meanings they assigned to taking a mood-stabilizing medication. The reviewers expanded on these issues with other supporting studies in Sections 5.2 and 5.3. These other studies were not included in this IR because they did not directly address patients' perceptions of medication adherence (Inder et al., 2008) or focus on patients with bipolar disorder (Shoemaker and de Oliveira, 2008). Importantly, no study provided perspective on how important self-perception, attitude, and belief were as contributors to nonadherence. Specific interventions, as discussed in Section 5.5, are not derived directly from the review itself; instead they represent the reviewers' attempts to offer practical advice from what is really scant and fragmentary research evidence. This IRR reveals how complex the issue of medication adherence/nonadherence is, particularly in persons with a chronic, mood-related disorder. Much more research is needed on this important topic.

http://go.jblearning.com/brown3e

REFERENCES

Chan, P. S., Jain, R., Nallmothus, B. K., Berg, R. A., & Sasson, C. (2010). Rapid response teams: A systematic review and meta-analysis. *Archives of Internal Medicine, 170*, 18–26. doi:10.1001/archinternmed.2009.424. Retrieved from http://archinte.ama-assn.org/cgi/reprint/170/1/18

Cleveland, L. M. (2008). Parenting in the neonatal intensive care unit. *Journal of Obstetric, Gynecologic, and Neonatal Nursing, 37*, 666–691.

Cochrane Consumer Network (2012). *Evidence-based health care: Using evidence to inform your decisions*. Retrieved from http://consumers.cochrane.org/evidence-based-health-care

Daniels, R., van Rossum, E., de Witte, L., Kempen, G. I., & van den Heuvel, W. (2008). Interventions to prevent disability in frail community-dwelling elderly: A systematic review. *BMC Health Services Research, 8*, 278. Retrieved from http://www.biomedcentral.com/content/pdf/1472-6963-8-278.pdf

Eden, J., Wheatley, B., McNeil, B., & Sox, H. (2008). *Knowing what works in health care: A roadmap for the National Committee on Reviewing Evidence to Identify Highly Effective Clinical Services*. Washington, DC: National Academies Press. Retrieved from http://www.nap.edu/catalog.php?record_id=12038.

Fink, H. A., Taylor, B. C., Tacklind, J. W., Rutks, I. R., & Wilt, T. J. (2008). Treatment intervention in nursing home residents with urinary incontinence: A systematic review of randomized trials. *Mayo Clinic Proceedings, 83*(12), 1332–1343.

Higgins, J. P. T. & Green, S. (Eds.). (2011). *Cochrane handbook for systematic reviews of interventions* (Version 5.1.0). The Cochrane Collaboration. Retrieved from http://www.cochrane-handbook.org

Institute of Medicine. (2011). *Finding what works in health care: Standards for systematic reviews*. Retrieved from http://www.iom.edu/Reports/2011/Finding-What-Works-in-Health-Care-Standards-for-Systematic-Reviews/Standards.aspx

Joanna Briggs Institute. (2011). *Reviewers' manual*. Adelaide, South Australia: Author. Retrieved from http://www.joannabriggs.edu.au/Documents/JBI-Reviewers%20Manual-2011%20HR.pdf

O'Keefe-McCarthy, S. (2008). Women's experiences of cardiac pain: A review of the literature. *Canadian Journal of Cardiovascular Nursing, 18*(3), 18–25.

Valido, T., Wilkes, L., Carter, B., & Jackson, D. (2010). Mothering disrupted by illness: A narrative synthesis of qualitative research. *Journal of Advanced Nursing, 66*(7), 1435–1445.

CHAPTER TEN

Evidence-Based Clinical Practice Guidelines

Earlier research findings were described as raw products that must be transformed into applied products that can be used in practice. Extending that metaphor, research findings are often summarized as conclusions of a systematic review (SR), then those conclusions in turn are used as the basis for the recommendations of an evidence-based clinical practice guideline (EbCPG). EbCPGs are generic in that they are not designed for a particular agency; rather, they are offered as guidelines for care in a variety of agency settings.

Forerunners to Clinical Protocols

Actually, clinical practice guidelines are not quite the end product. Rather, clinical practice guidelines usually undergo a final transformation when they are translated into practice standards for a particular agency or health system. These agency-endorsed standards are often called clinical protocols because they serve as guides for clinicians regarding the care they should give to patients in their care. Thus EbCPGs, like SRs, are an intermediate step on the road from individual studies to evidence-based practice. To an agency developing a clinical protocol, the advantages of working with an EbCPG rather than a systematic review are that it saves time and usually brings greater expertise to the formulation of recommendations. Clinical protocols will be discussed at length in the next part of the book.

EbCPGs, if translated into agency protocols and integrated into practice, have the potential to:

1. Reduce undesirable variation in practice.
2. Increase the use of clinical actions that are effective.
3. Reduce the use of actions that are of minimal value.
4. Target actions to the population most likely to benefit from them.

Having made a distinction between clinical practice guidelines and clinical protocols, it must be acknowledged that some agencies and healthcare systems refer to protocols specific to their agency as clinical guidelines. However, for the purpose of clarity in this book, the term *clinical practice guideline* is used to refer to a set of *generic* recommendations, whereas clinical practice protocol, or more simply clinical protocol, refers to standards for care endorsed by a healthcare-providing agency. The various forms of clinical protocols are discussed later; for now I will just refer to them as *clinical protocols*.

There is another bit of confusion arising from the fact that any government agency, professional association, or health system can produce clinical practice guidelines using whatever process and standards it wishes. Increasingly, the standard in all healthcare professions is that clinical

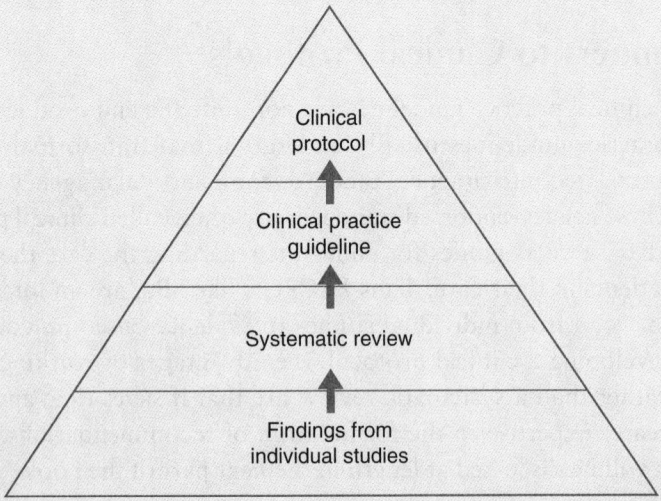

Figure 10-1 Knowledge Transformations

practice guidelines be research based to the extent possible. In this chapter, I use the abbreviation *EbCPG* to make it clear that the guidelines to which I refer are based on research evidence complemented by expert opinion when necessary.

Many guideline developers recognize expert opinion as evidence—albeit a low level of evidence—because it is subjective. It is much like the testimony of a reliable eyewitness of an event—better than no witness but not as strong as physical evidence. The fact that expert opinion is the opinion of the whole guideline development panel, not just one individual, adds to its credibility.

EbCPG Production Process

Multidisciplinary groups and professional associations in many countries provide manuals regarding the development of clinical practice guidelines (AGREE Collaboration, 2010; Institute of Medicine, 2011; Registered Nurses' Association of Ontario, 2006; Scottish Intercollegiate Guidelines Network (SIGN), 2010). Perhaps a good place to start in getting a sense for how high-quality, trustworthy EbCPGs are produced is with SIGN's description of its methodology:

> SIGN guidelines are developed using an explicit methodology based on three core principles:
>
> - Development is carried out by multidisciplinary groups
> - A systematic review is conducted to identify and critically appraise the evidence
> - Recommendations are explicitly linked to the supporting evidence (Scottish Intercollegiate Guidelines Network, 2008)

These principles capture in broad brushstrokes most of the standards put forth by other groups, and thus they can serve as the structure for a description of EbCPGs.

Panel Composition and Expertise

The government organization or professional association commissioning the development of a guideline typically provides specific goals for the development panel and decides on the composition of the development panel. Some groups such as SIGN design for an international audience, whereas others develop the guideline for a national audience or a discipline-specific audience. The important point is that all stakeholders, that is, those who will be affected by the EbCPG, should be represented on the development panel. Members are also chosen to ensure that the needed expertise is at the table. That would include the following:

- Clinical expertise in the various issues the guideline will address
- Research expertise to help appraise study quality and interpret the study results
- Evidence-based practice expertise to ensure sound transfer of knowledge from science to clinical recommendations
- Information search and retrieval expertise to help locate research evidence
- Group process expertise to facilitate the development process, group dynamics, and consensus decision making

Strength of the Body of Evidence

The development panel starts by identifying existing systematic reviews or conducting one or more systematic reviews themselves. The SRs serve as the basis for the recommendations included in the EbCPG. If the panel does their own SR, it should meet the standards set forth earlier in Chapter 9. In either case, the panel then makes a judgment about the strength of the body of evidence related to each of the recommendations it is considering making.

In the recent past, systems for rating the strength of evidence on which a recommendation was based considered only the type of design used. These systems, which were developed with evidence related to intervention or treatment effectiveness in mind, were hierarchical and conveyed graphically as pyramids with five to eight levels. A meta-analysis or systematic review of randomized controlled trials was considered the highest/best form of evidence; nonexperimental/observational studies were ranked at a lower level; and expert opinion was classified as the weakest form of evidence. Scores, alphabetical or numerical, were assigned to each level; the scoring readily conveyed the kinds of study designs that comprised the evidence. There are numerous such evidence ranking systems still in use.

Currently, there is recognition that design is not the only issue that needs to be considered when evaluating a body of evidence. Many other considerations should go into the evaluation (Australian Government National Health and Medical Research Council, 2009; IOM, 2011; Owens et al.,

2009). These other considerations are listed in **Box 10–1**; most are self-explanatory, but several need explanation. The overall quality of the studies means the extent to which the studies were soundly conducted, in particular free of bias and conclusion error. A precise estimate of treatment effect in the population consists of a sample statistic (e.g., difference in means or relative risk) with narrow confidence intervals around it, which usually results by having a large sample or by combining data from several studies. See **Box 10–2** for an example of a precise population estimate.

BOX 10–1 Strength of a Body of Evidence

- **Are the studies of the best design type for the issue being considered?**
- **The quality (risk of bias) of the studies and/or SRs**
- **The consistency of the findings across studies**
- **The number of studies**
- **Were enough patients studied to be confident in the findings?**
- **If an intervention, was the size of the estimated benefit in the population reasonably precise?**
- **Directness to health outcomes**

BOX 10–2 Example of Precise Population Estimate

In a systematic research review of interventions for preventing falls in older people living in the community (Gillespie et al., 2009), it was reported that pooled data from 14 studies of group exercise involving several types of exercise showed a reduction in the rate of falls. The relative risk (RR) was 0.78, 95% CI = 0.71 to 0.82. This result means that the fall risk of those in the 14 exercise groups was 78% that of those in the 14 usual activity groups; although in the population, persons who exercise would have 71% to 82% of the risk of those who do not exercise. (If the RR were 1, the risk of the two groups would be equal; a RR value less than 1 indicates lower risk and a value higher than 1 indicates greater risk.) This confidence interval is narrow (11% points), thus it provides the clinician-reader with a fairly precise estimate of the risk reduction that might be expected from exercise programs in the population.

A strength-of-evidence-grading system that incorporates several of the considerations is shown in **Box 10–3**; it would work well when evaluating a body of evidence related to an intervention. A simpler system that relies more on an overall judgment about the body of evidence rather than on conveying the details of the evidence is shown in **Box 10–4**. This scale has the advantage of being concise and yet conveying the strength of the evidence overall.

BOX 10–3 Evidence Grading

Scheme for Grading the Strength and Consistency of Evidence in the Guideline

A1 = Evidence from well-designed meta-analysis or well-done systematic review with results that consistently support a specific action (e.g., assessment, intervention, or treatment)

A2 = Evidence from one or more randomized controlled trials with consistent results

B1 = Evidence from high-quality evidence-based practice guideline

B2 = Evidence from one or more quasi-experimental studies with consistent results

C1 = Evidence from observational studies with consistent results (e.g., correlational, descriptive studies)

C2 = Evidence from observational studies or controlled trials with inconsistent results

D = Evidence from expert opinion, multiple case reports, or national consensus reports

Source: Courtesy of Research Translation & Dissemination Core. University of Iowa College of Nursing (NIH Grants P30NR03979, PI. Toni Tripp-Reimer). Used with permission.

BOX 10–4 Strength of a Body of Evidence Scale

High ↑ ↑ ↑

There are consistent results from good-quality studies. Further research is very unlikely to change the conclusions.

Moderate ↑ ↑

Findings are supported, but further research could change the conclusions.

Low ↘

There are very few studies, or existing studies are flawed.

Insufficient ○

Research is either unavailable or does not permit estimation of a treatment effect.

Source: AHRQ: Owens et al., 2010.

Clearly, there is no standardized way of representing the supporting evidence for the recommendations in a clinical practice guideline. Neither is there a uniform standard for determining how strong the evidence should be to make a recommendation—although work is underway to produce some degree of standardization regarding these issues (IOM, 2011).

Grading the Recommendations

In addition to rating the quality of the evidence, guideline developers should also grade the recommendations provided in the guideline.

> "When CPG developers are confident that the beneficial effects of a recommendation outweigh the harms, a strong recommendation can be made. A strong recommendation commonly depends on high-or moderate-quality and consistent evidence regarding patient outcomes" (IOM, 2011, p. 113).

The considerations that go into having confidence that the recommendation will produce desired patient outcomes without undue risk of harm are numerous (IOM, 2011). They are listed in **Box 10–5**. Again, there is no agreement about exactly how this should be done, and quite a few different systems are in use. The system shown in **Box 10–6** is used by the Oncology Nursing Society for their Putting Evidence Into Practice guidelines.

BOX 10–5 Grading of Recommendations Considerations

- The strength of the supporting evidence.
- The size of the benefit likely to be achieved by the recommendation, i.e., it is clinically significant.
- The balance of benefits and the risk of harm.
- Whether patients value the outcomes likely to be achieved and/or support the actions and trade-offs involved.
- It is clear to whom the recommendation would apply.

BOX 10–6 Strength of Recommendation Grading

Recommended for Practice. Interventions for which effectiveness has been demonstrated by strong evidence from rigorously designed studies, meta-analyses, or systematic reviews, and for which expectation of harm is small compared to the benefits.

Likely to be Effective. Interventions for which effectiveness has been demonstrated from a single, rigorously conducted controlled trial, consistent supportive evidence from well-designed controlled trials using small samples or guidelines developed from evidence and supported by expert opinion.

Benefits Balanced With Harm. Interventions for which clinicians and patients should weigh the beneficial and harmful effects according to individual circumstances and priorities.

Effectiveness Not Established. Interventions for which insufficient or conflicting data or data of inadequate quality currently exist, with no clear indication of harm.

Effectiveness Unlikely. Interventions for which lack of effectiveness has been demonstrated by negative evidence from a single rigorously conducted controlled trial, consistent negative evidence from well-designed controlled trials using small samples, or guidelines developed from evidence and supported by expert opinion.

Not Recommended for Practice. Interventions for which lack of effectiveness or harmfulness has been demonstrated by strong evidence from rigorously conducted studies, meta-analyses, or systematic reviews, or interventions where the costs, burden, or harm associated with the intervention exceed anticipated benefit.

Source: Oncology Nursing Society, 2012.

Formats

Many guidelines are quite long. There are several reasons for this, including the following:

1. The broad nature of a guideline's purpose.
2. The inclusion in the guideline of details about the research evidence.
3. Inclusion of a description of the guideline production process.
4. Recommendations for practice, education, and organizations.

The presentation of the details about the supporting evidence and discussion of the body of evidence is usually displayed in a separate document; this is done to keep the guideline document itself of reasonable length. However, sometimes supporting studies and SRs are indicated in the guideline document. An example of this format is shown in **Box 10–7**.

BOX 10–7 Recommendations with Grades and Supporting References

In a guideline on acute confusion/delirium in the elderly, the following recommendations were among those offered regarding assessment. The grades indicated are based on the grading system in Box 10–3.

- **Nurses should maintain a high index of suspicion for delirium in the older adult, specifically for those with more predisposing factors that increase risk for delirium (Inouye et al., 1993; Registered Nurses Association of Ontario [RNAO], 2003. Evidence Grade = B1).**
- **Nurses must recognize that delirium may be superimposed on dementia and differentiate baseline from more acute changes in cognitive function (Fick & Foreman, 2000; Fick, Agostini, & Inouye, 2002; RNAO, 2003; Royal College of Physicians, 2006. Evidence Grade = A1).**
- **Assessment for predisposing/vulnerability factors for delirium should occur on hospital admission and are the most powerful factors for identifying patients at greatest risk for developing delirium (Inouye & Charpentier, 1996; Inouye et al., 1993; Pompei et al., 1994; Schor et al., 1992; Williams-Russo et al., 1992. Evidence Grade = C1).**

Source: University of Iowa Gerontological Nursing Interventions Research Center, Research Translation and Dissemination Core (Sendelbach & Guthrie, 2009).

Although there is no standardized format for EbCPGs, the one that follows is typical:

I. Title
II. Producing agency (date)
III. Table of contents
IV. Copyright statement
V. Background context
VI. Purpose and scope
VII. Practice recommendations
VIII. Levels of evidence
IX. Definitions
X. Discussion of evidence
XI. Evidence tables
XII. Production process
XIII. Plans for updating
XIV. Implementation strategies
XV. References

To make guidelines more convenient and usable for clinicians, some EbCPG producers issue a quick-reference guide separate from the full version of the guideline. Quick-reference guides typically list the recommendations and indicate a level of support for each recommendation. Notably, neither the production process nor details of the research evidence is presented in these shortened guides but is available elsewhere from the producer. The Joanna Briggs Institute produces two- to six-page *Best Practice Sheets*, which are designed for clinicians; some are free to nonsubscribers. Recently, the Registered Nurses' Association of Ontario (2010) began making available abbreviated versions of its guidelines for personal digital assistants (PDAs).

In light of the fact that organizations and associations around the world are producing EbCPGs, it is becoming more common for several guidelines to exist about the same topic. In responses to this, several organizations have begun to produce syntheses of several guidelines. These syntheses lay out areas of agreement and difference and compare the recommendations. I suggest you look at the guideline synthesis about prevention of venous thromboembolism (VTE) following total hip and knee replacement at the U.S.

National Guideline Clearinghouse (http://www.guideline.gov/syntheses/synthesis.aspx?id=16473). This synthesis compares three guidelines on the topic. Unfortunately, few syntheses of nursing-specific guidelines have been produced, although in the guideline development process, many nursing guideline developers do incorporate earlier guidelines on the topic or on a subtopic.

Comorbidity

Recently, attention has been given to the reality that most guidelines address a single condition whereas real-world patients often have several conditions (Boyd & Fortin, 2010). Few guidelines take into account that many patients have several conditions (comorbidity) that could limit the applicability of a particular guideline to their care. An attempt to apply several guidelines to the care of a person with several conditions could result in the clinician being confronted by conflicting recommendations (IOM, 2011). Ultimately, addressing this dilemma will require changes in how research is conducted, how guidelines are developed, and the ability of the healthcare systems to support patient-centered care.

Exemplar

Reading Tips

The version of the EbCPG you are about to read is a reduction of the full guideline. The reprinted sections introduce the guideline, the full set of recommendations, and the evidence relative to exercise and lifestyle modification. Large sections about psychological therapies, self-help, alternative therapies, and herbal therapies are not included in the reprint.

To truly get a sense for this guideline, it is best to establish a link to the SIGN methodology website (http://www.sign.ac.uk/guidelines/fulltext/50/index.html) so you can refer to it as suggested in the guideline and in my commentary.

The abbreviation *CBT* stands for cognitive behavioral therapy, and the ☑ symbol indicates a Good Practice Point, which is a non–research-based recommendation based on the clinical experience of the guideline development panel.

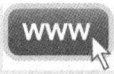

Non-pharmaceutical Management of Depression in Adults: A National Clinical Guideline

SCOTTISH INTERCOLLEGIATE GUIDELINES NETWORK (2010).
RETRIEVED FROM HTTP://WWW.SIGN.AC.UK/PDF/SIGN114.PDF

KEY TO EVIDENCE STATEMENTS AND GRADES OF RECOMMENDATIONS

LEVELS OF EVIDENCE

1^{++}	High quality meta-analyses, systematic reviews of RCTs, or RCTs with a very low risk of bias
1^{+}	Well conducted meta-analyses, systematic reviews, or RCTs with a low risk of bias
1^{-}	Meta-analyses, systematic reviews, or RCTs with a high risk of bias
2^{++}	High quality systematic reviews of case control or cohort studies High quality case control or cohort studies with a very low risk of confounding or bias and a high probability that the relationship is causal
2+	Well conducted case control or cohort studies with a low risk of confounding or bias and a moderate probability that the relationship is causal
2–	Case control or cohort studies with a high risk of confounding or bias and a significant risk that the relationship is not causal
3	Non-analytic studies, e.g., case reports, case series
4	Expert opinion

GRADES OF RECOMMENDATION

Note: The grade of recommendation relates to the strength of the evidence on which the recommendation is based. It does not reflect the clinical importance of the recommendation.

A	At least one meta-analysis, systematic review, or RCT rated as 1^{++}, and directly applicable to the target population; *or* A body of evidence consisting principally of studies rated as 1^{+}, directly applicable to the target population, and demonstrating overall consistency of results
B	A body of evidence including studies rated as 2^{++}, directly applicable to the target population, and demonstrating overall consistency of results; *or* Extrapolated evidence from studies rated as 1^{++} or 1^{+}

C A body of evidence including studies rated as 2^{+}, directly applicable to the target population and demonstrating overall consistency of results; *or*

Extrapolated evidence from studies rated as 2^{++}

D Evidence level 3 or 4; *or*

Extrapolated evidence from studies rated as 2^{+}

GOOD PRACTICE POINTS

☑ Recommended best practice based on the clinical experience of the guideline development group.

* * *

NHS Quality Improvement Scotland (NHS QIS) is committed to equality and diversity and assesses all its publications for likely impact on the six equality groups defined by age, disability, gender, race, religion/belief and sexual orientation.

SIGN guidelines are produced using a standard methodology that has been **equality impact assessed** to ensure that these equality aims are addressed in every guideline. This methodology is set out in the current version of SIGN 50, our guideline manual, which can be found at **www.sign.ac.uk/guidelines/fulltext/50/index.html** The EQIA assessment of the manual can be seen at **www.sign.ac.uk/pdf/sign50eqia.pdf** The full report in paper form and/or alternative format is available on request from the NHS QIS Equality and Diversity Officer.

Every care is taken to ensure that this publication is correct in every detail at the time of publication. However, in the event of errors or omissions corrections will be published in the web version of this document, which is the definitive version at all times. This version can be found on our web site **www.sign.ac.uk**

Contents

1 Introduction 1
1.1 Background 1
1.2 The need for a guideline 1
1.3 Remit of the guideline. 1
1.4 Defining the patient group 2
1.5 Outcomes 3
1.6 Target audience 3
1.7 Statement of intent. 3
2 Summary of recommendations 4
2.1 Psychological therapies. 4
2.2 Self help 4
2.3 Structured exercise 4

3 Psychological therapies . . . 5
3.1 Introduction . . . 5
3.2 Behavioural activation . . . 5
3.3 Cognitive behavioural therapy . . . 5
3.4 Counselling . . . 6
3.5 Couple-focused therapy . . . 6
3.6 Family therapy . . . 6
3.7 Hypnotherapy . . . 6
3.8 Interpersonal therapy . . . 7
3.9 Mindfulness based cognitive therapy . . . 7
3.10 Music therapy . . . 7
3.11 Problem solving therapy . . . 8
3.12 Psychodynamic psychotherapy . . . 8
3.13 Reminiscence therapy . . . 8
3.14 Other psychological therapies . . . 8
3.15 Common factors in psychological therapies . . . 8
4 Self help . . . 9
4.1 Self help support groups . . . 9
4.2 Guided self help . . . 9
4.3 Computerised self help . . . 9
5 Exercise and lifestyle modification . . . 10
5.1 Exercise . . . 10
5.2 Lifestyle modification . . . 11
6 Herbal remedies and nutritional supplements . . . 12
6.1 Introduction . . . 12
6.2 Folate . . . 12
6.3 *Hypericum* extract (St John's wort) . . . 12
6.4 Inositol . . . 13
6.5 Polyunsaturated fatty acids . . . 13
6.6 S-adenosyl-L-methionine . . . 13
6.7 Other nutritional supplements and herbal remedies . . . 13
7 Complementary and alternative therapies . . . 14
7.1 Acupuncture . . . 14
7.2 Animal assisted therapy . . . 14
7.3 Homeopathy . . . 14
7.4 Light therapy . . . 14
7.5 Massage therapy . . . 14
7.6 Yoga . . . 14
7.7 Other complementary and alternative therapies . . . 15

8 Provision of information 16
8.1 Checklist for provision of information 16
8.2 Sources of further information 17
9 Implementing the guideline 20
9.1 Resource implications of key recommendations 20
9.2 Auditing current practice 20
9.3 Advice to NHS Scotland from NHS Quality Improvement Scotland . . . 20
10 The evidence base 21
10.1 Systematic literature review 21
10.2 Recommendations for research 21
10.3 Review and updating 21
11 Development of the guideline 22
11.1 Introduction 22
11.2 The guideline development group 22
11.3 Consultation and peer review 23
11.4 Acknowledgements 25
Abbreviations 26
Annexes 27
References 35

1 Introduction

1.1 Background

Depression is a significant health problem. It affects men and women of all ages and social backgrounds. Around one in five of the population of Scotland will experience depression at some point in their lives.[1] Prevalence is higher in women than men.[1] It can range in severity from a mild disturbance to a severe illness with a high risk of suicide. The impact of the disorder will also be experienced by family, friends and colleagues.[2] In Scotland in 2006/07 there were around 500,000 general practitioner consultations with depression and other affective disorders.[3] Over half of those with depression do not seek formal treatment.[4]

As well as the personal and social consequences of depression there are also negative economic effects. Depression is associated with sickness absence and prevents many people seeking, maintaining or returning to employment. In an economic analysis the total loss of output due to depression and chronic anxiety in England in 2002/3 was estimated at £12 billion.[5]

The most common intervention for depression is prescribed antidepressant medication. A total of 3.65 million items of antidepressant medication were prescribed in Scotland during 2006/07 at a cost of £43.7m. It is estimated that 8.8% of the Scottish population aged 15 and over make daily use of antidepressant medication.[6]

1.2 The Need for a Guideline

Depression Alliance Scotland proposed the development of this guideline based on feedback from service users who were seeking information about interventions, other than prescribed antidepressants, which could be helpful in treating depression. This highlighted the need for accessible and robust information about the alternatives to prescribed antidepressants to be available to both GPs and service users.

The Scottish Integrated Care Pathway (ICP) for depression sets standards for appropriate care and treatment of people with depression. This includes a standard that requires an offer of matched self help and signposting to other services. It also states that for those who choose a non-pharmacological approach, or for whom medication is not effective, there should be the offer of a brief depression-focused psychological intervention.[7]

A small qualitative primary care study (n = 60) of patients with depression found that almost two thirds had attempted to use self chosen therapies, although few had discussed their use with health practitioners. A broad range of therapies was identified. The most commonly reported were St John's wort, counselling, relaxation tapes and gym, walking or other leisure interests.[8]

1.3 Remit of the Guideline

The focus of the guideline is to examine the evidence for depression treatments which may be used as alternatives to prescribed pharmacological therapies. Interventions were prioritised for inclusion by the guideline development group if they were known to be delivered, or be under consideration for delivery, by NHS services in Scotland or if, based on the experience of group members, they were interventions which patients asked about or sought outside of the health service.

Depression is often a multifactorial illness with biological, social and psychological factors all contributing to the development, severity and length of a depressive episode. During a period of depression, people typically report symptoms in all three domains: at a biological level, e.g., sleep disruption, appetite changes; at a psychological level, e.g., impaired concentration and memory, increased negative thinking; and at a social level, e.g., loss of self confidence, withdrawal from social contact. Recovery in one of these domains may be reflected in concurrent improvement in the others; thus the interventions for depression examined in this guideline are wide ranging, covering both biological and psychosocial modes.

This guideline examines psychological therapies, exercise and lifestyle interventions, and complementary and alternative treatments, many of which are not routinely available within the NHS. This guideline provides an assessment of, and presents the evidence base for, the efficacy of these interventions for depression in adults aged 18 years and over. Therapies commonly available to patients without prescription in Scotland were selected for inclusion and are described in Annex 1. The key questions on which the guideline is based are outlined in Annex 2.

This guideline focuses on systematic review and randomised controlled trial (RCT) evidence of effectiveness, with searches extended to identify observational studies only where appropriate.

Unless otherwise stated, recommendations apply to adults aged 18 years and over with no upper age limit.

Depression in children and young people is a significant issue but is beyond the scope of this guideline development project.

1.4 Defining the Patient Group

The evidence base for depression presents several difficulties including the wide range of diagnostic and severity definitions and the heterogeneity and lack of equivalence between measures. The guideline development group adopted a pragmatic definition of depression. Given the nature of the treatment approaches studied, study populations tended to be patients with mild to moderate depression. Many studies either do not make clear the severity of depression studied and/or use diagnostic systems that do not include severity descriptors.

Studies were excluded where there was no formal diagnosis by International Classification of Disease (ICD) 9, ICD 10, Diagnostic Statistical Manual (DSM)-III or DSM-IV, or use of a recognised, validated and reliable measurement scale specifically for depressive symptoms.

Studies in patient groups with clear indicators of severe depression or with significant psychological comorbidities were excluded as below:

- psychotic depression
- depression in the perinatal period (which includes postnatal depression)
- bipolar disorder
- personality disorder
- dysthymia
- seasonal affective disorder
- primary addiction
- significant cognitive impairment (brain injury or dementia)
- learning disability.

Studies in patients with significant physical comorbidities were also excluded.

A large number of studies of depression had mixed patient groups, typically with anxiety disorders and personality disorders. Individual studies were excluded unless there was clear analysis of the depression subgroup. Where recommendations were based on systematic reviews which included studies with mixed patient groups this was taken into account when grading recommendations.

The guideline development group recognised the limitations of adopting such specific diagnostic criteria in terms of applicability to routine care populations, but required a clear remit to assure rigour in study selection and analysis.

1.5 Outcomes

The primary outcome of interest was reduction in depressive symptoms as measured by a recognised depression scale. Short term outcomes and longer term benefits were examined.

Where appropriate, secondary outcomes including illness duration, relapse, quality of life, and patient satisfaction were considered.

1.6 Target Audience

This guideline will be of particular interest to those developing mental health services, healthcare professionals in primary and secondary care, and patients with depression and their carers. It may also be helpful to voluntary organisations and exercise professionals working in exercise referral schemes, public or private fitness centres, and promotion of physical activity.

1.7 Statement of Intent

This guideline is not intended to be construed or to serve as a standard of care. Standards of care are determined on the basis of all clinical data available for an individual case and are subject to change as scientific knowledge and technology advance and patterns of care evolve. Adherence to guideline recommendations will not ensure a successful outcome in every case, nor should they be construed as including all proper methods of care or excluding other acceptable methods of care aimed at the same results. The ultimate judgement must be made by the appropriate healthcare professional(s) responsible for clinical decisions regarding a particular clinical procedure or treatment plan. This judgement should only be arrived at following discussion of the options with the patient, covering the diagnostic and treatment choices available. It is advised, however, that significant departures from the national guideline or any local guidelines derived from it should be fully documented in the patient's case notes at the time the relevant decision is taken.

1.7.1 Patient Version

A patient version of this guideline is available from the SIGN website, www.sign.ac.uk

2 Summary of Recommendations

2.1 Psychological Therapies

A Behavioural activation is recommended as a treatment option for patients with depression.

A Individual CBT is recommended as a treatment option for patients with depression.

A Interpersonal therapy is recommended as a treatment option for patients with depression.

B Mindfulness based cognitive therapy in a group setting may be considered as a treatment option to reduce relapse in patients with depression who have had three or more episodes.

B Problem solving therapy may be considered as a treatment option for patients with depression.

B Short term psychodynamic psychotherapy may be considered as a treatment option for patients with depression.

2.2 Self Help

A Guided self help based on CBT or behavioural principles is recommended as a treatment option for patients with depression.

A Within the context of guided self help, computerised CBT is recommended as a treatment option for patients with depression.

2.3 Structured Exercise

B Structured exercise may be considered as a treatment option for patients with depression.

5 Exercise and Lifestyle Modification

5.1 Exercise

Studies described relate to structured exercise interventions (*see Annex 1*).

The effects of both aerobic exercise (e.g., walking and jogging) and anaerobic exercise (e.g., weight training) have been examined in younger and older adults with depression, with a large variety of intervention types delivered across a range of settings.[45-58] There is a larger evidence base for aerobic exercise than for anaerobic exercise. Limitations of the evidence base include small sample sizes in many studies and the use of volunteer subjects who may be particularly motivated to adhere to an exercise programme.

A Cochrane meta-analysis of 23 trials from 1979–2007 (n = 907) found a large and statistically significant clinical effect of exercise (measured post-treatment) when compared to no treatment or control intervention. The effect was moderate when the five trials with long term follow up were analysed separately. Only three trials in the Cochrane review were assessed as high quality with respect to allocation concealment, intention to treat analysis and blinded outcome assessment. A meta-analysis of these trials (n = 216) found a moderate clinical benefit which was not statistically significant (standardised mean difference –0.42 (95% CI -0.88, 0.03).[59]	1++
Those trials which systematically reported adverse events found that adverse events were low in both the exercise and control groups. There was between 55% and 100% completion of exercise interventions.[59]	1++
In comparisons of effectiveness with antidepressant medication and CBT there was no difference between exercise and the established interventions.[59]	1++
The benefits of exercise have generally been shown to be independent of social group effect.[50-54]	1+
A small number of studies were identified which examined the duration, frequency and intensity of physical activity required to produce benefit.	1+
The results of one study support the following minimum requirements: three sessions per week; of 30-40 minutes duration each; and a total energy expenditure of 17 kcal/kg per week. Similar effects were also found for five sessions per week of 30 minutes at a lower intensity with similar total energy expenditure.[50,60] Other studies suggest a required intensity of exercise correlated to energy expenditure of 70-80% of heart rate reserve (*see Annex 1*).[45-47,49,56,61]	1++

B Structured exercise may be considered as a treatment option for patients with depression.

- ☑ Individuals who are interested in using structured exercise as a treatment intervention for depression should be referred to appropriate exercise counselling and activities in their local community that are relevant to the type of exercise they feel they will enjoy. This may include a range of community provision e.g., local gyms, swimming pools, and voluntary walking groups. If there are doubts about the individual's physical health they should be referred back to the GP for health/cardiovascular assessment.
- ☑ The physical activity readiness questionnaire (PAR-Q) provides a validated tool to determine whether individuals require screening investigations

ahead of commencing a structured exercise programme. (www.csep.ca /CMFiles/publications/parq/par-q.pdf).

- ☑ Patients should be made aware of factors which may improve and help maintain motivation. For example: setting realistic goals may allow individuals to monitor their progress; exercising with others; and an exercise class or buddy system can increase enjoyment.

Annex 3 outlines resources related to physical activity for health.

5.2 Lifestyle Modification

5.2.1 Reducing Alcohol Consumption

No good quality evidence was identified on the effect of reducing alcohol consumption on depressive symptoms.

Examination of alcohol consumption as a causative factor in depression was outside the scope of the guideline.

Primary care interventions for patients with alcohol dependence, hazardous or harmful drinking are described in SIGN 74.[62]

5.2.2 Reducing Caffeine Intake

No good quality evidence was identified on the effects of reducing caffeine intake on depressive symptoms.

5.2.3 Return to Work

No evidence applicable to the UK employment and benefits systems was identified on the effectiveness of return to work programmes in reducing depressive symptoms.

5.2.4 Good Practice in Lifestyle Advice for Patients with Depression

- ☑ General advice on following a healthy lifestyle is relevant in the management of patients with depression. Advice should address:
  - alcohol and drug use
  - diet and eating behaviours
  - maintenance of social networks and personally meaningful activities
  - sleep problems.

10 The Evidence Base

10.1 Systematic Literature Review

The evidence base for this guideline was synthesised in accordance with SIGN methodology. A systematic review of the literature was carried out using an explicit search strategy devised by a SIGN Information Officer. Databases searched include Medline, Embase, Cinahl, PsycINFO, AMED, and the Cochrane Library. The year range covered was 1998-2008 with variations depending on topic. Internet searches were carried out on various websites including the US National Guidelines Clearinghouse. A complete search narrative, including search strategies and date ranges for each key question, is available on the SIGN website. The main searches were supplemented by material identified by individual members of the development group. Each of the selected papers was evaluated by two members of the group using standard SIGN methodological checklists before conclusions were considered as evidence.

10.2 Recommendations for Research

For many of the interventions described in this guideline there was little or no robust published evidence. This was particularly the case for complementary and alternative therapies, nutritional therapies, alcohol reduction and self help groups. In addition to a lack of primary studies on such interventions a number of wider research themes were identified:

- validity of trial designs for psychological therapies
- dose-response studies for effective psychological therapies
- factors which contribute to drop-out
- non-specific treatment factors including patient/therapist interaction
- patient selection for psychological therapies
- long term effectiveness of non-pharmaceutical interventions
- contribution of unstructured exercise to beneficial effects on mood
- optimum type of exercise (aerobic, mixed or strength)
- how exercise programmes can best be facilitated through primary care.

10.3 Review and Updating

This guideline was issued in 2010 and will be considered for review in three years. Any updates to the guideline in the interim period will be noted on the SIGN website: www.sign.ac.uk.

Annex 1: Definitions of Interventions

Section 4 Self help	
Computerised self help	Online or computer based packages of self help material.
Guided self help	Self help interventions which incorporate some form of therapist support.
Self help interventions	Self help interventions cover a range of interactive packages, paper or web-based written self help materials. Interventions supporting access to self help books may be termed bibliotherapy or books on prescription.

Section 5 Exercise and lifestyle interventions

Exercise	Exercise is a subset of physical activity, which is any movement of the body that results in energy expenditure rising above resting level, and includes activities of daily living, domestic chores, gardening and walking.
Structured exercise	Exercise that is undertaken three or more times a week for 30–40 minutes at an intensity sufficient to provide an energy expenditure of 70–80% of heart rate reserve; this equates to the public health dose of accumulating 30 minutes of moderate intensity physical activity on most days of the week. Walking at a level of moderate intensity, slightly out of breath, most days of the week can achieve the public health dose. Heart rate reserve is a term used to describe the difference between a person's measured or predicted maximum heart rate and resting heart rate. Some methods of measurement of exercise intensity measure percentage of heart rate reserve. As a person increases their cardiovascular fitness, their resting heart rate will drop, thus the heart rate reserve will increase.

Annex 2: Key Questions Used to Develop the Guideline

This guideline is based on a series of structured key questions that, where possible, define the population concerned, the intervention under investigation, the type of comparison group, and the outcomes used to measure the effectiveness of the interventions. These questions form the basis of the systematic literature search.

The Key Questions Used to Develop the Guideline

Delivery of Care/Lifestyle and Self Directed Interventions

Compare with psychological therapies, pharmacological therapies, placebo or waiting list control. Consider short term effects and any longer term benefits.

Key Question	See Guideline Section
1. Do the following lifestyle changes reduce depressive symptoms,and are any reductions in symptoms sustained? • reducing caffeine intake • reducing alcohol consumption • increasing physical activity • return to work	5.2

(continues)

Key Question	See Guideline Section
2. What is the effectiveness of assisted return to work programmes in alleviating depression compared with no assistance? Include: • assisted return to employment/education/ meaningful activity • back-to-work treatment • condition management • recovery-based treatment • rehabilitation • REMPLOY	5.2
3. What is the evidence for the effectiveness of the following on depressive symptoms? • bibliotherapy • self help support groups • guided self help • psychoeducation	4.1, 4.2, 4.3
4. What is the evidence for the effectiveness of exercise (any structured physical activity) alone or in combination with psychological therapies, on depressive symptoms?	5.1

Profile & Commentary

TOPIC

The topic is clearly set forth in the guideline title. The key questions that guided the development of the guideline are set forth in Annex 2. Background information about depression and why there is a need for a guideline on this topic are set forth in Section 1. Although the background statement cites data from Scotland and England, there is no reason why the evidence used is not applicable in many other countries. The Contents page gives you a sense for the various nonpharmaceutical therapies considered and the format of the guideline as a whole.

METHODS

The methods used to produce the guideline are a bit difficult to get a handle on because they are not spelled out in the guideline itself. Instead, Section

10.1 says that the SIGN methodology was followed. I suggest you look at the *Guideline Development Handbook*. Chapter 6 ("Systematic Literature Review") and Chapter 7 ("Forming Guideline Recommendations") of the handbook are particularly important to understanding the guideline development process. The databases, websites, and dates used in the search for evidence for this particular guideline are briefly described in Section 10.1 but are spelled out in considerable detail in the file "search narrative," for which there is a link on the guideline's website.

The "Key to Evidence Statement" and "Grades of Recommendations" sections right at the beginning of the guideline links are important. The "Evidence Statements" ranked the various pieces of evidence in terms of type and quality of evidence. However, the discussion of the evidence goes beyond that to also note the consistency of findings, the size of the clinical benefit, and the number of patients in the three high-quality studies. The discussion of the evidence is broken down into subissues, e.g., aerobic versus anaerobic exercise, clinical benefit compared to no treatment, adverse effects, and clinical benefit compared to antidepressant medication.

The grades of recommendations were based mainly on the level of evidence, the consistency of results, and the directness of the evidence to the population of depressed persons. Although not listed in the definitions of the recommendation grades, the discussion of the evidence does indicate that adverse effects of exercise were considered, as was how many patients completed exercise interventions. In short, there is clear linkage between the recommendations and supporting evidence.

In Section 2, "Summary of Recommendations," all the recommendations are set forth. Notice the wording of the recommendations; some say: "is recommended" whereas others say "may be considered." This difference in vigor of the recommendations reflects the confidence in the recommendation resulting from varying strength of the supporting evidence and other considerations.

In Section 5, a summary of the evidence related to exercise is provided. It is 1^{+} or 1^{++} level evidence. (Note that most of the statements about the evidence also have references.) Two major findings of the meta-analysis were that the three high-quality studies of clinical benefit showed that exercise produced only a slightly more modest clinical benefit than no treatment or control treatment, and no additional benefit when compared to other established interventions. The meta-analysis also revealed low levels of adverse events related to exercise. The rather weak evidence related to benefit in combination with the low level of adverse events led the panel to issue a rather tentative recommendation, "Structured exercise may be considered," and three Good Practice Points.

For lifestyle modification (Section 5.2), the research is almost nonexistent. This is extremely unfortunate because these are probably suggestions that are frequently given to patients by healthcare providers. This impression is confirmed by the fact that the reviewers' experience led them to issue a Good Practice Point about alcohol and drug use, diet, maintaining social activities, and sleep problems.

Wrap-Up

Going back and forth between print and online documents makes it somewhat difficult to put the whole picture together. However, most guidelines these days are quite long, ranging from 20 pages to a few hundred pages, so it was not feasible to reprint one in its entirety in this text. Ergo, this reprint is somewhat of a patchwork quilt.

At the other end of the length spectrum, you might want to take a look at the *Quick Reference Guide,* which provides a one-page summary of the main recommendations of this guideline. Also, a *Patient Booklet* is available on the guideline's website.

http://go.jblearning.com/brown3e

References

AGREE Collaboration. (2010). Introduction to AGREE II. Retrieved from http://www.agreetrust.org/about-agree/introduction0/

Australian Government National Health and Medical Research Council. (2009). *HMRC levels of evidence and grades for recommendations for developers of guidelines.* Retrieved from https://www.nhmrc.gov.au/_files_nhmrc/file/guidelines/developers/nhmrc_levels_grades_evidence_120423.pdf

Boyd, C. M., & Fortin, M. (2010). Future of multimorbidity research: How should understanding of multimorbidity inform health system design. *Public Health Review, 32*(2), 451–474. Retrieved from http://www.publichealthreviews.eu/upload/pdf_files/8/PHR_32_2_Boyd.pdf

Institute of Medicine (IOM). (2011). *Clinical practice guidelines we can trust.* Retrieved from http://www.iom.edu/Reports/2011/Clinical-Practice-Guidelines-We-Can-Trust.aspx

Oncology Nursing Society. (2012). *ONS PEP(r)—Putting evidence into practice.* Retrieved from http://www.ons.org/Research/PEP

Owens, D. K., Lohr, K. N., Atkins, D., Treadwell J. R , Reston J. T., Bass, E. B., et al. (2009). Grading the strength of a body of evidence when comparing medical interventions. In Agency for Healthcare Research and Quality, *Methods guide for comparative effectiveness reviews.* Rockville, MD: Agency for Healthcare Research and Quality. Available at http://www.effectivehealthcare.ahrq.gov/index.cfm/search-for-guides-reviews-and-reports/?pageaction=displayproduct&productid=318

Registered Nurses' Association of Ontario. (2006). *BPG development methodology.* Retrieved from http://rnao.ca/bpg/guidelines/methodology

Registered Nurses' Association of Ontario. (2010). *Condensed guidelines for personal digital assistants (PDAs).* Retrieved from http://rnao.ca/bpg/pda

Scottish Intercollegiate Guidelines Network. (2008). *SIGN 50: A guideline developer's handbook.* Retrieved from http://www.sign.ac.uk/guidelines/fulltext/50/index.html

Scottish Intercollegiate Guidelines Network. (2010). *Non-pharmaceutical management of depression in adults: A national clinical guideline.* Retrieved from http://www.sign.ac.uk/guidelines/fulltext/114/index.html

Sendelbach, S., & Guthrie, P. F. (2009). *Acute confusion/delirium.* Iowa City, IA: University of Iowa Gerontological Nursing Interventions Research Center, Research Translation and Dissemination Core. Retrieved from http://www.guideline.gov/content.aspx?id=14340&search=delirium+iowa

PART II

Evidence-Based Practice

11 Asking Clinical Questions

12 Searching for Research Evidence

13 Appraising Research Evidence

14 Appraising Recommendations of Clinical Practice Guidelines

15 Appraising Conclusions of Integrative Research Reviews

16 Appraising Findings of Original Studies

17 Evidence-Based Practice

18 Evidence-Based Practice Participation Scenarios

19 Research-Informed Practice

From Part I, hopefully you have acquired an appreciation of and basic knowledge about the different kinds of research studies that are used to study nursing phenomena and the desirable features of each. You also have basic knowledge about how integrative research reviews are done and how evidence-based clinical practice guidelines are produced. **Figure P2–1** graphically portrays the ground that is covered in the first part of the book. This knowledge is essential to using research evidence in your own nursing practice and to participating in evidence-based practice (EBP) projects in your work setting.

However, research knowledge is not enough; you also need to be able to find research evidence, appraise it, and strategically use it in practice—and that is what this part of the book addresses. To this point, the focus has been on research evidence, and that will continue to be the focus in the remaining chapters, albeit from the consumer of research evidence perspective. In Chapter 17, the lens is opened up and you will learn how research evidence is used in combination with other types of evidence. As a result, evidence-based practice in a broader sense and in a practical context will come into view.

The Evidence-Based Practice Impact Model

The Evidence-Based Practice Impact Model shown in **Figure P2–2** depicts the major steps in achieving effective evidence-based practice. Importantly, each step should be carried out using explicit and

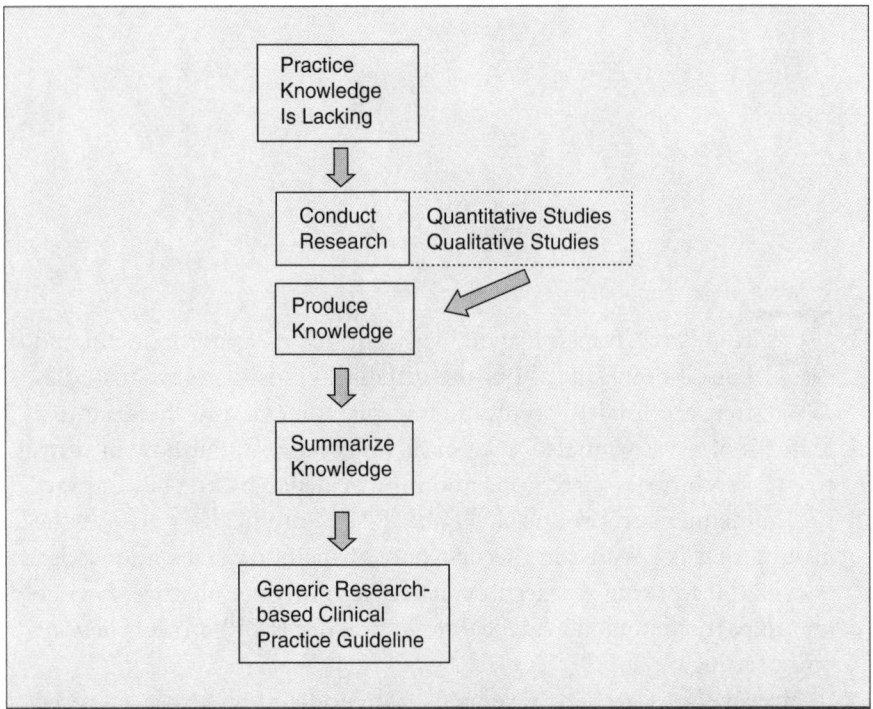

Figure P2-1 Scientific Nursing Knowledge Production

rigorous methods. Discipline in doing so ensures that the agency protocol produced is truly evidence based and that the implementation of the protocol has the desired effect on patient outcomes. To achieve this level of translation of evidence into practice, EBP projects are conducted by units, service lines, or agency teams. The E-B Practice Impact Model portrays how EBP plays out in everyday activities and serves as a map for this part of the book.

In Chapter 19, the individual nurse's use of research evidence, research-informed practice (RIP), is described. The steps individual nurses use to incorporate research evidence into clinical decision making for individual patients and to refine their own methods of practice are similar to those of EBP, albeit performed with less rigor (Eddy, 2005).

Not all writers differentiate between agency evidence-based practice and the individual's use of research evidence, but I think a

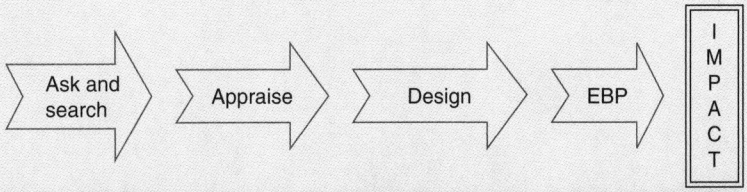

Figure P2-2 EBP Impact Model

distinction is important. A distinction between the two ways of using research evidence retains high standards for translating research evidence into clinical protocols while recognizing the value of individual nurses seeking better information when agency protocols are lacking or are not applicable to a particular patient situation. A distinction also recognizes that EBP is an organizational activity, whereas RIP is the individual professional nurse's responsibility. Maximally effective nursing care requires research utilization at both levels.

The EBP Impact model is similar to several other models that are used as working frameworks for the evidence-based practice programs of healthcare agencies (Rycroft-Malone & Bucknall, 2010). If these more detailed and comprehensive models are of interest to you, see the paper, *Evidence-Based Practice Models,* on the companion website for this book, which can be accessed at **go.jblearning.com/brown.**

References

Eddy, D. M. (2005). Evidence-based medicine: A unified approach. Two approaches to using evidence to solve clinical problems and how to unify them. *Health Affairs, 24*(1), 9–17.

Rycroft-Malone, J., & Bucknall, T. (Eds.). (2010). Models and frameworks for implementing evidence-based practice: Linking evidence to action. Hoboken, NJ: Wiley-Blackwell.

CHAPTER ELEVEN

Asking Clinical Questions

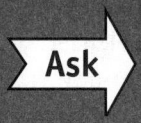

The starting point for a clinical team embarking on a project to develop an evidence-based protocol is to formulate a clinical question in a way that will guide the search for research evidence and keep the project on mission. First, we need to consider how an issue might have risen to the level of the agency deciding to develop a care protocol regarding it. Clinical questions for which research evidence has a high probability of providing answers (or at least partial answers) arise while giving care, are revealed by agency quality-monitoring data, or are brought to the forefront in professional dialogue. Sometimes they arise out of problematic patient care situations, such as a family complaint, an adverse event, or even a lawsuit. In the Iowa Model of Evidence-Based Practice, these initiators are referred to as *triggers* (Titler et al., 2001).

Triggers

Information pointing to a problem with care can come from various places in the agency and trigger an initiative to find more effective approaches. Sources of triggers can be a staff member, quality management monitoring, risk management, financial reports, infection control monitoring, or a discharge planning coordinator. The trigger can also come from outside the agency in the form of new standards of care from a professional association, regulatory agency, or accrediting organization.

Clinical Practice

Care providers who are thoughtful and not robotic while giving care see what, in spite of good intentions, could be done better and find themselves asking questions such as the following:

- What groups of people should we be screening in the emergency department for domestic violence?
- Should I recommend once-a-day vitamin supplements to my elderly patients?
- Should we be using bladder scans to determine urinary residual on all patients who have had an indwelling/Foley catheter removed?
- What nonpharmacologic measures can we use to prevent and treat muscle spasms in persons who have had cervical fusion surgery?
- Is acetaminophen or ibuprofen more effective and safer in treating fever in young children?
- Why do some adolescent girls in poor, urban neighborhoods aspire to good diet, exercise, good grades, and sexual abstinence?
- What factors determine whether middle-aged men working in an industrial plant follow recommendations regarding how to avoid back injury?

These kinds of questions can be answered in part by examining the knowledge produced by research.

Quality Data

All healthcare agencies collect a great deal of information to prove to third-party payors, accrediting agencies, and the public that important aspects of care are being given consistently and that their patients are attaining the appropriate outcomes. For example, for people with an ischemic stroke, a hospital might keep track of the following: mortality, global disability status at discharge, discharge destination, special after-hospital services required, and readmission within 30 days. Based on these outcomes, if a hospital's poststroke patients who were discharged on warfarin had more emergency care visits for bleeding than similar patients discharged from other hospitals, the clinical staff would be obliged to reevaluate their discharge protocol for patients taking anticoagulants. If the current protocol was found to not represent current evidence-based standards of care, an EBP project to design a new protocol might be initiated.

Thus, quality monitoring data often sheds light on a deficiency in care and thereby serves as a trigger for an EBP project. Quality monitoring and its relationship to EBP are discussed more extensively later in Chapter 17.

Professional Standards

When national professional associations and organizations issue evidence-based guidelines, agencies are obligated to take notice and decide if they should change the way they are giving care. Similarly, when licensing and accrediting agencies, such as the Centers for Medicare and Medicaid Services or the Joint Commission set forth new standards of care, agencies have to decide how they will meet them, and this initiates a search for research evidence to help develop a new protocol. This was the case when the Joint Commission and the CMS required inpatient psychiatric settings to report data regarding their use of holding patients in seclusion rooms.

At a less formal level, a staff nurse might see an article or a research report in a clinical journal about a care approach that seems promising. Or she may learn about a new approach in a session at a conference or workshop. After thinking about the matter, she may come to the conclusion that this aspect of care as it is being done in her setting is of dubious effectiveness. Taking the concern and idea to a nurse leader, clinical nurse specialist, or case manager might lead to a search for research evidence about the alternative approach to care.

Questions Not Answerable by Research Evidence

Before looking at how to formulate a focused clinical question for an evidence-based project, it might be helpful to address the issue of the kinds of questions that cannot be answered by research evidence.

One type of question that often cannot be answered with research evidence is a question involving new technology. If studies are available about a new technology, they may have been conducted by the manufacturer and therefore should be appraised carefully. An example would be if scientists were able to produce an external device that senses seizures a minute before they occur; the early users of such a device would most likely have very little research evidence to go on.

Another question for which research evidence may not be available is the application of an existing intervention to a new population. There may be considerable evidence regarding the intervention in the population in which it was developed but none in the population with whom the agency is considering using it. A digital device that teaches people how to correctly use their asthma inhaler may have been tested in adults and found effective but may not have been tested in children. Another example is that a body of research about the use of an intervention with white women may be available but no research about the use of the intervention with women of color. In these situations, the research available is informative but clinical protocols for the new population cannot be truly based on the available evidence.

A third type of question that cannot be definitively answered with research evidence is a question pertaining to the care of an individual patient. The ethical principle is that each competent patient has the right to determine what happens to his or her person and body, and this principle must be respected regardless of what research evidence shows. Questions about what care should be given to an individual must be decided by the patient and his or her care providers (which providers depends on the care issue and the setting). Research evidence can provide useful information to consider in the discussion, but ultimately the decision is the patient's; there are exceptions to this, such as when the patient is not competent to make a decision or when the well-being of others is endangered.

In light of the ethical principle just described, research evidence is also of limited use in questions having to do with values or deciding what is a moral or ethical course of action. The question, "Should we treat pneumonia in nursing home residents older than 90 years of age who have cognitive deficits?" is a moral question. Research may shed some light on the question by providing data regarding the percentage of this population that has an uncomplicated recovery and return to their former functional status when treated with antibiotics, but research cannot answer the question. In fact, the question cannot be answered in general. It must be answered on a case-by-case basis because the answer depends on how cognitively compromised the person was prior to the onset of the pneumonia, whether intubation is a likely possibility, and what the patient's end-of-life wishes were when last expressed—again, the ethical principle of self-determination. These reminders are necessary to assure that research evidence is used for the purposes it inherently serves and not as a means of controlling individual lives.

Forming a Useful Project Question

To keep the project on target and to avoid spending a lot of time searching for and sifting through a large number of citations, it helps to formulate a focused project question—as opposed to a very broad or vague one. One of the previously listed questions asked about doing an ultrasound bladder scan on patients who have an indwelling catheter removed. This is a legitimate question, but it is vague and requires more focus. Let us assume that in the process of developing a postoperative order set for adults after abdominal surgery, a medical–surgical practice council decides to consider the research on this issue.

The council might use an approach that many healthcare providers have found useful in focusing their evidence-based clinical projects; it is referred to by the acronym PICOTS (Sackett, Straus, Richardson, Rosenberg, & Haynes, 2000; Stillwell, 2010). The PICOTS format helps clinicians zero in on specific elements of a question that are of interest.

P Patient population
I Intervention/Issue
C Comparison intervention
O Outcomes
T Timing
S Setting

Generally, when using PICOTS, the patient population can be characterized by attributes such as age, illness experience (e.g., shortness of breath), disease, or risk, to name a few. The intervention of interest can be specified by naming a clinical intervention, a particular approach, or a group of interventions (e.g., school-based programs regarding weight loss). For some questions, the *I* could stand for an issue rather than an intervention; this would be the case if the question was about mobility obstacles associated with foot drop. A comparison of the intervention to another intervention or to usual care may be of interest; alternatively, the effectiveness of just one intervention may be what is under consideration. Patient outcomes are almost always of interest, particularly outcomes that are important to patients, such as improved functional ability or fewer episodes of hypoglycemia. The timing, in terms of clinical status, duration, and frequency of treatment or length of follow-up, may be relevant. Specifying the setting of care can often help focus the question and reduce the number of studies retrieved that are not relevant. Managing urinary incontinence in home care is quite different than managing it in hospital.

Getting back to the council developing a bladder scanning protocol, the PICOTS question would be the following.

In patients who have an indwelling bladder catheter removed after surgery (P) (implies acute care setting S), does bladder scanning (I) after the first voiding (T) identify persons who have a large urine residual (O) and require further monitoring of their urination (O)?

If you were to state this question specifying the population as patients who have had repair of a hip fracture, you probably would not find studies pertaining to it. So, it is possible to get too specific; sometimes some trial and error is required to get the question just right.

A similar question pertains to the use of bladder scanning in patients who have had a catheter in for a long time and who after its removal cannot void. That question would be one of the following:

With patients who have had an indwelling catheter removed after its being place for a minimum of 3 weeks (P), does bladder scanning (I) after 8 hours (T) avoid the need for straight catheterization (O) and reduce urinary tract infections (O)?

What nonpharmacologic measures should nurses use (I) to reduce pain, discomfort, and agitation (Os) with full-term newborn infants (P) before, during, and after venipuncture and insertion of intravenous lines (T)?

In neither question is a comparison intervention suggested. The intervention (nonpharmacologic measures) is somewhat open ended and could result in examining studies comparing the effectiveness. A more focused question would be: "Is oral sucrose pacifier or swaddling more effective (I and C) in controlling pain (O) during and after venipuncture (T) of full-term newborns (P)?" Note that the population specified in all the questions is newborns, so the team looking into this issue would not retrieve or review studies done on premature infants or infants older than 28 days.

Although not every clinical question about an intervention will have every element, it is useful to at least consider each one. Generally, PICOTS works best for questions about intervention effectiveness. Questions regarding patients' experiences, the meaning of illness, relationships among clinical variables, and risk require modification of the PICOTS format.

Nonintervention questions typically seek background information useful in developing assessment guides, teaching protocols, plans of care, or even whole programs. The I then represents *Issue* or *Issues*, instead of

Intervention. An example would be the question used by a project team at a military hospital opening a department to treat soldiers with traumatic brain injury.

In soldiers returning from combat with traumatic brain injury (P), what rehabilitation setting characteristics (Issue and S) promote partner support and renewal of family relationships (Os)?

Sometimes project teams seeking evidence about background issues find it better to have two closely related questions rather than cramming the issues of interest into one question. For instance, a protect team developing a support program for men with urinary incontinence might look at qualitative and descriptive studies about the experience of urinary incontinence and self-management strategies these men find helpful. The project questions could be:

1. **What experiences and self-management issues (I) do men with urinary incontinence (P) find stressful or difficult to manage (Os)?**
2. **What self-management actions and strategies help (I) these men (P) adjust to and cope with urinary incontinence (Os)?**

Together these questions could result in retrieval of research evidence that would be useful in developing a clinical program that is patient centered and evidence based. Both questions have population, issue, and outcome elements but no comparison or time element.

Another example would be a project group developing a care protocol to support chronically ill mothers of young children; the questions guiding the project would be as follows:

1. **When mothers of young children develop a chronic illness that affects physical functioning (P), how is their ability to mother their children affected (O)?**
2. **When mothers of young children become chronically ill (P), how do they and their partners (or immediate family) adjust to the situation (O)?**

This project team was not interested in intervention, rather in understanding how these mothers are affected by the illness and how the family unit adjusts to it.

A focused question pertaining to risk could be formulated as follows:

In home-dwelling older adults who take two or more prescriptions medications (P and S), how prevalent are major drug–drug interactions (O) between prescription medications and over-the-counter drugs or natural remedies? (I)?

Okay, hopefully you get the idea: Make the project as focused as possible by developing a specific question. Consider using the PICOTS elements in the question. If it turns out to be too specific (i.e., you cannot find any studies about it), you can either broaden one of the elements or drop it altogether. Doing so may open it up just enough that relevant studies can be identified.

One last piece of advice: If a project team has difficulty focusing its question, it sometimes helps to have several members spend a half hour muddling around in a database looking at various abstracts and articles about the issue. This muddling may help formulate a more focused question and help identify the terminology that will result in a productive search for studies.

Moving on, assuming the protocol development team has a focused question that is consistent with the agency's commitments and resources, the next step is to conduct a search for research evidence related to that question—next chapter.

http://go.jblearning.com/brown3e

References

Sackett, D. L., Straus, S. E., Richardson, W. S., Rosenberg, W., & Haynes, R. B. (2000). *Evidence-based medicine: How to practice and teach EBM* (2nd ed.). Edinburgh, Scotland: Churchill Livingstone.

Stillwell, S. (2010). Asking the clinical question: A key step in evidence-based practice. *American Journal of Nursing, 110*(3), 58–61.

Titler, M. G., Kleiber, C., Steelman, V. J., Rakel, B. A., Budreau, G., Everett, L. Q., et al. (2001). The Iowa model of evidence-based practice to promote quality care. *Critical Nursing Clinics of North America, 13*(4), 497–509.

CHAPTER TWELVE

Searching for Research Evidence

Ellen F. Hall

In this chapter we will look first at how to locate evidence-based clinical practice guidelines (EbCPGs) and systematic reviews (SRs), covering just those that are widely recognized by clinicians and broadly available. In the second part of this chapter we will consider techniques for finding high-quality research evidence when EbCPGs and SRs are not available for the clinical issue you wish to investigate.

Searching for EbCPGs and SRs

The first step in your search is to have your population and intervention or issue in mind. The second step is to explore the principal sources of EbCPGs and SRs. They save you time because finding, reading, evaluating, and synthesizing research results from original studies have already been completed. However, there are over 12,000 known diseases, most of these with several possible interventions. EbCPGs and SRs do not exist for each of these population–intervention combinations. SRs are most likely to have been developed for those conditions that have a high incidence and a high cost to third-party payers. Consider obesity. According to the Centers for Disease Control and Prevention, 33% of adults in the United States are obese. EbCPGs and SRs are broadly available regarding interventions to help adults lose weight. However, when there is not a substantive body of original studies, there is no basis on which a team can develop an SR. For instance, there is limited research and no SRs for some of the complementary health therapies.

Sources of EbCPGs and SRs

Fortunately there are now a number of organizations producing EbCPGs and SRs on a wide variety of topics. These organizations systematically and consistently apply stringent criteria in their selection and appraisal of evidence; they are your best sources of evidence. There are also organizations that index EbCPGs or SRs and provide abstracts and links to them. What follows is a mix of producers and indexers.

Registered Nurses' Association of Ontario

The Registered Nurses' Association of Ontario (RNAO; www.rnao.ca) sponsors the Nursing Best Practice Guidelines program. To date there are nearly 50 patient care guidelines. Examples of current guidelines include *Establishing Therapeutic Relationships*, *Nursing Management of Hypertension*, *Primary Prevention of Childhood Obesity*, and *Stroke Assessment*.

These excellent guidelines are freely available at the RNAO website by clicking on the Best Practice Guidelines tab, then Guidelines in the left column. The RNAO now also offers condensed guidelines for PDAs.

Joanna Briggs Institute

The Joanna Briggs Institute (JBI; www.joannabriggs.org) is a collaboration of nurses, medical and allied health researchers, clinicians, academics, and quality managers in 40 countries. The JBI promotes evidence-based health care by conducting and disseminating systematic reviews and the evidence-based Best Practice Information Sheets. Its nursing content enables nurses to see which of their practices are supported by evidence. Besides evidence related to nursing practice, it has a special interest as well in systematic reviews of economic, qualitative, and policy research.

To date the JBI offers about 2,300 continuously updated reports in three series.

1. Systematic Reviews provide extensive summaries of the best research on selected clinical topics.
2. Evidence Summaries provide short extracts of research literature on selected clinical topics that are based on structured searches of the

literature and selected evidence-based healthcare databases. They focus on the characteristics of the evidence, the clinical bottom line, and best practice recommendations.

3. Best Practice Information Sheets summarize the findings of systematic reviews of evidence.

Most JBI resources are available only by subscription from OvidSP or Lippincott Nursing Center, so nursing students typically access these resources through their library. If your library does not subscribe to one of these, you may still access JBI's Best Practice Information Sheets at its website. Most JBI resources are now designed for download to mobile devices.

Cochrane Collaboration

The Cochrane Collaboration (http://www.cochrane.org) is an international organization that develops and distributes high-quality systematic reviews of interventions for use by many healthcare professions. Its reviews integrate findings, pool data, and generate overall results. Most of these have been based on randomized controlled trials that investigate the effects of interventions. Increasingly, however, other kinds of study designs are being included in their reviews.

The Cochrane database contains over 7,000 reviews, many with relevance to nursing care. Happily, Cochrane is becoming an even more valuable resource for nursing practice with the 2009 establishment of the Cochrane Nursing Care Field (CNCF) within the collaboration. The CNCF is specifically charged with supporting the conduct, dissemination, and utilization of systematic reviews relevant to nursing. Most importantly, the CNCF identifies priority topics related to nursing that are not currently covered by existing Cochrane reviews. Access to the full text of Cochrane's systematic reviews requires a subscription. Check with your librarian to see if your library subscribes to the Cochrane Collaboration. If your library does not subscribe to Cochrane, you can search for findings directly at its website. This free access will enable you to read abstracts, and often plain-language summaries, of the findings. Cochrane also now makes mobile-optimized versions of its reviews available.

National Guideline Clearinghouse

The National Guideline Clearinghouse (NGC) is principally a database of thousands of clinical practice guidelines, which are provided free at its website (www.guideline.gov). It should be noted that the NGC does not write or appraise guidelines. Nor is there a requirement that the guidelines be evidence based. It is a disseminator of guidelines developed by others. The NCG includes levels of evidence only if they are submitted by the guideline developer. Thus, the quality of guidelines posted on this site varies widely.

The Advanced Search choice on the homepage enables the user to enter a disorder. It will then display options to limit the results in several ways, including the gender and age range of the population group; the intended user group, for example, nurses, dieticians, occupational therapists, physicians, or social workers; and the methodology used to analyze the evidence, for instance, a systematic review. One can also create side-by-side comparisons of several guidelines using the guideline comparison tool. Points of comparison include description of methods used to collect/select evidence; assess quality and strength of evidence; analyze evidence; formulate recommendations; and validate guidelines.

National Institute for Health and Clinical Excellence NICE Guidelines

Similar to the U.S. National Guideline Clearinghouse, the excellent NICE Clinical Guidelines (http://guidance.nice.org.uk/CG/Published) provide access to authoritative clinical evidence and best practice. The NICE is a part of the National Health Service in the United Kingdom.

Nursing Reference Center

The Nursing Reference Center (http://www.ebscohost.com/pointOfCare/nrc-about) is a subscription resource providing nurses with the rigorously reviewed Evidence-based Care Sheets. These are a distillation of current best practice on well over 700 clinical conditions and interventions. Ask your librarian if your institution subscribes to this excellent product.

Database of Abstracts of Reviews of Effects

The Database of Abstracts of Reviews of Effects (DARE; www.crd.york.ac.uk/crdweb) is one of several databases produced by the Centre for Reviews and Dissemination (CRD), an agency within the United Kingdom's National Institute for Health Research. This database of SRs can be used for answering questions about the effects of health and social care interventions. While the search interface offers no feature to efficiently limit the database's 21,000 abstracts of systematic reviews to those addressing nursing practice, over 1,300 of the reviews do mention nurses or nursing. A useful feature of this database is the History link located on the left side of the screen. It records your search activity and it creates sets of abstracts for each of your search statements. These sets can be combined for highly targeted searching. There is no charge for searching this database online.

Centre for Evidence-Based Physiotherapy

The Centre for Evidence-Based Physiotherapy (CEPD; www.pedro.org .au) sponsors the Physiotherapy Evidence Database, also known as PEDro. All trials on PEDro are independently assessed for quality and are of more value to nursing practice than the title at first might suggest. Certainly it is an excellent source of EbCPGs and SRs for use with any of the movement disorders. A surprisingly broad range of other medical conditions is included as well, such as COPD and asthma. The reviews and guidelines are available free online.

Journal Databases and Specialty Nurses' Associations' Websites

CINAHL, Medline, and PubMed can also be used to find systematic reviews and practice guidelines. A fuller introduction to the use of these databases to find systematic reviews and practice guidelines as well as original studies will follow later in this chapter. Although PubMed (www.ncbi.nlm.nih.gov /pubmed/) is available free online, CINAHL and Medline are available only by subscription. CINAHL is the most broadly available database at universities or colleges with nursing programs. Many hospitals subscribe to both CINAHL and Medline. Look for access via your library's website or ask your librarian.

Specialty nurses' associations (e.g., American Association of Critical-Care Nurses, American Psychiatric Nurses Association, Emergency Nurses Association, Oncology Nursing Society, etc.) are also excellent sources for systematic reviews and practice guidelines. Many make these documents available through their websites, usually through a tab. You can also search for them by using their website's search box and typing in *practice guidelines*. Browse a list of over 30 specialty associations with links at the American Nurses

Association website (www.nursingworld.org/AffiliatedOrganizations). Or go to the International Council of Nurses (www.icn.ch/about-icn/about-icn/) to access links to member and affiliate organizations from almost every country.

Searching Databases

We now move on to discover how to find high-quality evidence when EbCPGs or SRs have not yet been developed for your chosen topic. Because reviews and guidelines do not exist for every issue you wish to investigate, it is important for you to know how to efficiently find original research studies (DiCenso, Bayley, & Haynes, 2009). This part of the chapter will help you develop these important skills. A later chapter will address methods of appraising the studies you find.

Databases are best understood as a tool for communication. I think of them as another form of what clinicians frequently refer to as the "hallway consult." Picture yourself in the hospital hallway saying to yourself, "I wonder why . . .?" or "I wonder if . . ." Another clinician approaches, one whom you trust with your question. We all do this frequently in our everyday lives as well. The discourse can be as simple as asking a friend which website they used to get that low ticket price. In fact, a study of clinicians found that they generate about 3 questions for every 10 patients seen (Ely et al., 1999). Health sciences databases are constructed to facilitate this transfer of information from research to clinical practice. Unlike the hallway consult, in which you are limited to the expertise of your immediate associates, you can use a database to pose your question to a much more extensive group of experts. And, in a sense, you can even ask them how they came to their conclusion. For the most part, databases allow access to original research studies, although many include book chapters, letters to the editor and even cartoons as well. We will focus on research studies published as articles in professional journals for the purposes of this chapter.

What's in a Database?

First, no database includes all studies. Even Google only provides access to about 10% of the information delivered over the Internet. Databases, such as Medline/PubMed, CINAHL, and PsycINFO, each provide access to the contents of a defined group of journals. For instance, there are about 20,000 journals in the biomedical sciences. Medline indexes almost 5,000 of these, concentrating on those of greatest benefit to physicians, dentists, veterinarians, and health planners. It indexes some of the major nursing journals as well. CINAHL looks at slightly more than 3,000 journals in the fields of nursing and allied health. There is some overlap between the journals covered by these two databases, but most of what you might find will be unique to that particular database. Similarly, PsycINFO, which covers articles from thousands of psychology journals, is often of value to nurses and has some overlap with Medline and CINAHL. Before database developers decide to include a particular journal, they carefully consider the typical quality of the articles the journal accepts. The very fact that a journal, for instance *Cancer Nursing*, is included in CINAHL is an indicator of CINAHL's perception of that journal's quality. Once a journal is selected, a record is created for each article in that journal. This record is made up of searchable fields, including the author's name, the title of the article, the name of the journal, the words in the abstract, and the date of publication. An indexer also reads the article and tags it with at least five subject headings to describe the content of the article (e.g., asthma, therapeutic exercise) and the nature of the population under study (e.g., female, adolescent). These headings are searchable. Just how they enable very powerful, precision searches will be demonstrated in the sections on intermediate and advanced techniques.

Are All the Articles in a Database Available in Full Text?

Because of the U.S. Copyright Law, databases cannot legally distribute the full text of all the articles in all the journals they index. They may include only those for which they have been able to negotiate access with the copyright owner, typically the journal's publisher. Libraries and hospitals, in turn, purchase access to these databases through a vendor, like Ovid or EBSCOhost. Many vendors work very hard to negotiate access to as much full text as possible, knowing that clinicians prefer those databases providing the greatest amount of full text.

I Know How to Search Google. Can I Use Those Same Skills to Search CINAHL or Medline?

The short answer is yes. We search Google by using text words, otherwise known as everyday or natural language. If you searched Google for the common cold it would list over 2,000,000 websites containing the phrase *common cold*. However, if an author used a different word to discuss the common cold, let us say rhinitis, Google would not retrieve these for you. Google is very good at giving you what you ask for, but not necessarily at giving you what you want.

You can also use text words to search CINAHL and Medline. When you enter the text words, the search engine will scan all titles, authors' names, and words in the abstract for those text words. If you type in the word *AIDS*, it will return all the articles with that word, including those that are not about the disease, such as the following: "Electronic Aids for Daily Living," "A Comparison of Hearing Aids," "Assessment Aids Learning," and "Pain Management Aids in Rapid Recovery." These are called false hits. Again, they are examples of getting exactly what you asked for but not what you wanted.

A further challenge in looking for clinical information is that medical terminology is a rich mix of Greek, Latin, and Anglo-Saxon terms. Consequently we often have three different words for the same organ. Consider the words and prefixes *eye*, *opti-* and *ophthalm-*, as well as *kidney*, *renal*, and *nephr-*. Because Medline and CINAHL are meant to support efficient investigation, they enable you to search by subject headings in addition to a specific text word. I will show you how this works in the sections on intermediate and advanced searching. While these are more advanced techniques, in many ways they make your search so much easier. Certainly searching with subject headings helps avoid the pitfalls described previously. But let us first concentrate on simple text word searching.

Just the Basics

Please recall that CINAHL is available only by subscription. Check with your librarian regarding its availability at your institution. CINAHL (http://www.ebscohost.com/biomedical-libraries/the-cinahl-database) offers you several search boxes that you can use to start your search. It is best to first consider your question and its component parts. Let us try something simple like nursing assessment of children with cancer. Using PICOTS terminology, the *P* element would be children with cancer and the *I* element would be assessment.

The first concept in our search is *cancer*, so we type that word in the first box. I will show you how we focus on the pediatric segment of the cancer population further later. Our second concept is *nursing assessment*, so we type those words into the second box, and then hit the Search command. We combine these sets with the Boolean operator *and*. This enables us to identify just those articles discussing both cancer and nursing assessment. The following schematic illustrates the process and resulting number of journal articles:

1. Cancer	106,148 articles
2. Nursing assessment	15,657 articles
3. 1 *and* 2	864 articles

Now, let us take our search a few steps further. Let us say we are only interested in research studies from the last 5 years, and since the patient is in grade school we are specifically interested in the 6- to 12-year-old population.

Locate Refine your results on the left side of the screen and click on Show More. Here we find that CINAHL offers options for limiting the results of our search.

4. Results limited to research studies	243 articles
5. Results limited to last 5 years	86 articles
6. Results limited to ages 6–12 years	5 articles

You can see that as we begin to consider the specifics of our patient population and our interest in current research, our group of articles on nursing assessment quickly shrinks to a modest size. Following are some sample titles from this group of five studies: "Pain in Children with Central Nervous System Cancer," "Assessing Procedural Pain in Children with Cancer," and "Exploration of Social Support Available to Mothers of Children with Cancer."

Intermediate Techniques

Now let us move on to some intermediate level skills and consider a slightly different clinical situation. This time we will look for recent research on supporting the patient with breast cancer. Using PICOTS terminology, the *P* element would be people with breast cancer and the *I* element would be support.

If we type *breast cancer* in the search box, CINAHL will retrieve nearly 22,000 articles. Each of these articles will contain both the word *breast* and the word *cancer*. Let us look instead at what happens if we use a very powerful tool for precision searching, the CINAHL Headings tab. We can use this tool to search by concept, that is, by the headings assigned by the indexer, and to free ourselves from the constraints of text word searching.

You will spot this tab near the top of the search screen. When we click on this tab, a browse box opens and we can type in the words *breast cancer*. The database will then advise us that all the articles on breast cancer are identified with the heading, Breast Neoplasms.

If we run this search using this subject heading, we find over 29,000 articles. How can using a subject heading find so many more articles than the 22,000 produced by our text word search? The answer is that not all articles about breast cancer use the words *breast* and *cancer*. The following three titles of articles in nursing journals are examples: "Barriers to Follow-Up of Abnormal Screening Mammograms," "Advances in Symptom Management: Lymphedema," and "Mastectomy and Lumpectomy Offer Equal Chances of a Cure."

We return to the CINAHL Headings tab and type the word *support* into the browse box. CINAHL returns a list of possible headings, including Support, Psychosocial, which is the one we will select for this exercise. CINAHL identifies over 29,000 articles on this topic. When we combine these two sets we see the following results:

1. Breast neoplasms	29,940 articles
2. Support, psychosocial	29,389 articles
3. 1 *and* 2	968 articles

Combining these two sets with the Boolean operator *and* means that each of the resulting articles discusses both breast neoplasms and psychological support.

Let us take our search a few steps further. You may recall from the first part of this chapter that the CINAHL database can be used to find EbCPGs and SRs. Once you have created a set of articles on a specific population and intervention, as we have with the previous search, click on the Show More link. You may also see an Edit icon on the right side of the screen. Clicking on either of these will result in a screen with a number of ways to limit your results. One of these is a drop-down menu called Publication Type. Among the various types listed under Publication Type are Systematic Review and Practice Guidelines. Selecting either or both of these will limit your results to just those articles that are systematic reviews or contain practice guidelines. But this section of the chapter is not simply an introduction to the use of databases, but how to use databases in the absence of available EbCPS and SRs. This means we are interested in finding original research studies, and specifically those that include the outcomes of a process or an intervention.

Let us consider our current PICOTS search where *P* stands for breast cancer and *I* for support. Let us now try to determine if this intervention enables a reduction in the anxiety level of the patient. In other words, we are looking at anxiety reduction as the outcome, or the *O* element using PICOTS terminology. Following the process previously discussed, we enter *anxiety* into the browse box available through the CINAHL Headings tab, and then combine this set of articles (set 4) with the previous set (set 3.) Using either the Show More or Edit link, we further refine our results to research articles. Then, because we are interested in the psychosocial support provided by nurses, we finally narrow our results to articles in nursing journals.

4. Anxiety	11,984 articles
5. 3 *and* 4	58 articles
6. Results limited to research	46 articles
7. Results limited to nursing journals	23 articles

Our assumption in narrowing our results to nursing journals is that if the study is published in a nursing journal, the clinician most likely to be providing the psychological support would be a nurse. You can narrow your results to nursing journals by using the drop-down menu Journal Subset, then clicking on Nursing. Be sure to select Nursing rather than Core Nursing, as the latter is a much smaller group of nursing journals. What we know about these remaining 23 articles is that each is a research study published in a nursing journal and addressing anxiety, psychosocial support, and breast neoplasms. A few titles from our resulting 23 articles are "Effect of Supportive Care on the Anxiety of Women with Suspected Breast Cancer," "Coping with a Possible Breast Cancer Diagnosis," and "Identifying the Educational Needs and Concerns of Newly Diagnosed Patients with Breast Cancer after Surgery."

You may note that we have not tried to include the *C* or *T* or *S* elements of PICOTS terminology in our search strategies. Finding comparative studies (*C*) involves additional techniques that are outside the scope of this chapter, and there are numerous indexing inconsistencies in capturing the timing (*T*) or setting (*S*) concepts, so I generally do not recommend including them in a search strategy.

Advanced Techniques

In this section we look at three additional features available in the CINAHL and Medline databases. These are the Explode, Subheading, and Citation features, and they deserve a bit of explanation first. To understand the Explode feature, I will share an example I use in class. Let us assume there is a subject heading Dogs, and, in addition, there are the following subject headings, Airedale, Basset Hound, and Cocker Spaniel. In fact, let us assume there is a separate subject heading for every major breed of dog.

What if you were interested in finding studies researching the extent to which dogs reduce the level of loneliness in nursing home residents? It would be so much easier if you could use the subject heading Dogs and automatically retrieve all the articles about dogs, even if the articles were specific to a certain breed. The Explode feature allows you to do just that.

Consider the following results in our dog search. Our search on the subject heading Airedale would retrieve just those articles about that breed. If we did a search on the subject heading Dogs without using the Explode command, we would retrieve only those articles about dogs in general, articles that are not about a specific breed. But when we use the Explode command we retrieve all the articles about dogs, those that are specific to particular breeds that have their own subject headings, and those that are about dogs in general.

Airedale	22 articles
Basset	90 articles
Cocker	230 articles
Dogs	15,338 articles
Explode dogs	262,232 articles

Let us now apply the Explode command to our search on breast cancer. In the following image we have just completed a subject heading search for breast cancer and we see the preferred term *Breast Neoplasms*. If we click on the Breast Neoplasms link, the image shown in **Figure 12–1** appears.

As in our dog breed example, we notice that there are several different kinds of breast cancer (male breast neoplasms and ductal carcinomas), each with its own subject heading. We know from our intermediate level example that a search for Breast Neoplasms will retrieve over 29,000 articles. But if we click on the Explode box on the right side of the screen, and then the Search box, we will get this group of articles plus all those about breast ductal carcinomas and male breast neoplasms. Thus a comparison of results looks like this:

Breast neoplasms	29,940 articles
Explode breast neoplasms	30,189 articles

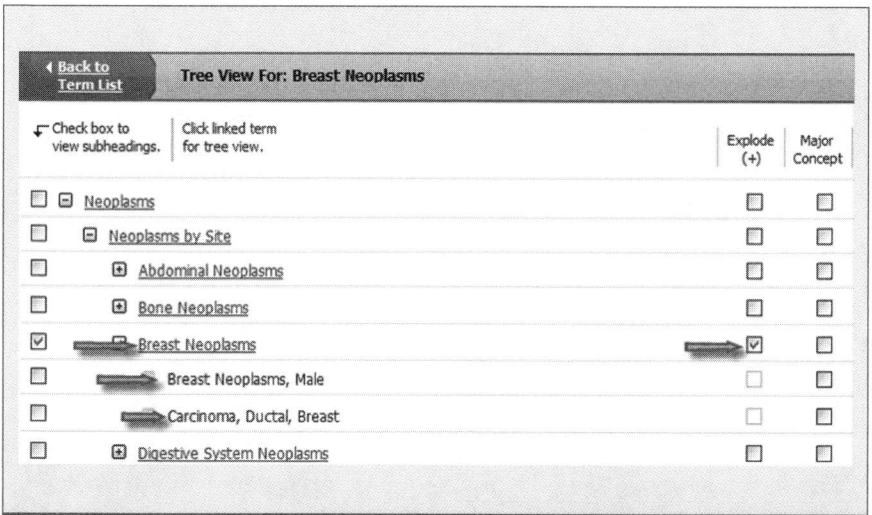

Figure 12-1 Using the Explode Feature
Source: Reproduced from CINAHL with Full Text database with permission from EBSCO Publishing.

If we repeat this process, exploding Support, Psychological, and Anxiety, we find the following differences in the number of resulting articles:

Support, psychological	29,389 articles
Explode support, psychological	31,657 articles
Anxiety	11,984 articles
Explode anxiety	12,790 articles

It should be noted that not all subject headings can be exploded. For instance, there is no Explode box featured with the subject heading, Patella. Using the Explode feature will increase the size of your sets and therefore may retrieve valuable results that you would have otherwise missed.

The second advanced technique we will consider is the Subheading feature. While going through the Explode example, you may have noticed the note in the upper left hand corner of the screen that said, "Check box to view subheadings." Checking the box will produce a column of subheadings (**Figure 12–2**). Think of these as subgroups of your search. In Figure 12–2 we see a subject heading search for Anxiety on the left and some of its associated subheadings in the column on the right. Clicking the box for Prevention and Control will narrow the search to articles about the prevention and control of anxiety.

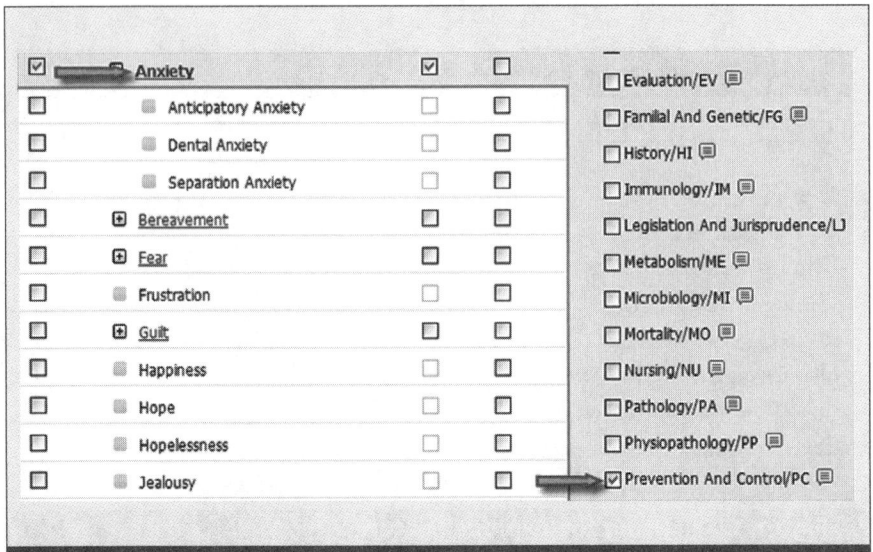

Figure 12-2 Using the Subheading Feature

Source: Reproduced from CINAHL with Full Text database with permission from EBSCO Publishing.

There are in fact over 1,600 articles on the prevention and control of anxiety. If we added our set of breast neoplasm articles, we would then have over 30 resulting articles and our PICOTS search would look like this: the *P* element for patients with breast neoplasms, the *I* element for prevention and control, and the *O* element for anxiety. We then use the Show More or Edit feature to further narrow our results to research articles and nursing journals. Titles of some of these research studies about control measures used by nurses include "Effects of Exercise Intensity and Self-Efficacy on State Anxiety with Breast Cancer Survivors," "The Effect of Supportive Care on the Anxiety of Women with Suspected Breast Cancer," and "Virtual Reality; a Distraction Intervention for Chemotherapy." Think of subheadings as another way of identifying interventions.

- **The use of the Explode feature will always make your results larger and more inclusive.**
- **The Subheading feature will always make your results smaller and more targeted.**

The final advanced feature is available in CINAHL but not Medline. It tracks citations forward in time. What does this mean? You have all probably heard an instructor suggest that you look at the list of references at the end of an article to find more articles on the same topic. If we were to take our breast neoplasm and psychosocial support search and investigate the references at the end of any of the articles from our results, we would be going back in time. The author can only reference the older work he/she read while preparing to write the article.

But what if you could go forward in time? What if you found an article that was very useful and you were able to find newer articles that referred to your useful article? Well, this in fact is possible. Consider the citation image shown in **Figure 12–3**. It is a description of one of the three articles mentioned in our breast neoplasm search. Note the link, Times Cited in this Database. This link will lead to 13 newer articles (i.e., newer than the article's August 2005 publication date) that cite this article; whereas the link, Cited References takes us to 56 older articles (i.e., older than August 2005).

1. Coping with a possible breast cancer diagnosis: demographic factors and social support.
(includes abstract); Drageset S; Lindstrøm TC; Journal of Advanced *Nursing*, 2005 Aug; 51 (3): 217-26 (journal article - *research*, tables/charts) ISSN: 0309-2402 PMID: 16033589 CINAHL AN: 2009005455
Aim. This paper reports a study examining the relationships between demographic characteristics, social support, anxiety, coping and defence among women with possible breast cancer. Background. A...
Subjects: Breast Neoplasms; Coping; Support, Psychosocial; Adult: 19-44 years; Aged: 65+ years; Middle Aged: 45-64 years; Female
Database: CINAHL with Full Text
Add to folder | Cited References: (56) | Times Cited in this Database: (13)
PDF Full Text
Check For Full Text

Figure 12-3 Using the Citation Feature
Source: Reproduced from CINAHL with Full Text database with permission from EBSCO Publishing.

What About Medline and PsycINFO?

While the aforementioned results all come from searches on the CINAHL database, Medline is used the same way. Recall that Medline is searching, for the most part, through a different set of journals. It also searches a greater number of journals. Some database vendors, like EBSCOhost, make it very easy to switch between databases, allowing you to use the same search strategy without having to type your search terms again. This seems quite tempting, but it only works if Medline and CINAHL use exactly the same subject headings. For instance, both databases use Anxiety, Breast Neoplasms, and Patella, but where CINAHL uses Support, Psychological, Medline uses Social Support. If either database encounters a subject heading it does not recognize in your search strategy, it will return zero results. This can be most misleading!

Because Medline is produced by a federal agency, the National Library of Medicine, it is also available for free through the Internet under the name PubMed (http://www.ncbi.nlm.nih.gov/pubmed). If you search it this way, that is, without going through your library's website, it is likely to come with significantly less full text attached. Nevertheless, using PubMed is a great way to begin a search and get a sense of the current research from home.

PsycINFO and its companion database, PsycArticles, are broadly available at college libraries, even at those schools with no health sciences programs. These databases are of value to nurses investigating psychological disorders as well as the psychosocial aspects of nursing practice. Patient self-image, treatment compliance, and the therapeutic relationship are examples of topics that are well covered in the psychological literature.

A Final Word and a Few Tips

Looking for research evidence is by its nature an iterative process. You may not find the answers to your question on your first try. Experimenting with different approaches is a normal part of the process. You may need to restructure your search strategy several times. Medline, PubMed and CINAHL have a function that keeps track of your search formulations each time you hit the Enter key. On CINAHL and some versions of Medline, this is labeled Search History. It is a good idea to print out this history of your searches before exiting the database. It will help you remember what worked well and will keep you from a return trip up those blind alleys. Similarly, after clicking the Search History link, you will find another feature called

Save Searches. This feature allows you to set up a user profile whereby you can save your search strategy for easy rerunning at a later date. Finally, most databases allow you to email your results to yourself and others.

In summary, these databases have many powerful features, and there is a learning curve to using them effectively. As with any other nursing skill, proficiency comes from practice! You can speed up the process by signing up for a searching class at your library or making an appointment with a nursing or health sciences librarian for an individual session. Many libraries are now creating their own online tutorials for CINAHL, Medline, and PubMed. Ask if these are available.

http://go.jblearning.com/brown3e

References

DiCenso, A., Bayley, L., & Haynes, R. (2009). Accessing pre-appraised evidence: Fine-tuning the 5S model into a 6S model. *Evidence-Based Nursing, 12*(4), 99–101.

Ely, J., Osheroff, J., Ebell, M., Bergus, G., Levy, B., Chambliss, M., & Evans, E. (1999). Analysis of questions asked by family doctors regarding patient care. *British Medical Journal, 319*(7206), 358–361.

CHAPTER THIRTEEN

Appraising Research Evidence

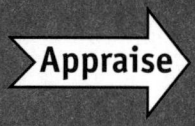

Assuming that your database searches resulted in retrieval of at least one clinical practice guideline, systematic review, or report of an individual study, the next step is to appraise its quality to determine if you can have confidence in it. Published guidelines, reviews, and individual study reports cannot be accepted on face value, even when they are issued by professional associations and published in clinical journals. Reports of flawed research do get published. Therefore, an agency or individual considering using research evidence as the basis for care must appraise it and decide whether it is trustworthy as the basis for clinical decisions and actions.

Appraisal is a step beyond extracting the *why*, *how*, and *what* of a study. It involves not just understanding how the study was done but also making a judgment about how well it was done. It involves not just understanding the results but judging whether the findings are credible, meaningful, and applicable to a particular setting. It requires seeing the relationship between how the study was conducted and what was found, and between what was found and how it might be incorporated into the agency's practice.

Just to be clear: appraisal is not equivalent to a thesis or dissertation. Most of the time invested will be in reading the evidence report or document and marking it up for later reference. As a novice reader of research reports, reading for true understanding and extracting essential details can be a slow go. Even as an experienced reader, it often takes me quite awhile to get a good grasp of a systematic review or complex study.

The time required for the appraisal itself is typically much less. At first it may take you an hour or so to complete it, but again, with a bit of practice, you can get the appraisal time down to 15 minutes in many cases. However, consideration of the applicability of the recommendations/conclusions/findings is quite variable. Thoughtful deliberation is required, but the applicability issues are usually done by a project group, so you initially may just need to give some thought to them prior to the working session.

Appraisal Systems

Numerous appraisal systems for evaluating the quality of guidelines, systematic reviews, and studies exist. The ones used in this book were developed specifically for students who are encountering evidence-based practice appraisal for the first time. They require a level of research knowledge appropriate to what a BSN nurse should possess. Therefore, you should be able to answer the questions in the appraisal guides with the knowledge you acquired in reading the first part of the book. Importantly, these appraisal guides will help you develop basic appraisal skills so that you can use more demanding appraisal guides in the future.

Appraisal guides are discussed in the next three chapters; the guides themselves are in the appendices. The same template is used in all four guides, although the specific questions are different from one guide to another. The chapters are deceptively short because the real work of getting a handle on appraisal requires that you actually use the appraisal guides—and that will take considerable time.

Appraisal in General

The goal of critical appraisal of any type of research evidence is to systematically and thoughtfully judge whether the research evidence is:

- Credible
- Clinically significant
- Applicable (Brown, 1999)

What follows is a brief introduction to each area of appraisal—synopsis, credibility, clinical significance, and applicability. In the following three chapters, each area will be discussed in greater detail—as it pertains to the particular forms of research evidence.

Synopsis

The starting point for appraisal of all forms of research evidence is identifying why the guideline/systematic review/study was done, how it was produced, and what was found. Here you are on familiar ground; this is what you learned earlier in Part 1 of this book. Actually, you could write a useful synopsis using *why*, *how*, and *what* as a template. However, in the appraisal guides provided, you are asked more specific questions about each type of research evidence.

Writing a synopsis not only ensures that you have understanding of the evidence, but it also provides a brief to refer back to later. Importantly, a synopsis contains just the facts—no judgments or interpretations. Research articles typically are very dense, meaning that every sentence contains important information—there is little fluff. Consequently, you may find that to complete the synopsis you have to refer to the article quite a few times to answer the synopsis questions.

Credibility

Question–Design Match

The first issue related to credibility is whether the research design and methods match the research question. A one-group before-and-after study cannot answer the question of whether an intervention or treatment is effective. There simply are not enough controls in place to zero in on the cause–effect relationship that is the essence of effectiveness. Natural improvement over time, patients' perceived empathy from the person who delivers the intervention, or just the fact that something is being done for them can all affect clinical outcomes. Thus, when evaluating intervention effectiveness, a comparison group, randomization, and other controls are essential to avoid bias.

"The art of medicine consists in amusing the patient while nature cures the disease."
—Voltaire

Similarly, a descriptive design using several measurement instruments cannot access understanding of what receiving a new, aggressive form of treatment means to patients. Only qualitative methodology, which allows the patients to identify the issues important to them and express them in their own words, can truly get at what the treatment experience means to them. The bottom line question regarding the match between the research question and the methods used is whether the researchers can legitimately make the claim they are making based on the methods they used.

Produced by Sound Methods

Without a doubt, the most important issue in regard to credibility is making a judgment as to whether the findings are trustworthy because they were produced by sound research methods. In Part I of the book, features of good studies, systematic reviews, and e-b were set forth; now that information will be used to make a thumbs-up or thumbs-down judgment about the methods. Thus, most of the credibility questions in the appraisal guides drill down on the control of bias and error.

Appraising credibility requires an answer to the bottom line question: Was the guideline/review/study produced using methods that were sound enough that you can trust its recommendations/conclusions/findings? If the production process was seriously flawed, its end products are not credible; therefore, they should not be considered as a basis for practice.

This linkage between the soundness of production method and the credibility of the end products is the reason you will notice in the guides provided that some questions pertain to the guideline, the review, or the study, whereas others pertain to the individual recommendation, conclusion, or finding. Generally, use of a sound production process confers credibility on the end product, but each recommendation of a guideline, each conclusion of an integrative review, and each finding of a study stands on its own and must be appraised separately. That is because one of these end products might be credible, clinically significant, and applicable, whereas another may come up short in one or more appraisal categories. Ultimately, the recommendation, conclusion, or finding is what is incorporated into practice, not the whole guideline, review, or study.

Similar to Findings from Other Studies

The credibility of findings is also judged by whether they are similar to findings from other studies conducted in the field of study. Findings that are different are not automatically assumed to be not credible; however, they are held to a high level of rigor—even skepticism. The researcher should acknowledge differences and similarities between the findings of the study being reported and findings from other studies; reasons why her findings might be different should be set forth.

Clinical Significance

In general terms, clinically significant findings are those that have enough impact or substance to make a difference in patients' health outcomes or life experiences should they be used as a basis for practice. Appraising clinical significance would lead you to ask questions such as the following:

- Is the average increase in patients' coping abilities found in the study sizeable enough to make practical differences in patients' everyday lives?
- Is a change in women's attitudes regarding osteoporosis prevention likely to produce a change in their dietary, exercise, or smoking behaviors?
- Are the insights revealed by the study about the process of living with a history of breast cancer after successful treatment informative enough to provide clinicians who see these women for follow-up with a fresh perspective?
- Is the lower end of the 95% confidence interval around a difference in the means of an outcome variable enough of a difference that intervention A is likely to be more effective than intervention B in the population?

In short, how strong are the findings from a clinical perspective? Is the treatment effect strong enough to make a difference in patient outcomes or well-being? Is the relationship between two variables strong enough that it can be built on in some way to design patient assessments differently?

Regrettably, the clinical significance of research evidence is often not explicitly discussed in the report. The clinical implications paragraph in the discussion section of some reports does address the clinical meaning of the findings, but other times it consists mainly of opinions about the ways the findings could be used—not discussion of whether the findings would make a practical difference to patients. As a result, sometimes you will have to piece together your judgment about the clinical significance of the findings from what is reported in combination with your clinical knowledge. The fact that clinical significance is a bit more nebulous than credibility is not a reason to gloss over it in appraisal—it is an important consideration.

Applicability

If a recommendation/conclusion/finding is judged credible and clinically significant, you will then proceed to determine whether it is applicable to your setting, its patients, and its resources. If it is not credible and clinically significant, you need not proceed to appraising applicability because the recommendation/conclusion/finding should not be used as a basis for practice.

The applicability questions that should be asked will vary depending on the nature of the evidence being translated into a clinical protocol and the nature of the change or changes that need to be made. Generally, the questions fall into four categories:

1. Fit of the evidence to the setting's patients.
2. Safety.
3. Expected benefit.
4. Feasibility of incorporating the change.

Fit of the Evidence

The recommendations/conclusions/findings being considered were based on data from study samples. The fit question then is, "Were the persons who made up the samples of the studies similar to those in our setting?" If all the studies were done on white suburban women, the applicability to a multiethnic, inner-city group of women may be quite limited. Making a judgment regarding this fit will require taking note of the profile of persons who participated in the study and the characteristics of the setting(s) in which the study was conducted.

Safety and Expected Benefit

Safety and expected benefit are important considerations. If a protocol is likely to produce meaningful benefits to patients and has few associated risks, the other hurdles can usually be overcome. Both safety and expected benefit must be thoughtfully considered prior to deciding to introduce a new protocol or make a major change in practice. The expected benefit, be they attainment of optimal outcomes or avoidance of adverse events and complications, should actually be quantified. The quantification of the expected benefit is informed by what was found in the research studies. The agency then collects data to determine if their patients achieved the expected level of benefit.

Let's say a new protocol for patient self-monitoring of blood glucose and administration of insulin is being introduced in a clinic. The goal is to have fewer patients whose blood glucose is not in optimal range. Based on findings from the research studies and on data indicating patients' current level of control, the expected benefit might be stated as, "We expect an absolute decrease of 5% in the percentage of patients whose hemoglobin eAG values are above 154." Such a specific target in combination with data about the percentage of patients not meeting the target would quantify the impact of e-b protocol.

Feasibility

The ability of the setting to implement a clinical intervention in a way that is quite similar to the way it was delivered in the study or studies is another important consideration. If major changes have to be made because of limited resources or political forces, then the question could be raised as to whether the intervention being implemented will indeed be evidence based.

Feasibility also involves asking whether the change required could be implemented and maintained in the agency. Does it have the resources? Does it have the will? The project team should also consider whether their setting has the professional skills, support services, equipment, financial resources, and support of key persons to make the change and sustain it over time. A change that involves high cost or effort on the part of direct care providers or support services faces an uphill road to successful implementation.

The applicability questions set forth in the guides are directed at making an organizational change in practice; that is, implementing a new care protocol. Making a change in individual practice would involve fewer issues; however, risk, resources needed, and people affected should still be considered.

The guides for individual studies do not include applicability questions. That is because the applicability of findings from any single study should always be undertaken with caution, particularly when the current approach to care is not causing major problems and is thought to be at least somewhat effective. The assumption is that before a change in practice is made, several studies will be considered and applicability will be appraised based on across-study conclusions, not on findings from just one original study. Across-study analysis of findings is addressed later in Chapter 16.

In summary, four areas (synopsis, credibility, clinical significance, and applicability) serve as a template for the appraisal questions set forth for the recommendations of clinical practice guidelines, for the conclusions of integrative research reviews, and for the findings of original studies. The end point question of an appraisal is: Should we use the recommendation, conclusion, or finding to develop a unit or agency clinical protocol?

Practical Considerations

Even though appraisal of a piece of evidence is done using a set of objective criteria, appraisal inevitably involves a bit of judgment. Not infrequently, two appraisers using the same set of criteria will reach different judgments about the overall quality of a piece of evidence. The difference occurs for a variety of reasons, including the following:

- One appraiser may view a methodological weakness as minor whereas the other appraiser may view it as a critical flaw that undermines the credibility of the recommendations/conclusions/findings.
- One appraiser may consider bias or failure to control confounding influences in the way a study was done to be a major detractor from its credibility, but the other appraiser may view the same circumstances as inherent in the situation.
- One appraiser may conclude that the findings of several studies are similar, while the other appraiser may see an important difference in them.

For these reasons, most panels that produce an appraisal of a body of research require that two or more appraisers rate each piece of evidence and reach consensus about its quality.

In a related issue, when appraising research evidence, you have to strike a balance between identifying crucial flaws and being overly critical. There is no such thing as a perfect guideline/review/study. The goal is not to identify every weakness in the guideline/review/study; rather, you want to detect methods that introduce the possibility of bias to the point that they put in doubt the credibility of the end products. Ultimately, this is a judgment. When researchers design guidelines, reviews, or studies, they often have to make trade-offs between the ideal and the possible or conduct their work with limited resources. Thus, you should reject only recommendations, conclusions, or findings that were produced in a seriously flawed way. Sometimes it is a fine line between being seriously flawed and weak-but-acceptable quality. Appraisal guides can help you make that differentiation.

http://go.jblearning.com/brown3e

Reference

Brown, S. J. (1999). *Knowledge for health care practice: A guide to using research evidence*. Philadelphia, PA: Saunders.

CHAPTER FOURTEEN

Appraising Recommendations of Clinical Practice Guidelines

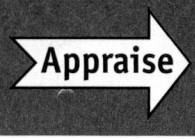

The healthcare literature (electronic and paper) includes an abundance of clinical practice guidelines—produced by professional associations, healthcare systems, specialty centers, and government agencies. Most of them are research based to the maximum extent possible. However, some were produced with little effort to systematically and widely examine the relevant research bases and to use an unbiased production process. Even when a guideline carries a title indicating it is evidence based, a measure of skepticism is needed.

As described earlier in Chapter 10, producing an evidence-based clinical practice guideline (EbCPG) involves quite a few steps, and each step has the potential for bias or error to creep in and distort the translation of the research evidence into clinical action recommendations. Thus, when considering using a clinical practice guideline as a basis for an agency protocol or as a guide for the care of an individual patient, the user should appraise the credibility, clinical significance, and applicability of the guideline's recommendations. In this chapter, you will be: (a) revisiting the clinical practice guideline about nonpharmaceutical management of depression in adults that you read in Chapter 10, (b) appraising it, and (c) comparing your appraisal to one a colleague and I did. First, a bit of background.

AGREE and GRADE

The AGREE Trust is an international organization that produced and validated an evaluation instrument for appraising the process of practice guideline development and the quality of reporting (AGREE Trust, 2012). The AGREE II instrument consists of 23 criteria organized under 6 domains:

1. Scope and purpose.
2. Stakeholder involvement.
3. Rigor of development.
4. Clarity.
5. Applicability.
6. Editorial independence. (Brouwers et al., 2010)

A score for each domain and a total score are calculated; these can be compared to the maximum and minimum points possible to determine if a sound development process was used to produce it. The appraiser using the AGREE II tool is also asked to make two overall judgments, one regarding the quality of the guideline and a second about whether or not s/he would recommend the guideline to others. However, the instrument does not grade the evidence base or the actual recommendations other than to require that there be an explicit linkage between recommendations and supporting evidence.

Another appraisal system, the GRADE system, grades both the body of evidence and the strength of the recommendation (GRADE Working Group, 2010). The grading takes into account the design of studies, quality of studies, and consistency of findings. When assigning a grade to recommendations nine different factors are taken into account, several of which are: (1) certainty regarding the benefits, risks, and inconvenience; (2) size of the benefit produced; (3) importance of the benefit produced; (4) precision of the benefit estimate; and (5) cost (http://www.gradeworkinggroup.org/FAQ/factors_rec.htm). Several nursing organizations are represented in the GRADE working group; still, the applicability of the GRADE system to the appraisal of nursing guidelines remains to be seen.

An Appraisal Guide for Use by the Nurse with a BSN

The AGREE and GRADE appraisal instruments for clinical practice guidelines clearly set forth specific and comprehensive standards for clinical practice guidelines. However, performing appraisals using these instruments requires advanced research knowledge and training, so they are not advisable for use by novice appraisers. The more basic appraisal guide provided in Appendix A includes the most important elements of the AGREE instrument and the GRADE system as well as the standards of the Institute of Medicine (2011).

Synopsis

The first step in the appraisal of a clinical practice guideline is to get a grasp of the health condition the guideline was designed to manage, the issues addressed, the recommendations that were made, and the process used to produce the recommendations. You want to summarize this information in brief so that you can refer to it throughout your project. At this point, I suggest you look at the synopsis questions in the appraisal guide for clinical practice guidelines (Appendix A).

Credibility

In broad terms, appraising the credibility of a guideline involves examining the following aspects of the guideline:

- Determine if the organization and persons that produced the guideline had the expertise to do so.
- Determine if the recommendations are based on sound evidence.
- Decide if the process used to produce the guideline was systematic and free of bias.
- Determine the confidence the developers have in the recommendations.

Production Process Description of the production process allows the potential adopter to determine if the search for evidence was extensive and if steps were taken to avoid bias during production. First, the composition of the panel that produced the guideline should be noted as well as the credentials of the persons on the panel. The panel members are often required to sign a document indicating they have no other involvements that would bias their participation in the development of the guideline; we say, "They are free of conflict of interest." This may or may not be explicitly stated in the guideline document. The composition of the panel should cover the issues addressed by the guideline. For instance, if the guideline makes reference to medications, a pharmacist, nurse practitioner, or physician in the field of practice should be included on the panel.

Then, the production process should be described in some detail. Unfortunately, some guidelines do not include any description at all of the development process. Omission of information about the development process makes appraising the credibility of a guideline almost impossible. Do note, however, that it is not uncommon for the production standards of the producing agency to be described elsewhere—often on its website.

The important steps of the process that should be described are:

1. How the search for evidence was conducted.
2. How the quality of evidence was evaluated.
3. The inclusion and exclusion criteria that were applied to what was found.
4. How decisions were made regarding whether or not to include a recommendation.
5. How differences of opinion were resolved (AGREE, 2010). Ideally, the guideline will have been reviewed by outside experts and field tested.

Linkage to Evidence Basing recommendations on research evidence is a major determinant of the credibility of a clinical practice guideline. Therefore, during appraisal, you should note whether the systematic reviews used or conducted by the panel were of high quality; there should be either indication that existing SRs passed a quality filter or a description of the process the panel used to conduct the SR.

The supporting evidence sources should also be indicated. Footnote citations indicating the supporting SR or studies would be the minimum, but a discussion of the research evidence or a detailed table setting forth the evidence relevant to each recommendation would be better. Details about the relevant evidence may be included in the guideline itself or in an accompanying document.

The strength of the evidence and the nature of the evidence serve as a basis for the rating of the recommendations themselves. The rating or grading of recommendations (as discussed in Chapter 10) reflects how much confidence the panel has that the recommendation will bring about desired patient outcomes with acceptable levels of risk and burden to the patient.

If the strength and quality of the evidence for each recommendation and the degree of confidence the panel has in the recommendation are evident in the guideline document, you can be reasonably confident that the recommendations are credible (IOM, 2011).

FEATURES INDICATING SOUNDLY DEVELOPED RECOMMENDATIONS

- **Grading of the evidence in support of each recommendation**
- **The source of the evidence and a discussion of the evidence are available to the user**
- **Grading of the confidence the panel has in the recommendation**

Current Status If a guideline was produced 4 or more years ago, it certainly would be advisable to search for more recent research evidence that might update the recommendations of the guideline. In 2001, a study of clinical practice guidelines produced by the U.S. Agency for Healthcare Research and Quality found that half of their 17 guidelines were outdated in 5.8 years (Shekelle et al., 2001). Research on some clinical topics (such as management of the blood sugar levels of diabetics) is being done at a fairly fast rate; thus, a guideline or review done even 2 years earlier could be out of date. In contrast, other clinical topics receive much less research attention so that a guideline is stable for quite a few years.

Clinical Significance

Evaluating the clinical significance of a guideline recommendation requires consideration of the following:

- Importance of the health benefits expected.
- Likelihood of health benefits.
- Side effects and risks.
- Practicality and acceptability to patients.

Consideration of these issues helps decide whether the recommendation would make a difference in patient outcomes. The clinical significance of a recommendation is often reflected in the strength of the recommendation grade given to it.

In addition, to be clinically significant, the set of recommendations that make up the guideline should address all the issues that are important to patients as well as all the important decisions nurses make while delivering the care. Some guideline producers pilot test their guidelines prior to releasing them. If this is done, it addresses the clinical significance issue by providing future users with information about how patients and providers view the value and practicality of the recommendations and whether following the guidelines actually resulted in the presumed outcomes.

Applicability

In the final section of the appraisal tool, "Applicability," you will be asked to make a judgment regarding the fit between the recommendations and the setting in which you intend to implement them. As a student, if you are familiar with one agency or hospital, you should try to envision what would be involved in making the changes in practice that a new care protocol requires. The applicability questions will help you think through some of those requirements. At the very least, you should consider the applicability questions and appreciate what is involved in making an organizational change in care practice. The issue of implementation of a research-based change in practice receives more attention later in the text.

A guideline can be soundly produced and make credible and clinically significant recommendations, but it may not be feasible for the setting in which a protocol project team intends to use it. Perhaps the population of patients or providers in the setting is not similar to those for whom the guideline was intended. Perhaps implementation of the protocol would require expenditure for training that is beyond what the setting can afford. Thus, one possible bottom line judgment resulting from appraisal of a guideline may be, "The guideline's recommendations are credible and clinically significant but are not applicable to our setting." Alternatively, some recommendations may be applicable but others may not be.

Your Turn

First, read through the appraisal questions in the Appendix A: *Appraisal Guide: Recommendations of a Clinical Practice Guideline*. Note the format. The questions are stated so that a *Yes* answer indicates compliance with a standard for that type of research evidence. Thus, a column of *Yes* answers in an area of appraisal indicates high quality and will probably lead you to a positive bottom line conclusion for that area of appraisal—the three bottom line conclusions are in **BOLD UPPERCASE** font. Although all the criteria are important, especially important ones are noted with an asterisk (*).

Then re-read the SIGN clinical practice guideline, *Nonpharmaceutical Management of Depression in Adults* reprinted in chapter 10 and complete an appraisal of its conclusions using the criteria in the appraisal guide (it can be completed on paper or interactively on the book's companion website). Although most questions on the appraisal guide ask for a yes/no answer, for most purposes, but particularly for student learning, a one- to three-sentence rationale for the yes/no answer should also be given. To get various perspectives, you might want to do the appraisal with one or several classmates. Afterwards, look at how a colleague and I appraised the guideline (Appendix B) and compare our judgments to yours.

As noted when you first read this guideline, the reprint contains only part of the guideline. In doing the appraisal, you may find that you prefer to work with the full online document and move between the full SIGN guideline at http://www.sign.ac.uk/pdf/sign114.pdf and the SIGN 50 *Guideline Developer's Handbook* at http://www.sign.ac.uk/guidelines/fulltext/50/index.html.

http://go.jblearning.com/brown3e

References

AGREE Trust (2012). Retrieved from http://www.agreetrust.org/

Brouwers, M., Kho, M. E., Browman, G.P., Burgers, J.S., Cluzeau, F., Feder, G., et al. for the AGREE Next Steps Consortium (2010). AGREE II: Advancing guideline development, reporting and evaluation in healthcare. *Canadian Medical; Association Journal* 182:E839-842; doi:10.1503/090449

GRADE Working Group. (2010). Retrieved from http://www.gradeworkinggroup.org/index.htm

Institute of Medicine (IOM). (2011). *Clinical practice guidelines we can trust.* Retrieved from http://www.iom.edu/Reports/2011/Clinical-Practice-Guidelines-We-Can-Trust.aspx

Shekelle, P. G., Ortiz, E., Rhodes, S., Morton, S. C., Eccles, M. P., Grimshaw, J. M., & Woolf, S. H. (2001). Validity of the Agency for Healthcare research and quality clinical practice guidelines: How quickly do guidelines become outdated? *Journal of the American Medical Association, 286*(12), 1461–1467.

CHAPTER FIFTEEN

Appraising Conclusions of Integrative Research Reviews

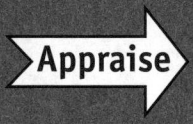

A systematic review (SR) is an important resource when designing an evidence-based care innovation. The comprehensive and systematic synthesis SRs provide is essential to a complete understanding of clinical topics. However, research evidence in the form of the conclusions of SRs, like the recommendations of clinical practice guidelines, must be critically appraised before using them as the basis for nursing care protocols or care of an individual patient. SR conclusions are a bit easier to appraise than are guideline recommendations because the translation of evidence into recommendations is not an issue. Still, there is much to consider because the move from individual findings to across-studies conclusions is susceptible to bias.

The appraisal framework discussed in this chapter uses the format introduced in Chapter 13: synopsis, credibility, clinical significance, applicability. The questions in the guide provided are specific to integrative research reviews (IRRs), the most common type of SRs seen in clinical nursing journals. The IRR from Chapter 9 about medication adherence in persons with bipolar disorder is used to demonstrate appraisal of an IRR.

There are many appraisal guides for systematic research but none as widely recognized as those for clinical practice guidelines. However, several premier review organizations have recently spelled out standards for conducting systematic reviews (Cochrane Collaboration, 2010; Institute of Medicine, 2011; Joanna Briggs Institute, 2008). The set of appraisal questions for IRRs presented in this chapter (see Appendix C) is representative of, albeit more basic than, the criteria of the premier producers and policy setters.

Synopsis

I have already made a case for completing a synopsis of the various forms of research evidence, so now I will just suggest looking at the synopsis questions specific to IRRs in the appraisal guide.

Credibility

IRR synthesis is prone to bias because it is all too easy for the reviewers to introduce their own predilections and beliefs into the review and synthesis process (Oxman & Guyatt, 1988). For this reason, the standards for IRRs include the requirements that the reviewers: (1) set out the evidence from the individual studies; and (2) be explicit about how important steps in the review were done (IOM, 2011; Steinberg & Luce, 2005). This requires that IRR reports include the following elements:

- A clear objectives statement.
- A description of how the search for relevant study reports was performed.
- A description of the criteria for including or excluding studies.
- A description of how the quality of individual studies was appraised and considered in the analysis.
- Tables or narrative that describe the population, methods, and findings of the individual studies.
- For each conclusion, the evidence that led to it should be clear, including the quality of studies, the quantity of studies, and the consistency of findings across the supporting studies (AHRQ, 2002; IOM, 2011).

When the research reviewers include these elements in their report, the reader is provided with information that can be used to decide if the conclusions are indeed derived from the across-studies synthesis of individual studies and are unbiased. If the reviewers do not provide this information, the reader is placed in the position of having to trust the reviewers' interpretation of the evidence, which is not in keeping with the explicit nature of scientific decision making.

The reviewers should be careful not to reach conclusions that are beyond what the evidence shows. This would be the case if the conclusions were applied to elders, but the studies had been done mainly with elders living in nursing homes. For many issues, the findings would not, or may not, apply to seniors living in their own homes or apartments, in assisted living facilities, or with family. Another example of going beyond the findings would be overstating the importance of the findings from several weak studies.

Importantly, when the evidence is inconclusive—that is, inconsistent across studies or from weak studies—the reviewers should not conclude that there is no effect, no difference, or no association. Rather, the conclusion should be that definitive evidence for or against an effect is lacking. A conclusion of *no effect* or *no association* assumes a clear finding of no effect based on consistent evidence, whereas a conclusion of *inconclusive evidence* or *insufficient evidence* recognizes that the evidence does not provide a clear and consistent answer regarding effect—two very different conclusions.

Clear connectivity between findings of the individual studies and the conclusions is established when the reviewers demonstrate a deep analysis of the data. The reviewers should convince you that they looked for patterns and similarities in findings and reasons for the differences. Reasons for different findings from one study to others would include differences in the samples studied, the form of an intervention, the outcomes studied, how the variables were measured, different measurement intervals, or length of follow-up. In short, conclusions based on a deep analysis give you, the consumer of the conclusions, confidence in their credibility.

Clinical Significance

To be clinically significant, the conclusions of a review should reflect issues that are important in everyday practice and that if incorporated into practice would make a difference in patient safety, comfort, or health outcomes. For reviews of interventions, this would include a conclusion that the treatment effect is large enough to be of benefit given costs and any burden to patients or staffs, as reflected in absolute benefit improvement (ABI), numbers needed to treat (NNT) findings, and economic analysis (if available). Clinical significance is more difficult to appraise in IRRs of issues other than intervention effectiveness, although the consistency of the findings across the studies, the strength of the relationship between variables across the studies, and the informativeness of the conclusions can be considered.

Applicability

The judgment regarding whether the conclusions of a review are applicable to a particular setting is determined in part by the setting and patients that were included in the original studies reviewed. If they are similar, or the reporting is such that you can identify a subset of studies that were conducted in a setting similar to yours, then the results of that subset would be applicable to your setting. For instance, an emergency department in a rural hospital would have to consider whether the conclusions of a review about triage systems is applicable to their setting if all the studies included in the review were from inner-city or suburban emergency departments. The issues for the rural emergency department are very different—for instance, no option to close to admissions and divert ambulances elsewhere, and fewer clinical services available 24/7. Beyond the settings and patients studied, the feasibility of implementing, resources required, and costs of implementing should also be taken into account.

Your Turn

I suggest that you reread the Crowe, Wilson, & Inder (2011) article about medication adherence in bipolar disorder that is reprinted in Chapter 9. Then complete an appraisal of it using the "Appraisal Guide: Conclusions of an Integrative Research Review" (Appendix C) or interactively on the book's website). Afterwards, look at the completed appraisal in Appendix D. You could further practice appraisal of IRRs by appraising one of the systematic reviews listed on the text's website. I suggest that readers new to appraisal not attempt appraisal of a meta-analysis or metasynthesis at this point.

http://go.jblearning.com/brown3e

References

Agency for Healthcare Research and Quality (AHRQ). (2002). *Systems to rate the strength of scientific evidence: Summary*. Retrieved from http://www.ncbi.nlm.nih.gov/bookshelf/br.fcgi?book=erta47

Cochrane Collaboration. (2010). For authors and MEs. Review production resources for Cochrane Review authors and managing editors. Retrieved from http://www.cochrane.org/training/authors-mes

Crowe, M., Wilson, L., & Inder, M. (2011). Patients' reports of the factors influencing medication adherence in bipolar disorder—An integrative review of the literature. *International Journal of Nursing Studies, 48*, 894–903.

Institute of Medicine (IOM). (2011). *Finding what works in health care: Standards for systematic reviews*. Washington, DC: National Academy of Science.

Joanna Briggs Institute. (2008). 2008 JBI reviewers manual. Retrieved from http://www.joannabriggs.edu.au/About%20Us/JBI%20Approach/Systematic%20Reviews

Oxman, A. D., & Guyatt, G. H. (1988). Guidelines for reading literature reviews. *Canadian Medical Association Journal, 138*, 697–703.

Steinberg, E. P., & Luce, B. R. (2005). Evidence based? Caveat emptor. *Health Affairs, 24*(1), 80–92.

CHAPTER SIXTEEN

Appraising Findings of Original Studies

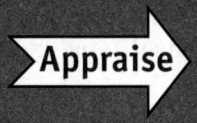

If your project group cannot find a sound and recent research-based clinical practice guideline or systematic review, you may decide to locate and appraise the findings of individual studies—first one study at a time and then as a group of findings from several studies (assuming more than one study was located). A finding of a single research study is like one block or stone in a wall—it is one piece contributing to knowledge about a topic. At some point there may be findings from only one or two studies about an issue, but gradually more studies are done and the knowledge about the topic becomes a more complete structure. Therefore, this chapter starts with a description of how to appraise the findings of individual studies and ends with a description of how to appraise findings across a group of studies.

Two appraisal guides are offered for the findings of individual studies: one for qualitative studies (Appendix E) and one for quantitative studies (Appendix F). Of course, this differentiation requires that you be able to determine which type of study you are appraising. Often, the research report will inform you, but you should be able to make the determination on your own. Most often, determining if you are reading a qualitative study report or a quantitative one is quite straightforward. However, if you are not sure, the questions in **Box 16–1** should help you decide what kind of study you are reading.

BOX 16–1 Deciding What Type of Research Article You Are Reading

Is the study qualitative, quantitative, or was a mixed approach used?

- **If the data consists of words, quotes, verbal descriptions, and/or themes, the study is a qualitative study.**
- **If the data consists of scores, scales, numerical data, percentages, graphs, and/or statistics, the study is a quantitative study.**
- **If both qualitative and quantitative data was presented, the study has a mixed design.**

After you have determined the type of study you are reading, you will know which appraisal guide to use. If the study used a mixed design, you should use a combination of both guides.

Broad Credibility Issues

Appropriateness of Design

The credibility of findings of both qualitative and quantitative studies depends on the researcher having used study methods that were appropriate to answer the research questions. So far, you have read about five different research designs but were not asked to challenge whether the researcher used the right design. Short of obtaining a doctoral degree, you may not be able to do this with 100% accuracy; however, there are a few things you should know. The study design used is determined by the question being asked—for some questions there is not a best design, but rather several that would be good although providing a slightly different perspective on the question.

If the question has to do with understanding the decision-making process used by parents of a child with severe mental retardation when deciding whether to keep the child at home or place the child in residential care, a study using qualitative methods would get at the complexities of this very personal decision process and how that thinking evolves over time.

A related but different question, "What are the characteristics of families that keep a child with severe mental retardation at home over at least a 5-year period?" could be studied using research methodology that quantifies characteristics such as number and ages of other children, ages of the parents, size of the extended family, social support, income, educational level, community services available, and housing situation. Such a study could produce a descriptive, quantitative profile of families who keep children with severe retardation at home.

If, instead of just quantifying family and community variables, the researcher also wanted to look for relationships among the variables, a correlation design could be used. This would be the case if the researcher looked for relationships between quantifiable family characteristics and the coping level of families who kept children with severe mental retardation at home. A more complex correlational design would examine a group of family and community variables to determine which ones are the best predictors of successfully keeping a child at home.

If the question was, "Does a day care service for children with mental retardation result in fewer children being placed in residential care than if families are paid to take care of their child 24 hours a day, 7 days a week with periodic paid respite?" neither a qualitative study, a descriptive study, nor a correlational study would get at the effectiveness of one intervention vis-à-vis the other. An experimental study would be best. Having said that, random assignment may not be possible, and a quasi-experimental design may have to be used.

Peer Review

You will note that the first question under credibility of both appraisal guides asks whether the research report was published in a journal requiring that all published articles be reviewed by peers. In asking this, the assumption is that research reports published in peer-reviewed journals are of higher quality than those published in journals that do not require review by peers prior to acceptance. Actually, opinions vary about whether this fact should affect judgment regarding the credibility of the findings. However, peer review does assure the nonresearcher reader that the report has been reviewed by two or three other persons in the field and was deemed worthy of publication.

Unfortunately, it is not always easy to determine if a journal requires peer review. If you cannot find a statement regarding peer review in the front material of the journal, you could check the journal's website—most have them. Research articles published on electronic sites are equally difficult to evaluate. In general, the absence of a statement on the website indicating that articles are peer reviewed should raise the possibility that they are not, which should cause you to be particularly careful in your appraisal of the study's credibility.

Appraisal of the Findings of a Qualitative Study

Credibility

When considering the credibility of the findings of a qualitative study, the main consideration is the rigor of the study's methods. Yet, the criteria for rigor of qualitative studies are diverse, numerous, and not widely agreed upon (Dixon-Woods, Shaw, Agarwal, & Smith, 2004; Mackey, 2007). Given the many criteria of rigor, several frequently mentioned ones were incorporated into the qualitative appraisal guide of this chapter. In general, the findings and interpretations of qualitative studies are considered credible if:

- The sampling of participants and observations served the purposes of the study (Fossey, Harvey, McDermott, & Davidson, 2002).
- Observation and/or interviewing were adequately prolonged and persistent (Lincoln & Guba, 1985).
- There was interaction between data collection and data analysis (Morse, Barrett, Mayan, Olson, & Spiers, 2002).
- The findings were rooted in the data (Dixon-Woods et al., 2004).

The findings of qualitative studies tend to be cohesive; that is, they hang together as a group rather than stand separately as findings of quantitative studies often do. Therefore, the findings of qualitative studies can be appraised as a group, although sometimes you might want to consider them separately.

Clinical Significance

Kearney (2001) made a strong case for evaluating the usefulness of findings from qualitative findings based on their richness and informativeness. Richness pertains to the demonstrated linking of findings into a web of connections and the creation of a truly new perspective on the phenomenon under study (Kearney, 2001, p. 146). Thus, the findings are informative to clinicians because they go beyond previous ways of thinking about the situation or experience. Vivid portrayal of the experience or situation and description of how context or events produce variations to the experience add to the usefulness of the findings to the clinician. As you read more qualitative studies you will see that some studies penetrate the experience or situation and produce new insights, whereas others fail to get much beyond what most clinicians in the field of practice already know. In brief, the clinical significance of qualitative findings pertains to their usefulness to clinicians. I suggest that now you look at the appraisal guide for findings of qualitative studies (Appendix E) and note how the issues just discussed were incorporated into the guide.

Appraisal of the Findings of a Quantitative Study

Credibility

In quantitative studies, the end products of the study are several, related findings, which are the researchers' data-based conclusions. Like all human conclusions, they can be right or wrong. In correlational and experimental studies, there are two possible correct conclusions and two possible erroneous conclusions.

The correct conclusions are the following:

1. Concluding that a relationship or difference exists in the population when in reality it actually does exist.
2. Concluding that no relationship or difference exists in the population when in reality it does not exist.

The two types of conclusion errors are the following:

1. Concluding that a relationship or difference exists in the population when in reality it does not exist (Type 1 conclusion error).
2. Concluding that no relationship or difference exists in the population when in reality it does exist (Type 2 conclusion error).

For a graphic of these possibilities, see **Table 16–1**.

Avoiding Conclusion Error The researcher is obviously aiming for correct conclusions and trying to avoid making conclusion errors. The ways in which she does this are as follows:

- Eliminate chance variation as an explanation.
- Avoid low statistical power.
- Control extraneous variables.
- Control bias.

Chance variation, which is always present to some degree when data is collected, can affect the statistical results of a study and lead to wrong conclusions. As you learned in Chapter 7, the researcher controls the role of chance

TABLE 16–1 Reaching Correct Conclusion

		Does a real difference exist?	
		Yes	No
Researcher's conclusion	Real difference	Correct	Type 1 error
	No difference	Type 2 error	Correct

variation by defining its limits. This is what is done when the researcher sets the maximal acceptable decision point *p*-level for significance at .05 or .01. In so doing, she is in essence saying, "I will accept only a low probability that my conclusion that there is a difference is due to chance variation." This in effect reduces the likelihood of a type 1 conclusion error.

Studies with small sample sizes can have statistical results indicating no relationship or effect when in fact the problem is that the sample size was not large enough (type 2 conclusion error). A too-small sample size results in insufficient statistical power to detect a significant difference; that is, the microscope was too weak, to use a metaphor employed earlier in Chapter 7. The problem is that there was insufficient data to allow the statistics to detect a relationship or a difference amid the chance variation that is inevitably present. The statistical result could lead the researcher to conclude that there is no relationship or difference, when in fact the problem is the low power of the study resulting from the too-small sample size. Using power analysis to determine sample size protects against type 2 conclusion errors. Remember that from Chapter 7?

Other aspects of the study also determine whether a conclusion is right or wrong. As you learned earlier, researchers use inclusion/exclusion criteria, random assignment, adherence to study protocols, and awareness of what is going on in the research setting to eliminate or isolate the influence of the extraneous variables. However, it may not be possible to control all extraneous variables, or the researcher may not have thought to control a particular influence. Some extraneous variables enter a study without the researcher's awareness in the form of an event or change in the research setting, whereas still others are introduced by the research activities themselves.

Uncontrolled extraneous variables distort study results by mixing with the study variables and producing a statistical result that is an illusion. For example, a statistical result of a study may indicate that there is a significant difference in the outcomes of two treatment groups but reality is that two treatments have equal effects. The statistical result leads the researcher to make a type 1 conclusion error. The reason underlying the misleading statistical result could be an uncontrolled extraneous variable, such as one treatment group had more persons with multiple comorbidities than the other group did. The higher level of comorbidities in one group could have caused that group to have a lower average score on the outcome than the other group, thereby producing a statistically significant difference. If the researcher does not recognize that a difference in comorbidity levels is present, she could wrongly conclude that one treatment is more effective than the other. Extraneous variables can also produce an illusion of no relationship or no effect when indeed there would have been one had a confounding variable not been at work (type 2 conclusion error). In short, when evaluating the credibility of findings, you want to ask, "Was anything else going on that could have produced the results obtained, other than what the researcher concluded?"

Bias, which can enter a study at various points in the form of preconceived ideas about what the results will be or unconscious preference for one treatment over another, is also a potential source of erroneous conclusions. In quantitative studies, bias is controlled by research methods such as random sampling, random assignment, checks on adherence to research protocols, blinding of study observers and/or staff, and use of placebo treatments. Generally, researchers will not speak to bias in their reports; rather, you as the reader have to be alert to the possibility of it and decide whether adequate means were taken to prevent bias from affecting study results, findings, and conclusions. Bias can produce either type 1 or type 2 conclusion errors.

Credible Versus Valid The appraisal questions in the guide should assist you in identifying possible sources of wrong conclusions. When the researcher's conclusions are trusted as the best explanation for the results, not chance, extraneous variables, low statistical power, or bias, the findings are deemed credible (Stoddard & Ring, 1993). Although the appraisal guides provided use the term *credible* to convey that the researcher's conclusions are likely to be trustworthy, other appraisal guides ask, "Are the findings valid?" When used to characterize findings from a study, *valid* means that the findings are judged to be trustworthy reflections of reality and not the result of how the study was conducted or the result of an extraneous variable at work. Note that this usage of the word *valid* is different from the way in which it was used to characterize measurement instruments (in Chapter 5). The term *valid* is more technical and more complex than the word *credible*. However, the word *credible* has more commonsense resonance and is an adequate substitute. I suggest that now you look at the credibility questions of the Appraisal Guide for Findings of a Quantitative Study (Appendix F) to see how the issues you just read about are incorporated into appraisal.

Clinical Significance

The clinical significance of the findings of a quantitative study is determined by the strength of the relationship between variables in correlational studies or the size of the difference in the outcomes of the two treatment groups in experimental or quasi-experimental studies. In a correlational study, one would consider the size of the r^2s, whereas in a study comparing interventions, one would consider: (1) the difference in the means of the two groups, (2) the absolute benefit increase (ABI), (3) the numbers needed to treat (NNT), or (4) the relative risk (RR). Therefore, in intervention studies, the clinical significance question is: Is the treatment effect found in the study large enough to make a clinical difference in patient outcomes or well-being?

Applicability

As mentioned earlier, no applicability questions are provided for single, original studies because the assumption is that *generally* a change in practice will not be made based on one study. Having stated the general principle that findings from a single study should not be used as the basis for a change in practice, two exceptions should be noted. One exception would be when a diligent search did not come up with another study and the basis for current practice is clearly not effective. Of course, the study should have been soundly conducted. In the rare case when the findings of a single study will be used as the basis for practice, the applicability questions from the integrative research review (IRR) guide can be used.

The second exception to not using the findings from a single study as a basis for change might be the findings from a soundly conducted qualitative study. Some would assert that findings from even a single qualitative study make unique contributions to health care in that they humanize it (Zuzelo, 2007, p. 497). Findings from single qualitative studies provide understandings of patients' experiences that are useful for assessment, anticipatory guidance, and coaching (Kearney, 2001)—and this information can be incorporated into clinical protocols as well as individual practice. The usefulness of the findings from single qualitative studies is derived from the fact that most qualitative researchers provide considerable detail about the study participants' thoughts and feelings, their experiences, and the contexts of their lives. Thus, it is often quite clear with whom the findings might be used.

Your Turn

At this point, I suggest you appraise the Evangelista et al. (2008) study reprinted in Chapter 6 using the appraisal guide for Quantitative Studies (Appendix F). Then read the appraisal of it that a colleague and I did, which is Appendix G.

You also should consider completing an appraisal of the Jacobson et al. (2008) study in Chapter 4 or one of the qualitative studies listed at the book's website to get some practice appraising qualitative studies. Alternatively, your instructor may ask you to appraise one of the other articles reprinted in Part 1. The more appraisals you do, the better you will get at using the questions to make a judgment regarding the credibility and clinical significance of study findings.

Across-Studies Analysis

Now that you have some skill in appraising individual studies, you need to at least be aware of what is involved in appraising several studies regarding a question or issue. This would have to be done when an agency team could not locate an evidence-based clinical practice guideline or systematic review, but did find several relevant studies. In addition to appraising each study separately, the several studies should be appraised as a body of studies; doing so is called across-studies analysis (Brown, 1999). In essence, the team has to do its own integrative research review before translating the evidence into an agency protocol (Stetler et al., 1998). This will require identifying, retrieving, and appraising studies, then bringing together the findings from all relevant and sound studies.

Doing an across-studies review and summary is not something an individual would be expected to do. It is an advanced skill and is best done by a group in which the individual members' interpretations and thinking regarding the findings of the various studies can complement and correct one another. Generally, project teams who do across-studies analysis have a few members with master's or doctoral education. You may, however, be asked to be a member of an evidence-based practice (EBP) project team, in which case you will learn by direct observation how across-studies analysis is done. To prepare you for that, I offer a brief description of what across-studies analysis involves.

The goal in looking at a body of evidence is to answer the question, "What findings earn our confidence because they are well supported by one or more sound studies?" To answer this question, the protocol development team must determine the following:

- How many studies addressed the issue?
- Were the studies of good quality?
- Was the finding consistently produced by several well-conducted studies?
- If an intervention was studied, was the size of the treatment effect or the relationship of similar magnitude across the studies?
- Can inconsistencies regarding a finding be explained by study differences in patient populations or research methods?

Thus, the essential across-studies issues are the quality, quantity, and consistency of evidence across studies. If the project team is appraising two or more studies, they may work with a findings table (see **Table 16–2**). If the clinical issue has several subissues, such as prevention and management, the team might use separate findings tables for each subissue. As mentioned earlier, the team may decide to weight studies with strong methodology or samples similar to their own population of patients more heavily than studies with weak methodology or samples that are very different.

Unlike the findings of single studies, for which the general recommendation was made that they not be used as the basis for clinical protocols,

TABLE 16–2 Findings Table

Topic			Date	
Author(s) and date	Questions, variables, objectives, hypotheses	Design, sample, setting	Findings	Notes

whenever clear conclusions are produced by across-studies analysis, the conclusions can be used as the basis for practice. The applicability questions in the IRR appraisal guide will assist in planning implementation of across-studies conclusions.

Appraisal of findings from several or many studies involves decisions about the credibility, clinical significance, and applicability of the body of evidence. Ideally, these decisions should be reached in a deliberative way by the consensus of the EBP project team (Lomas, Culyer, McCutcheon, McAuley, & Law, 2005). A deliberative process requires the following:

- Clear objectives.
- Careful extraction of information from reports by at least two persons.
- Clear criteria for appraising the evidence.
- Clear rules regarding how to handle studies of poor quality.
- Good analytical thinking.
- Broad participatory dialogue.
- Formal polling to resolve differences of opinion.
- Skillful chairing.

Appendix H is a completed findings table pertaining to fatigue in patients with congestive heart failure. Information from the study you read earlier in Chapter 6 is extracted onto this table along with several other studies about the issue. Be advised that this findings table is not inclusive of all studies on this topic; rather the studies are representative of what might be found.

Wrap-Up

Evaluating a body of evidence is definitely the long and labor-intensive way of establishing the state of the science regarding an issue. However, sometimes a project group will have to do it; when necessary, it is important that the group include a person with knowledge of research methodology—be it an in-house person or a consultant.

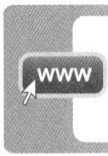

http://go.jblearning.com/brown3e

References

Brown, S. J. (1999). *Knowledge for health care practice: A guide to using research evidence*. Philadelphia, PA: Saunders.

Dixon-Woods, M., Shaw, R. I., Agarwal, S., & Smith, J. A. (2004). The problem of appraising qualitative research. *Quality & Safety in Health Care, 13*, 223–225.

Evangelista, L. S., Moser, D. K., Westlake, C., Pike, N., Ter-Galstanyan, A., & Dracup, K. (2008). Correlates of fatigue in patients with heart failure. *Progress in Cardiovascular Nursing, 23*(1), 12–17.

Fossey, E., Harvey, C., McDermott, F., & Davidson, L. (2002). Understanding and evaluating qualitative research. *Australian and New Zealand Journal of Psychiatry, 36*, 717–732.

Kearney, M. H. (2001). Levels and application of qualitative research evidence. *Research in Nursing and Health, 24*, 145–153.

Lincoln, Y. S., & Guba, E. G. (1985). *Naturalistic inquiry*. Beverly Hills, CA: Sage.

Lomas, J., Culyer, T., McCutcheon, C., McAuley, L., & Law, S. (2005). *Conceptualizing and combining evidence for health system guidance*. Canadian Health Services Research Foundation. Retrieved from http://www.chsrf.ca/migrated/pdf/insightAction/evidence_e.pdf

Mackey, M. C. (2007). Evaluation of qualitative research. In P. L. Munhall (Ed.), *Nursing research: A qualitative perspective* (4th ed., pp. 555–568). Sudbury, MA: Jones and Bartlett.

Morse, J. M., Barrett, M., Mayan, M., Olson, K., & Spiers, J. (2002). Verification strategies for establishing reliability and validity in qualitative research. *International Journal of Qualitative Methods 1*(2), article 2. Retrieved from http://www.ualberta.ca/~iiqm/backissues/1_2Final/html/morse.html

Stetler, C. B., Morsi, D., Rucki, S., Broughton, S., Corrigan, B., Fitzgerald, J., et al. (1998). Utilization-focused integrative reviews in a nursing service. *Applied Nursing Research, 11*(4), 196–206.

Stoddard, G. J., & Ring, W. H. (1993). How to evaluate study methodology in published clinical research. *Journal of Intravenous Nursing, 16*(2), 110–117.

Zuzelo, P. R. (2007). Evidence-based nursing and qualitative research: A partnership imperative for real-world practice. In P. L. Munhall (Ed.), *Nursing research: A qualitative perspective* (4th ed., pp. 481–499). Sudbury, MA: Jones and Bartlett.

CHAPTER SEVENTEEN

Evidence-Based Practice

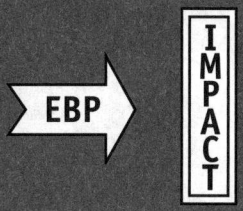

Now that you have some knowledge about how research is conducted and how to appraise research evidence for use as the basis of clinical practice, you need to learn how research evidence is translated into clinical actions with and for patients. In this and the next two chapters, the research–practice connection is explored in greater depth than it was early in the book. This chapter describes how healthcare agencies integrate evidence-based practice into clinical care protocols.

Professional Action

In an insightful book about the nature of professional practice (Schon, 1983), this very useful quote was offered: "All professional practice is centrally concerned with *design*, that is, with the process of changing existing situations into preferred ones" (Simon, 1969, p. 55).

This is a potentially powerful description of nursing. The image of a bridge is useful. One can visualize professional actions as spans of a bridge that link two sides of a river—on one side, a problematic or potentially problematic patient situation; on the other side, a better situation. Effective professional actions, which include acts of physical care and treatment, self-care teaching, and encouragement, help the patient get to a better state of health or wellness.

- In the hospital, when the patient is uncomfortable, the nurse repositions him or gives pain medication to make him comfortable; pain is

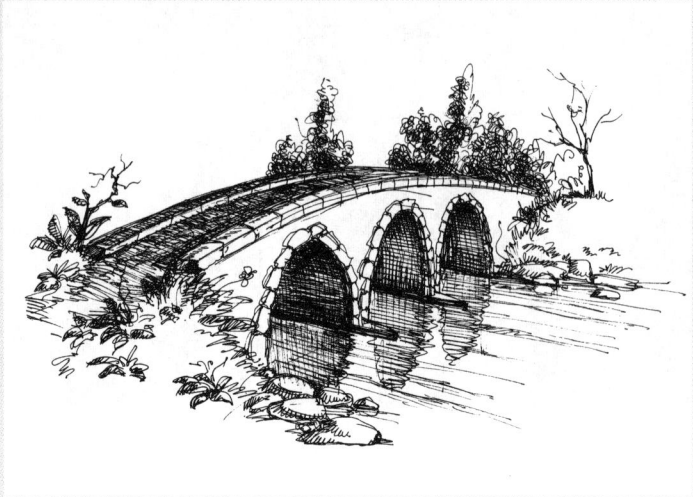

© Danussa/ShutterStock, Inc.

the existing situation, and comfort the preferred situation (discomfort → comfort).

- In the clinic, when a patient is at risk of hypertension, the nurse practitioner makes recommendations for lowering her blood pressure (existing level of risk → lower level of risk).
- At home, when the patient is not taking medications correctly, the nurse devises a system to promote more accurate medication taking (medication mistakes → fewer mistakes).
- In the ICU, when the patient has low oxygen saturation, the nurse suctions or repositions the patient to improve air exchange (low oxygenation → better oxygenation).

In all these situations, nurses help change problematic existing situations into preferred ones. Clearly, the ultimate goal of nursing, and indeed all of health care, is impact on patient outcomes.

Evidence-Based Care Design

The image of a bridge is applicable for another reason: A bridge is a designed structure. Bridges are not just put together at the site on a work-it-out-as-you-go basis. Rather, modern bridges are thoughtfully and carefully designed in advance using engineering knowledge that has been developed through research over the years. The same is true of professional nursing action—care should be designed in advance, to the degree possible, using scientific nursing knowledge.

Many providers work in clinical areas where most patients have health conditions that are seen over and over again. Thus, many aspects of care can be designed in advance of a particular patient. This is what is done when project teams develop clinical protocols for specific patient populations. Protocol development can be thought of as **prespecification design** in that the project team brings together knowledge about the issue and uses it as the basis for the protocol. Then, at the point of care,

> Clinicians combine the recommendation of the pre-specification care protocol with all they know about the individual patient. Based on their understanding of the patient and their own past experience dealing with similar patients, they make judgments about whether and how to alter the protocol. They decide how and when to deliver the pre-specified protocol and develop plans for clinical problems and issues not addressed by the protocol. (Brown, 2001, p. 5)

In brief, effective nursing care for individual patients requires sound prespecification design in the form of evidence-based clinical protocols and astute **point-of-care design** in the form of adapting clinical protocols to the individual patient.

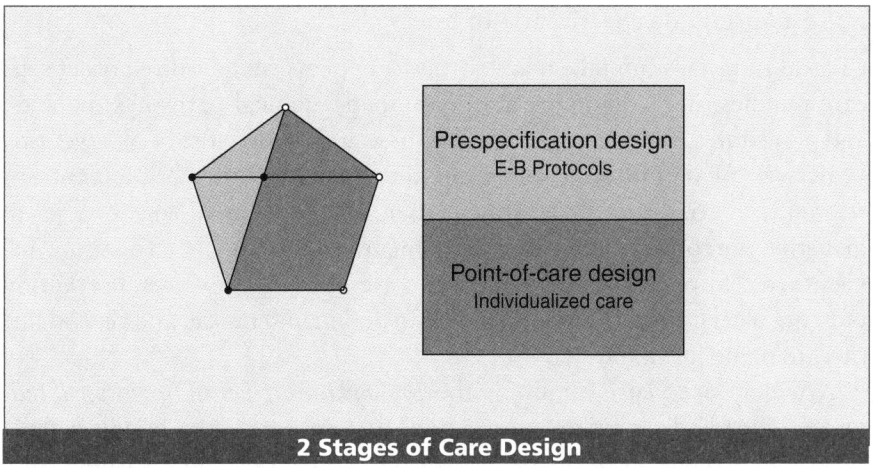

2 Stages of Care Design

Prespecification: Evidence-Based Care Protocols

There is general agreement that answers to the following kinds of questions should be based on the best scientific knowledge available.

- Does a combination of weekly tai chi and mindful meditation help obese middle-aged women lose weight?
- How should we carry out tight glucose control therapy with surgical patients?
- What is the best way to screen for domestic violence in the emergency department?
- Do peer support groups help preteens with chronic illness self-manage their illness and improve their integration into school activities?
- How can we differentiate between delirium, dementia, and depression in the elderly?

The practical hurdle to evidence-based practice is that practitioners engage in thousands of clinical actions each day. Obtaining and evaluating the research evidence for each action and each decision would be overwhelming for the individual practitioner. This is where agency-endorsed, clinical care protocols enter the picture—to support practitioners in their care planning and decision making. Clinical protocols serve two purposes:

1. They set forth standards of care to guide clinicians in giving care.
2. They promote consistency of patient care, that is, the care given by all providers to all patients in the population is similar; this ultimately benefits patients in terms of their experience of care and in terms of the effectiveness of care.

Clinical protocols can take many forms: care plans, standardized order sets, **care bundles**, decision algorithms, care maps, clinical pathways, policies, and procedures. References for each of these are listed on the book's website.

By way of definition, "a care bundle is a group of e-b interventions related to a condition or treatment that, when executed together, result in better outcomes than when implemented individually" (Institute for Healthcare Improvement, 2007). There are bundles for sepsis, preventing pressure ulcers, urinary catheter insertion and maintenance, and central line care, to name just a few.

A widely used care bundle is the *prevention-of-ventilator-associated-pneumonia* bundle; nursing interventions that are part of this bundle include elevation of the head of the bed, oral care, meticulous hand washing, suctioning secretions above the endotracheal cuff, and interruption of sedation

(Lawson, 2005). A review of six studies found that when used together, these practices decrease ventilator-associated pneumonia (O'Keefe-McCarthy, Santiago, & Lau, 2008).

An evidence-based bundle for the prevention and management of pressure ulcers was developed by a community hospital; it consisted of seven interventions: risk assessment, repositioning, minimal head-of-bed elevation, heel elevation, nutrition assessment, skin assessment, and sacral cleaning and moisturizing. They had good predata about their hospital-acquired pressure ulcer occurrences that served as a baseline for evaluating the impact of the bundle implementation (Gray-Siracusa & Schier, 2011).

Decision algorithms are step-by-step instructions for reaching a decision or solving a problem; they are often formatted as trees consisting of a series of yes/no questions leading to one of several possible decisions or actions. A clinical pathway, also called a care map, is a multidisciplinary specification of the actions to be implemented during the process of care for a well-defined group of patients over a specified period of time (DeBleser et al., 2006). A pathway explicitly sets forth time-specific goals, key elements and sequences of care, and specification of performance and coordinating roles.

Point-of-Care Design: Individualized Care

Care protocols help incorporate scientifically supported care actions into actual care and promote consistency of care. However, as noted earlier, most scientific evidence is based on what works best *on average*. Thus, even when the research evidence is strong in support of a care approach, we cannot expect everyone to benefit from it. Most certainly, scientifically based care has a high probability of benefiting patients in specified ways, but it is not a guarantee of effectiveness. Additionally, even though it is effective, the care approach may not be acceptable to some persons. For these reasons, a person's care ultimately should be individualized based on whether the care being offered is: (1) acceptable to him or her and (2) achieving its purposes. When care is adapted or modified to individual preferences and responses, it is considered individualized, personalized, or tailored to the individual.

Consider this example. A nurse saw a patient in a diabetes mellitus clinic. Noticing that he has some shortness of breath at rest, the nurse looked into his healthcare record to determine how his persistent asthma was being managed. He had a prescribed steroid inhaler (with a spacer) and a PRN inhaler for relief of shortness of breath. The nurse then asked the patient about how often he used the inhalers; he admitted that he did not use the steroid inhaler very often because "it has a bad taste, it dries out my mouth, and it ruins the taste of good food." He said he would rather use the PRN inhaler. The nurse explained the value of the steroid medication in preventing asthma symptoms and explained why it should be taken regularly, not when he needs more air. He said, "Yeah, I know." She also suggested gargling with warm water after using the steroid inhaler.

Two months later when the nurse saw the patient in the clinic, he was still noticeably short of breath. She asked about his use of the steroid inhaler. Again, he admitted that he was not using it very much. The nurse talked with him more and found out that he did not mind taking pills; she said she would talk with his physician about his medications and try to come up with an alternative approach for managing his asthma. Thus, even though the asthma protocol recommended inhaled steroid as a first-line treatment, his plan of care needed to be adjusted to take into account his rather strong aversion to using the inhaled steroid. This is individualized care. The nurse was attuned to how the patient was responding to protocol-recommended care and tried to help the patient get comfortable with it, but eventually she had to seek a different approach. As shown in **Figure 17–1**, at the point of care, the clinician and the patient together (whenever possible) decide if the evidence-based protocol endorsed by the agency or health system is appropriate, acceptable, and effective. The patient brings to this discussion responses, preferences, experiences, life goals, family support, and resources. The clinician brings clinical knowledge, prior experience with similar cases, and professional judgment. Through such an exchange, evidence-based protocols are tailored to the individual patient (Brown, 2001; Flynn & Sinclair, 2005; van der Weijden et al., 2010).

Goal: Quality Care

To state what is hopefully by now the obvious: The goal of evidence-based practice programs and projects is to improve quality of care by incorporating the best and most recent research evidence into the clinical care practices of the agency. An EBP program can be implemented as a series of projects to develop and introduce e-b clinical protocols, but generally this is not the most effective organizational strategy. There are several reasons why EBP projects should be embedded in a more dynamic way in a healthcare agency. The main reason is that EBP has a twin—another organizational program that also aims to improve the quality of care. The twin— fraternal, not identical—is quality improvement (QI).

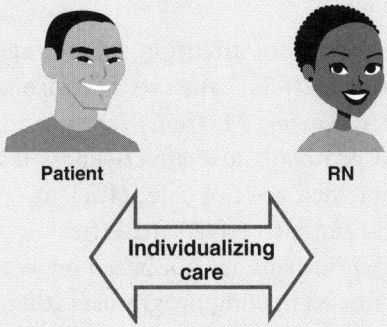

Figure 17-1 Tailoring Care to the Individual Patient
Art: Patient and RN illustrations © Moneca/ShutterStock, Inc.

Quality of care has several components: safety, effectiveness, patient-centeredness, timeliness, efficiency, and equity (Institute of Medicine, 2001). EBP programs and quality improvement programs work on different components of quality. EBP programs aim to improve the effectiveness and safety of clinical care by incorporating scientific evidence into care protocols and standards of care. QI programs aim to improve the performance of care delivery systems, which are made up of a network of logistics that support direct patient care services. That network includes patient movement in the system of care, scheduling, communications, product and equipment availability, role responsibilities, work patterns, and accountability structures. The aim of QI is to improve these operational activities and the connections among them with the goal of making care patient centered, safe, timely, efficient, and accessible.

An example of the difference: EBP uses knowledge produced by research to set standards for how patients are assessed for risk of skin breakdown during surgery and for steps that should be considered for various degrees and types of risk. In contrast, QI designs systems and collects data to assure that: (1) all patients are assessed for risk of skin breakdown, (2) appropriate bed surfaces are available, functional, and clean, and (3) the person in a particular job role is accountable for making sure that preventive measures against skin breakdown are taken for all patients but especially for patients at risk.

The difference in their foci of attention can be their strength (Batalden & Davidoff, 2007; Brown, 2006; Capuano, Davidson, & Hitchings, 2011; Ingersoll, 2005; Levin, Keefer, Marren, Vetter, Lauder, & Sobolewski, 2010. Evidence-based protocols lose effectiveness if the delivery systems in which they are embedded are not safe, efficient, and patient centered. In reverse, it makes no sense to have safe, efficient, and patient-centered delivery systems if care protocols are not based on available and sound science. QI and EBP are not competing programs; rather they can and should be complementary ones because they can achieve more together than either one can achieve by itself (Glasziou, Ogrinc, & Goodman, 2011). Each adds value to the other. Combining the two approaches leverages the strengths of both programs to ensure that the most effective clinical interventions are consistently provided to patients in a safe, efficient, timely, and patient-centered manner. Do be aware that quality improvement is just one of the names for programs aimed at improving safety and quality; other names are *performance improvement*, *continuous quality improvement*, *total quality improvement*, and *quality management*.

QI Programs

Quality improvement programs monitor indicators of safety and quality on an ongoing basis but also collect special-purpose data when a problem or potential problem is identified. Some of the data collected pertains to the processes of care, such as:

- In a home care agency, was the fall prevention assessment required by the protocol for patients over age 65 completed on the first visit?
- Did patients in the emergency department who had signs of a myocardial infarction receive aspirin at arrival?
- Did all patients admitted to the hospital with a subdural hematoma resulting from a fall at home receive a home care referral at the time of discharge as required by protocol?
- Were preoperative patients assessed specifically for skin allergies?

Other data is about patient outcomes such as:

- Infection rates with central lines.
- Self-harm events in inpatient psychiatry.

- Average hemoglobin A1c level for the population of patients seen in a clinic.
- Number of injuries related to the use of physical restraints or bed rails.
- Percentage of patients treated in a geriatric clinic who were on an antidepressant medication for 6 months or more.
- Readmission rates after acute care hospitalization.

Of course, the purpose of collecting this data is to identify weaknesses in the quality of care being given as a precursor to taking action to improve the care.

Standards of Care A great deal of ongoing data collection, analysis, and reporting is mandated by certifying agencies such as the Centers for Medicare and Medicaid Services (CMS) and by accrediting agencies such as the Joint Commission. At this point, the QI landscape is complex and has many players (e.g., the Agency for Healthcare Research and Quality (AHRQ), the National Quality Forum, the CMS, the Joint Commission, the American Nurses Association, the Institute for Healthcare Improvement, and the LEAPFROG Group). As a result, there are many sets of quality indicators, which may be referred to as accountability measures, performance measures, or effective care measures. Fortunately, the players are beginning to work together to reduce the indicators to those that:

1. Have strong research support.
2. Are closely connected to good patient outcomes.
3. Actually measure whether the evidence-based care has been provided.
4. Have few or no associate adverse effects (Joint Commission, 2012).

The AHRQ website has an inventory of quality measures from around the world. An example is the CMS/Joint Commission accountability measure, "Urinary catheter is removed on Postoperative Day 1 (POD 1) or Postoperative Day 2 (POD 2), with Day of Surgery Being Day Zero." The performance standard for this and similar measures is 85%. The rationale for this standard and the research evidence supporting the rationale are given on the AHRQ website (AHRQ, 2012).

It is beyond the scope of this book to go deeply into how quality measures are used to promote quality of care, but I will say that the influence of these national agencies and organizations on EBP is tremendous. By requiring compliance with e-b performance standards and by making information about compliance publicly available, they are infusing EBP into the healthcare patients receive—big time! One way this is being done is that quality measures are being used to provide reimbursement bonuses for hospitals that perform well or improve on certain quality goals (CMS, 2012).

Also, I do want to point out that *National Database of Quality Indicators* (ANA, n.d.) is aimed at improving patient outcomes by improving nursing care at the unit level. Nursing departments participating in this program collect data about nursing-sensitive indicators, which are aspects of care that are particularly influenced by the quality of nursing care (Montalvo, 2007). The indicators are comprised of specific performance measures pertaining to restraint use, IV infiltrations, falls, pain management, and incidence and prevalence of pressure ulcers. Participating hospitals submit data and get back an analysis of their data as well as comparisons to similar hospitals. This kind of comparison is called benchmarking, and it provides a hospital with a sense of what is achievable. The trend in the data is also important because it indicates whether changes aimed at improving an area of deficiency are working. For instance, a hospital might determine that the patient fall level on their medical unit is 2.8 falls per 1,000 patient days, whereas similar units in their benchmarking network have a fall rate of 1.9 falls per 1,000 patient days; the indicators also indicate which fall prevention activities are and are not being performed. Once the specific performance deficiencies related to fall prevention have been identified and corrective action taken, the nursing sensitive indicator data will hopefully show that nursing practice relative to this issue has improved and that the fall rate has declined.

Improving Care Delivery Systems In addition to improving performance by measuring care given against e-b standards of care and making changes in clinical practices, QI programs also work to improve the system of care delivery by reducing errors, improving efficiency and communication, improving scheduling, maximizing patient flow within the system, reducing patients admitted to off-service beds, and increasing the capacity of a specialty area such as the operating rooms. Again there are many methods for analyzing and redesigning delivery systems, but most rely heavily on collecting data and detailed analysis of work flow.

To really understand what is and is not working well in a system of care may require really digging deeply into the details of who does what, when, and how. Observation, data collection, brainstorming, surveys, tracking logs, activity counts, process maps, activity diaries, and flow diagrams (see **Figure 17–2**) are used to understand what could be done better and to design a revised process of care (Hemman, 2011; Nelson, Batalden, &

Godfrey, 2007). The kinds of process-of-care problems identified include weak communication among providers and with patients, inconsistency in care methods, delays and blockages in patient movement through the system, weak support systems, slow turnover between activities, lack of knowledge about standards of care, noncompliance with standards of care, and cost inefficiencies.

Although the data collected to make these kinds of determinations are usually retrospective, the goal is to make the improvement cycle as short as possible—from understanding the issues involved to designing changes in the delivery systems to making changes, and then to evaluating the impact of the changes. QI projects are increasingly carried out at the microsystem level; that is, by the people who work together to deliver care to a population of patients (Dartmouth Institute, 2011). This may be the unit, such as the mental health unit, or a service line, such as those providing care to patients with pulmonary diseases, or a home care agency.

QI methods for analyzing and improving care delivery processes include Lean, Six Sigma, and Plan-Do-Check-Act (Glasgow, 2011). There are similarities and differences in these approaches to quality improvement, and they can be used in combination with one another, but all have as a goal improving the safety, efficiency, timeliness, and patient-centeredness of care. It is highly likely that one of these quality improvement programs, or a combination of them, is being used in the agencies in which you are having

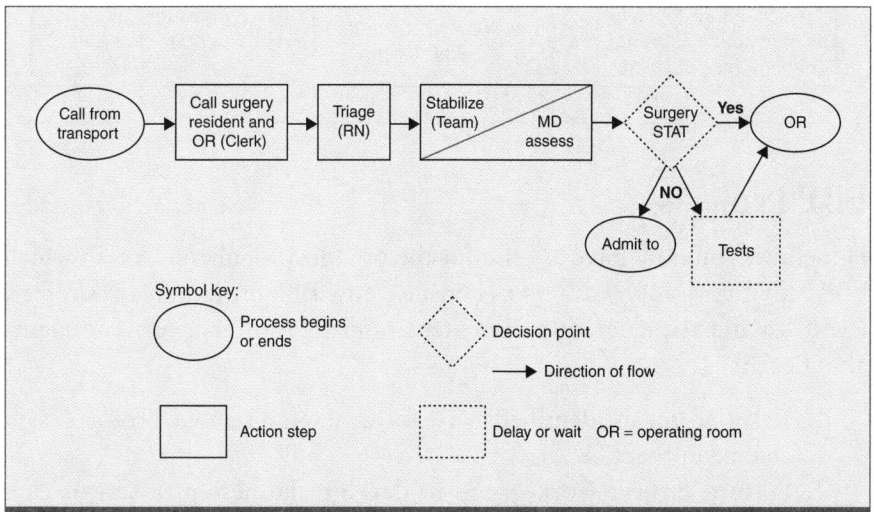

Figure 17-2 Example of a Flow Diagram

your clinical experiences. References about these programs are listed on the companion website.

QI and EBP Relationship

Quality improvement has a broader mission than EBP, which impacts quality in a very specific way. As acknowledged earlier, EBP projects can be undertaken independent of a broader QI effort or they can be part of a broader QI project. My bias toward the latter is clear. Either way, QI methods can serve as bookends to EBP projects. QI outcome monitoring is often the tool that identifies an area of weak practice and not infrequently the weakness is due, at least in part, to the lack of a clear, evidence-based standard of care. At that point, an e-b project to develop a new protocol or change in practice may be launched. Before beginning the project, however, it is often wise to use QI performance measurement methods to pinpoint the problem more exactly and to document baseline performance. Once the e-b protocol has been implemented, repeat QI measurement of performance and outcomes can help quantify the success of the implementation and the impact of the protocol. Thus QI measurement often bookends an EBP project. For specific examples of projects that used QI and EBP methods in combination, see the book's website.

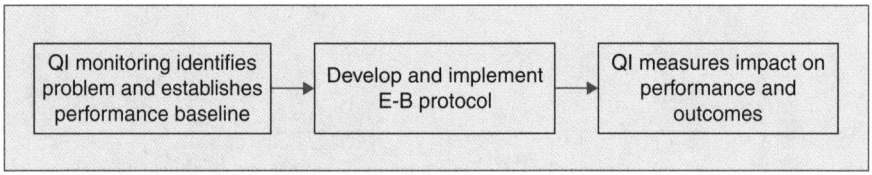

EBP Projects

Hopefully, you now have a sense for the organizational contexts in which EBP activities reside. Now, let us consider how EBP projects play out. First I will list the sequence of action steps, and then offer a few comments about each:

1. Respond to an identified need for a new or revised protocol or a change in practice.
2. Form a project work group to develop the new protocol or care innovation.

3. Search for relevant research evidence.
4. Extract information from relevant evidence reports.
5. Eliminate poor quality evidence.
6. Use recommendations/conclusions/findings from the qualifying reports to design a clinical protocol.
7. Plan implementation of the protocol.
8. Evaluate impact of the protocol.
9. If necessary, revisit and revise the protocol or its implementation.

Respond to an Identified Need

Common triggers for an EBP project are:

1. A person or persons within the organization recognize that care could be improved by introducing a new method or updating an existing one.
2. Quality monitoring data reveals that care methods used with a particular population of patient or some aspect of care is less effective than it could be.
3. An accrediting or certifying agency imposes a standard of care but leaves open the methods the agency uses to meet the standard.
4. A new component of care is going to be introduced (e.g., continuous oxygen saturation monitoring or a new body-cooling device).

Form a Project Work Group

The EBP project requires a team with knowledge and skills in the following areas:

- Familiarity with how the work of unit or service line is done.
- Searching citation databases for relevant e-b guidelines, SRs, and reports.
- Familiarity with collection and analysis of data in the organization.
- Critically appraising guidelines, summaries, and individual research reports.
- Designing evidence-based protocols.
- Working within the larger system of care to implement organizational change.

To possess the full complement of skills, the team may be comprised of direct care providers, advanced practice nurses, managers, a health science librarian, a quality improvement staff person, and an EBP specialist (e.g., nurse researcher).

Search for Relevant Research Evidence

Searching for evidence was addressed extensively in Chapter 12; however I will reiterate the mantra that finding evidence-based clinical practice guidelines and systematic reviews can greatly reduce the time required to develop an agency protocol. As important, the use of EbCPGs and SRs increases the likelihood that the evidence used includes all important evidence sources.

Extract Information

Generally the accuracy of the information used to develop a clinical protocol can be increased if at least two persons read the report and extract the information. An extraction guide and findings tables are valuable tools in producing accurate and useful evidence displays.

Eliminate Poor Quality Evidence

The evidence must be appraised to eliminate poor, noncredible, or nonapplicable sources. Ergo, the chapters on appraisal you have just read.

Design a Clinical Protocol

The actions that comprise the protocol should be faithful to the available evidence. This requires that the project team proceed systematically, objectively, and logically—with considerable attention to detail. Committing to achieving consensus prior to including each action in the protocol will also help produce an agency protocol that is truly based on the evidence.

Most assuredly, there will be times when the project group feels the need to include a clinical action for which no research evidence exists. If the project team feels it is important, it should be included (Goode, Fink, Krugman, Oman, & Traditi, 2011).

Plan Implementation of the Protocol

Here we are on new ground and very difficult ground indeed. Even when clinicians value research evidence and strive to practice in an evidence-based way, a new protocol may be difficult to incorporate into a busy day. There are many reasons why staff may not follow an evidence-based protocol. Among them: the needed supplies may not be readily available, the protocol may not fit in with the work flow, or a learning curve may be associated with some aspect of the new protocol.

Research in the area of translating research into practice has determined that the adoption of an evidence-based innovation in practice depends on many factors. These factors can be grouped as:

a. Characteristics of the e-b innovation itself.
b. Facilitation strategies used to introduce the innovation.
c. Characteristic of the targeted adopters.
d. The work dynamics of the setting into which the practice is introduced (Kitson et al., 2008; Titler, 2008).

Each of these factors is complex in itself.

Characteristics of the Evidence-Based Innovation Some innovations or changes in practice ask little of the clinicians, but others ask a great deal. Leaders introducing an evidence-based innovation should be sensitive to what the innovation is asking of busy clinicians. Clinicians will be more receptive to innovations that they see as important to patients' well-being, as opposed to what they view as change for change's sake.

Facilitation Strategies Facilitation involves making it as easy as possible for practitioners to make the needed change in practice but also working with them to make sense of the evidence leading to the change (Rycroft-Malone, 2004). It involves creating convincing communication, a smooth path to change, and support while making the change to new care behaviors. Strategies found to be persuasive in promoting adoption of a care innovation include:

- Analyzing how the innovation fits into the clinical process and workflow of those who will have to change how they do things and making it as easy as possible to incorporate the innovation (e.g., pocket checklist, clinical information system reminders, easy reference guides).
- Creating awareness and interest in the innovation through staff meetings, posters, continuing education, and reminders of the clinical information system.

- Providing practice or interactive learning with any new equipment being introduced.
- Having influential persons in the peer group lead the rollout of the innovation and troubleshoot its implementation.
- Having persons with recognized expertise on the topic present the science underpinning the innovation (also called academic detailing).
- Sustaining the innovation through feedback sessions, fine tuning the innovation based on feedback, patient outcome reports, celebrating unit progress, public recognition, and individual performance evaluation (Cullen & Adams, 2012).

Making a change in practice typically encounters both enthusiasm and resistance. Cullen, Greiner, Greiner, Bombei, and Comried (2005) described the *tag-flag-nag* approach to supporting EBP innovation. Tagging involves identifying and visibly recognizing staff nurses who adopt the practice change. Flagging involves identifying less compliant staff and discussing with them how they can incorporate the change into their care. Nagging is the way of dealing with persistent noncompliers; it involves recruiting opinion leaders on the unit to talk with the noncompliers about their failure to adopt the new standard of care, and, if necessary, more firm ways of dealing with their resistance to change. Thus, leaders use a variety of carrot and stick strategies to convey that quality of care is the goal and that persons who detract from that goal will be held accountable for their failure to meet unit standards (Stetler, Ritchie, Rycroft-Malone, Schultz, & Charns, 2009).

In a sense, a care system is like an ocean liner in that quite a bit of energy has to be put forth to make even a small change in course. So, introducing a change in practice is a real all-hands-on-deck situation.

The Targeted Adopters The probability of the users being receptive to an innovation in practice is greater if they have been oriented to the organization's QI and EBP goals and exposed to them on an ongoing basis such as in orientation, nursing grand rounds, journal clubs, and professional development programs. How-are-we-doing reports that inform staff about their progress in meeting performance targets also promote buy-in to evidence-based changes (Rees, Leahy-Gross, & Mack, 2011). One very helpful strategy is for new staff to have a preceptor who helps smooth their adjustment to their job but who also mentors them in understanding organizational goals, the QI and EBP programs, and innovations being implemented in their immediate setting. Over time the nurse being mentored hopefully will come to see the value of QI and EBP and want to become more active in projects in his unit or work group.

Work-Setting Dynamics The reality is that some units or service lines are more committed to e-b care than others. In part that is because the leaders value e-b improvement and encourage the staff to identify clinical care that is not being done in an effective manner. Support from nurse executives and directors can take the form of creating a culture of quality, taking interest in individual projects, committing resources (like dedicated time away from direct care responsibilities to work on the project), and recognition once the project is completed (Cullen & Adams, 2012). Some larger agencies are able to create a job position that is specifically devoted to leading and supporting QI and EBP innovation. However, enthusiasm for EBP doesn't just come from leaders; it can bubble up from one or two staff members. And sometimes it just takes just one project to produce good results and thereby set the stage for others.

Most clinicians are working in complex environments where many standards of care must be kept in mind. In addition, changes in standards, technology, and medication are introduced at a rapid pace. There is no settling into a groove. Clinicians have to stay informed about changing standards that affect them and be flexible to meet new standards.

Remember from the study about endotracheal suctioning in Chapter 5 how many specific action standards the nurses had to keep in mind for just that one procedure. Another health system found that in one of its medical ICUs, 38% of their patients were on two or more care bundles (Hurd, 2011); each bundle included a set of specific actions that must be incorporated into care. That means the nurse giving care to those patients had to give care in accordance with quite a few specific action standards. Keeping many standards in mind puts quite a cognitive strain on the nurse in that she not only has to be fully immersed in the immediate care situation, but also has to be keeping in mind the actions required by the care standards (Krichbaum et al., 2007). In response to this complexity, real-time clinical information systems are being developed to prompt clinical staff in delivering care in accord with the many standards.

"Nurses have so much to think about!"
—Hurd, 2011

Evaluate the Impact

Even when an evidence-based protocol was carefully developed and introduced, there needs to be a check on its ultimate impact. If the introduction of the e-b protocol or innovation was part of a large QI project, evaluation will naturally be undertaken. Many of the measurements used to analyze the care system early on can be repeated to determine if the protocol has been adopted and is having the desired impact.

Note that the appraisal guides for clinical practice guidelines and integrative research reviews (IRRs) you learned about earlier include a question about how the protocol innovation will be evaluated. This question is included because the impact evaluation should be planned at the time the protocol is developed and introduced, not as an afterthought. Typically, measurement of performance and outcomes before, during, and after implementation of a change in practice is needed to be sure that the new protocol has resulted in the desired patient outcomes and that the change is being maintained over time. Too often improvements in performance and outcomes realized a few months after introducing an innovation are lost over time; thus monitoring of performance and outcomes should continue long term (Glasgow, 2011).

If Necessary, Revisit and Revise

If the anticipated results are not occurring, the protocol and the context in which it was embedded must be revisited to determine why it is not working, including the following questions:

- Was the evidence not interpreted correctly?
- Was the translation of the evidence into the agency protocol faulty?
- Was the implementation lacking in some way?
- Is the protocol unrealistic or in conflict with other job expectations?

The pursuit of quality care is indeed demanding and ongoing.

Organizational Integration of EBP

Some agencies and nursing department have integrated QI-EBP programs and see value in the integration (Capuano, Davidson, & Hitchings, 2011; Levin et al., 2010; Pardee & Rundquist, 2011). Others have chosen to have separate programs but recognize the need for strong communication and linkages between them (Newhouse, Dearholt, & Poe, 2007; Oman, 2011; Pardee & Rundquist, 2011). A nursing department or agency with integrated programs might have a Best Practice Council or a Quality of Care Council that combines both QI and EBP missions and goals. If the QI and EBP councils are separate, strong linkages could be built by something as simple as overlapping membership or just sharing of agendas between the EBP council and the QI council. Or the linkage could be more structured such as a Shared Governance Council or Coordinating Council made up of members of all councils. Another dynamic structural arrangement is to have a Nursing Practice Council whose mission is to "implement and maintain standards of clinical nursing practice and patient care consistent with evidence-based practice and requirements of regulatory agencies" (UNC Health Care System, 2012). Such an organizational structure could provide strong linkages between QI, EBP, and nursing care standard setting.

To get more specific about the importance of integrating QI and EBP deeply and dynamically into a nursing department or agency, a Nursing Practice Council should not revise nursing procedures and policies without referring to the research base relevant to the issue. A Quality Management Council should not develop a Foley catheter care protocol without considering the research evidence about insertion and maintenance of an indwelling catheter system (Batalden & Davidoff, 2007). A Research/EBP Committee in a home care agency should not develop an evidence-based program for managing polypharmacy in their elderly patients without data that sheds light on exactly what kinds of problems are actually occurring. In summary, the overlapping and multifaceted nature of QI and EBP efforts makes it wise to structure an organization in a way that creates dynamic linkages between QI, EBP, and practice (Cullen et al., 2005).

Then there is the related matter of supporting the conduct of research. Agencies that have few activities related to the conduct of research may find that a combined Research-EBP Council works well for them. Whereas larger nursing departments that engage in many activities related to the conduct of research may find it more productive to have separate research and EBP councils or at least separate subcommittees within a combined council. Clearly, there is no one best way to position EBP functions in an organization. Organization missions are overlapping, so there must be collaboration between councils (Oman, 2011).

Research–Practice Lag

A reality check is in order. In fact, many clinical care providers have been slow to incorporate research findings into clinical practice. A recent article detailed one such lag in research evidence uptake—the safety of allowing clear liquids until 2 hours before surgery (Crenshaw, 2011). Research evidence regarding the safety of allowing this has been available for 25 years, yet orders for *NPO after MN* persist. I highly recommend that you read Dr. Crenshaw's interesting and readable article.

Another interesting case in point is nurses' choice of intramuscular injection sites. In a 2007 study of 652 Canadian nurses, 71% preferred using the dorsal gluteal buttock site over the ventrogluteal hip site—even though the buttock sites carries a higher risk of nerve and muscle damage (Walsh & Brophy, 2011) and research evidence about the greater safety of the hip site has been available for more than 50 years!

Reasons for the slow uptake of solid research evidence are numerous. The following are among those most frequently cited:

- The way research questions are asked.
- The way research findings are communicated.
- Conflicting findings from several studies.
- Clinicians' limited ability to locate, understand, and assess research evidence.
- Clinicians' lack of time to find and read research reports.
- The cultural and structural characteristics of the work setting.

For those with an interest in the research–practice lag, there is a large body of literature on the barriers to and facilitators of research being adopted into practice (Chau, Lopez, & Thompson, 2008; Gale & Schaffer, 2009; Solomons & Spross, 2011).

Most assuredly, the access to research evidence is greatly improved in recent years; the formats are more clinician friendly; and the ability of clinicians to locate, read, and understand research articles is increasing. Moreover, government and privately funded initiatives in many countries are promoting evidence-based practice and funding studies about how to best translate research findings into practice.

In spite of initiatives aimed at making it easier for clinicians to learn about evidence-based clinical methods, studies have found that the percentage of patients receiving medical care recommended in e-b clinical practice guidelines is around 55%, although there is quite a bit of variability by condition and setting (Institute of Medicine, 2011, p. 146). This room for improvement makes studies about the effectiveness of various ways of introducing evidence-based changes in practice, i.e., translation research, very important going forward.

Recap

At this point, I suggest you pause to consider all that has been presented to this point in the book. **Figure 17–3** portrays the really big picture beginning with recognition that knowledge for practice is not adequate, proceeding through the steps of knowledge production and EBP, and finally to confidence that patients are being given the best care possible and as result are achieving good health outcomes. It is a long path, but we owe it to our patients, to society, to our profession, and to ourselves as professional nurses to walk the EBP walk.

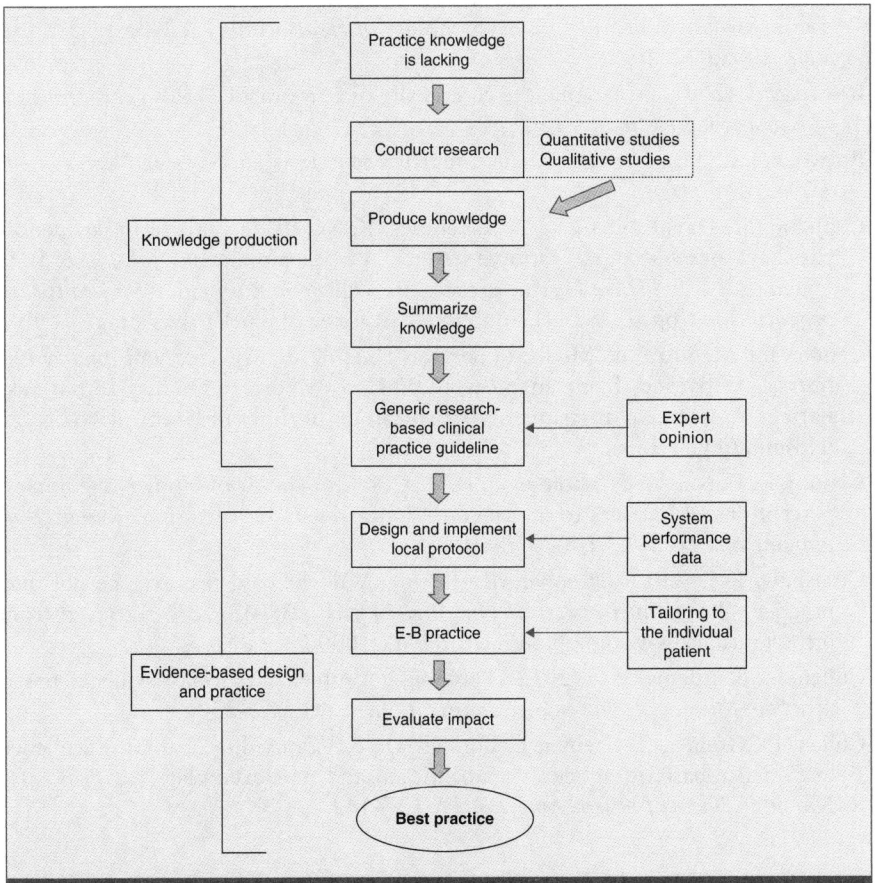

Figure 17-3 Really Big Picture

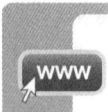

http://go.jblearning.com/brown3e

References

AHRQ. (2012). *Surgical care improvement project: Percent of surgical patients with urinary catheter removed on postoperative day 1 or postoperative day 2 with the day of surgery being day zero.* Retrieved May 24, 2012 from http://www.qualitymeasures.ahrq.gov/content.aspx?id=27416&search=surgical+care

American Nurses Association (ANA). (n.d.). The National Database of Nursing Quality Indicators. Retrieved May 24, 2012 from http://www.nursingworld.org/ndnqi2

Batalden, P. B., & Davidoff, F. (2007). What is "quality improvement" and how can it transform healthcare? *Quality & Safety in Healthcare, 16*, 2–3. doi:101136/qshc.2006.022046

Brown, S. J. (2001). Managing the complexity of best practice health care. *Journal of Nursing Care Quality, 15*(2), 1–8.

Brown, S. J. (2006). The performance improvement decision. *Nursing Management 37*(4), 16–17.

Capuano, T., Davidson, C. L., & Hitchings, K. S. (2011). Integrating evidence-based practice with organizational systems: A case example. In J. Houser & K. S. Oman (Eds.), *Evidence-based practice: An implementation guide for healthcare organizations* (pp. 231–247). Sudbury, MA: Jones & Bartlett Learning.

Centers for Medicare & Medicaid Services (CMS). (2012). *Hospital quality initiative.* Retrieved from http://www.cms.gov/Medicare/Quality-Initiatives-Patient-Assessment-Instruments/HospitalQualityInits/index.html?redirect=/HospitalQualityInits/

Chau, J. P., Lopez, V., & Thompson, D. R. (2008). A survey of Hong Kong nurses' perceptions of barriers to and facilitators of research utilization. *Research in Nursing and Health, 31*(6), 640–649.

Crenshaw, J. T. (2011). Preoperative fasting: Will the evidence ever be put into practice? *American Journal of Nursing, 111*(10), 38–43. Also retrieved from http://journals.lww.com/ajnonline/toc/2011/10000

Cullen, L., & Adams, S. L. (2012). Planning for implementation of evidence-based practice. *Journal of Nursing Administration, 42*(4), 222–230.

Cullen, L., Greiner, J., Greiner, J., Bombei, C., & Comried, L. (2005). Excellence in evidence-based practice: Organizational and unit exemplars. *Critical Care Nursing Clinics of North America, 17*, 127–142.

Dartmouth Institute. (2011). *Clinical microsystems*. Retrieved from http://clinicalmicrosystem.org/about/background/

DeBleser, L., Depreitere, R., De Waele, K., VanHaecht, K., Vlayen, J., & Sermeus, W. (2006). Defining pathways. *Journal of Nursing Management, 14*(7), 553–563.

Flynn, A. V., & Sinclair, M. (2005). Exploring the relationship between nursing protocols and nursing practice in an Irish intensive care unit. *International Journal of Nursing Practice, 11*, 142–149.

Gale, B. V. P., & Schaffer, M. A. (2009). Organizational readiness for evidence-based practice. *Journal of Nursing Administration, 19*(2), 91–97.

Glasgow, J. (2011). *Introduction to Lean and Six Sigma approaches to quality improvement*. Retrieved from http://www.qualitymeasures.ahrq.gov/expert/expert-commentary.aspx?id=32943

Glasziou, P., Ogrinc, G., & Goodman, S. (2011). Can evidence-based medicine and clinical quality improvement learn from each other? *BMJ Quality and Safety, 20*, i13–i17. Retrieved from http://qualitysafety.bmj.com/content/20/Suppl_1/i13.full.html

Goode, C. J., Fink, R. M., Krugman, M., Oman, K. S., & Traditi, L. K. (2011). The Colorado patient-centered interprofessional evidence-based practice model: A framework for transformation. *Worldviews on Evidence-Based Nursing* (2nd quarter), 96–105.

Gray-Siracusa, K., & Schier, L. (2011). Use of an intervention bundle to eliminate pressure ulcers in critical care. *Journal of Nursing Care Quality, 26*(3), 216–225.

Hemman, E. A. (2011). Cultivating quality: Meeting effective care measures. *American Journal of Nursing, 111*(12), 54–60.

Hurd, D. (2011). *Quality initiative and the concept of complexity compression*. Presentation at the Nursing Leadership Congress. Retrieved from http://sites.mckesson.com/nlcplc/documents/NLC%20Breakout%20Session_Quality%20Initiatives%20and%20the%20Concept%20of%20Complexity%20Compression_Presentation.pdf

Institute for Healthcare Improvement. (2007). What is a bundle? Retrieved from http://www.ihi.org/knowledge/Pages/ImprovementStories/WhatIsaBundle.aspx

Institute of Medicine. (2001). *Crossing the quality chasm: A new health system for the 21st century*. Retrieved from http://www.iom.edu/~/media/Files/Report%20Files/2001/Crossing-the-Quality-Chasm/Quality%20Chasm%202001%20%20report%20brief.pdf

Institute of Medicine (2011). *Clinical practice guidelines we can trust*. Retrieved from http://www.nap.edu/catalog.php?record_id=13058

Joint Commission. (2012). Facts about accountability measures. Retrieved from http://www.jointcommission.org/assets/1/18/Accountability_measures_7_1_111.PDF

Kitson, A., Rycroft-Malone, J., Harvey, G., McCormack, B., Seers, K., & Titchen, A. (2008). Evaluating the successful implementation of evidence into practice using the PARIHS framework: Theoretical and practical challenges. *Implement Science, 3*(1). Retrieved from http://www.implementationscience.com/content/pdf/1748-5908-3-1.pdf

Krichbaum, K., Diemart, C., Jacox, L., Jones, A, Koenig, P., Mueller, C, & Disch, J. (2007). Complexity compression: Nurses under fire. *Nursing Forum, 42,* 86–94.

Lawson, P. (2005). Zapping VAP with evidence-based practice. *Nursing 2005, 35*(3), 66–67.

Levin, R. F., Keefer, J. M., Marren, J., Vetter, M., Lauder, B., & Sobolewski, S. (2010). Evidence-based practice improvement: Merging 2 paradigms. *Journal of Nursing Care Quality, 25*, 117–126.

Montalvo, I. (2007). The national database of nursing quality indicators (NDNQI®). *Online Journal of Issues in Nursing, 12* (3). Retrieved from http://www.nursingworld.org/MainMenuCategories/ANAMarketplace/ANAPeriodicals/OJIN/TableofContents/Volume122007/No3Sept07/NursingQualityIndicators.aspx

Nelson, E. C., Batalden, P. B. & Godfrey, M. M. (2007). *Quality by design: A clinical microsystems approach.* San Francisco, CA: Jossey-Bass.

Newhouse, R. P., Dearholt, S., Poe, S., Pugh, L. C., & White, K. M. (2007). Organizational change strategies for evidence-based practice. *Journal of Nursing Administration 37*(12), 552–557.

Oman, K. S. (2011). Developing a structure for evidence-based practice. In J. Houser & K. S. Oman (Eds.). *Evidence-based practice: An implementation guide for healthcare organizations* (pp. 73-82). Sudbury, MA: Jones & Bartlett.

O'Keefe-McCarthy, S., Santiago, C., & Lau, G. (2008). Ventilator-associated pneumonia bundled strategies: An evidence-based practice. *Worldviews on Evidence-Based Nursing, 5*(4), 193–204.

Pardee, C., & Rundquist, J. (2011). Systems for identifying EBP opportunities. In J. Houser & K. S. Oman (Eds.), *Evidence-based practice: An implementation guide for healthcare organizations* (pp. 125–138). Sudbury, MA: Jones & Bartlett.

Rees, S., Leahy-Gross, K., & Mack, V. (2011). Moving data to nursing quality excellence. *Journal of Nursing Care Quality, 26*, 260–264.

Rycroft-Malone, J. (2004). The PARIHS framework—a framework for guiding the implementation of evidence-based practice. *Journal of Nursing Care Quality, 19*(4), 297–304.

Schon, D. A. (1983). *The reflective practitioner: How professionals think in action.* New York, NY: Basic Books.

Simon, H. (1969). *The sciences of the artificial.* Cambridge, MA: MIT Press.

Solomons, N. M. & Spross, J. A. (2011). Evidence-based practice barriers and facilitators from a continuous quality improvement perspective: an integrative review. *Journal of Nursing Management, 19,* 109-120.

Stetler, C. B., Ritchie, J., Rycroft-Malone, J., Schultz, A. A. & Charns, P. (2009). Institutionalizing evidence-based practice: An organizational case study using a model of strategic change. *Implementation Science, 4(1),* 78.

Titler, M. G. (2008). The evidence for evidence-based practice Implementation. In *Patient safety and quality: An evidence-based handbook for nurses* (chap 7). Rockville, MD: Agency for Healthcare Research and Quality publication no. 08-0043. Retrieved from http://www.ahrq.gov/qual/nurseshdbk/

UNC Health Care System. (2012). *Professional practice council bylaws.* Retrieved from http://www.unchealthcare.org/site/Nursing/sharedgov/profpractice/index_html

van der Weijden, T., Legare, F., Boivin, A., Burgers, J. S., van Veendaal, H., Stiggelbout, A. M., et al. (2010). How to integrate individual patient values and preferences in clinical practice guidelines? A research protocol. *Implementation Science (5)*10. Retrieved from http://www.implementationscience.com/content/5/1/10

Walsh, L., & Brophy, K. (2011). Staff nurses' sites of choice for administering intramuscular injections to adult patients in the acute care setting. *Journal of Advanced Nursing, 67*(5), 1034–1040.

CHAPTER EIGHTEEN

Evidence-Based Practice Participation Scenarios

There are several scenarios in which you might volunteer or be asked to participate in an evidence-based practice activity. I thought I could provide a bit of guidance in this regard. Five scenarios will be described, and suggestions will be made regarding participation:

1. As a member of a project team, you are asked to appraise one or several pieces of research evidence and give a short oral presentation about it.
2. You decide to submit an evidence-based poster to be displayed at an association congress.
3. You want to present an evidence-based clinical idea or concern to your nurse leader, clinical nurse specialist, or nurse manager.
4. As a participant in a patient care planning conference, you present research evidence relevant to the care of a patient with complex issues.
5. Evidence-based practice really interests you and you want to further develop you EBP knowledge and skills

In the first four scenarios, you want to be organized and carefully select what you present, so you need to do your homework.

Join a Project Team

First, let's imagine a context for this scenario. You work as a staff nurse on an orthopedic unit. The unit is looking at its use of special beds and bed surfaces for patients at risk of skin breakdown. The work group is charged with developing a decision algorithm or decision tree regarding the use of special beds and surfaces. The unit already uses a risk assessment scale to quantify patients' risk for skin breakdown. In PICOTS terms, this question would be outlined as follows:

P: Patients with orthopedic injuries and/or recovering from orthopedic surgery who are at risk for skin breakdown
I: Special beds and mattress overlays
C: Effectiveness of each and when to use one rather than another
O: Prevention of skin breakdown
T: Before breakdown occurs
S: Inpatient orthopaedics

The group decides to start by examining the effectiveness of various support surfaces aimed at preventing skin breakdown and then proceed to link risk assessment to the various surfaces. At the second meeting of this group, you are asked to appraise a systematic review regarding alternating air mattresses (Vanderwee, Grypdonck, & Defloor, 2008). The expectation is that you will extract information from the SR onto a findings table and at the next meeting give a less-than-5-minute summary and appraisal of the SR.

You could organize your talk in the following way:

- Give a summary of the SR along the same lines as the information in the synopsis part of the SR appraisal guide.
- State your overall impression of the credibility of the conclusions along with your reasons for confidence or concerns.
- State your opinion regarding the clinical significance of the conclusions.
- Address the applicability of the findings and conclusions to the patients seen on your unit and the resources that will be available.

Make a Poster

Professional conferences and congresses often issue calls for oral presentations or posters of research studies and EBP projects. A summary of evidence regarding a clinical question often makes a relevant and interesting poster. Posters are usually mounted on boards in specified areas at congresses, and people walk around and read them. Most congresses require that a person be present with the poster at specified times so people can ask questions.

So, let's say the bed surface-skin breakdown group's work is moving along well, and you notice a call from the National Association of Orthopaedic

Nurses (NAON) for posters at its spring congress. Because your work group has not finished its work on the algorithm/protocol, you decide to submit a poster regarding just the evidence used to produce the algorithm. Most associations allow submission of work-in-progress posters. You would first submit to NAON an abstract of your poster's content. Then, if it is accepted, you would proceed to create the poster using PowerPoint or similar presentation software and produce it using a poster-marking machine, which many agencies have on premises.

When making a poster, you have to be very selective about the information included. If it has too much information or if the information is presented in a disorganized way, people will avoid stopping to read it or will read part of it and walk away. The idea of a poster is to present the main ideas—it is like an abstract. If the person looking at the poster is interested in knowing more, she will ask you some questions. You (the person explaining the poster) are the real resource; the poster is mostly just a lure.

There are no ironclad rules for how to design a poster, but a few suggestions may help. In regard to design of the poster, information should be grouped in some logical way with a header for each block and three to five points under each header. You can use some abbreviations if you define them the first time you use them; of course this is not necessary if they are very common ones. You might want to have a list of the EbCPGs and SRs that are referenced in the poster for people who ask for them, or you could have interested persons write down their email address and after the congress you can send a list of references to them.

The poster could look like **Figure 18–1**. This is a low-budget poster, produced with only gray tones. Color would spruce it up considerably but would add to the cost. Note that the poster in the figure is fabricated—it does not represent an actual project or literature search.

Having a poster at a congress is a fun and informative experience. A lot of people will talk with you, and you will learn a lot. It's definitely a recommended step in your professional growth and development.

Present an Idea or Concern

Let us say while you were at the congress, you went to a session about preventing and managing mental confusion in elderly patients with hip fractures. You went to the session because this issue has recently been a challenge in caring for several patients on your unit. You decide to see what research evidence is available on the topic and to talk with the clinical

Evidence used as the basis for a clinical protocol
Special beds and surfaces for preventing skin breakdown

Phillips-Guarino Medical Center Wishville, MN ▸▸ Terry Winshaw

Project goal: Develop an evidence-based (e-b) decision tree for using special bed surfaces to prevent skin breakdown in at risk orthopaedic patients

Databases searched: CINAHL, MEDLINE, PEDRO (2000–2010)

Main recommendations from guidelines that will be built into the decision tree

Types of evidence found	
4 E-B clinical practice guidelines linking risk assessment and surface interventions	✓ ✓ ✓
4 Systematic Reviews (SRs) about effectiveness of various surfaces	✓
2 Reports of original studies about surface effectiveness (not in the SRs)	

Main conclusions from SRs and findings from studies that will be built into the decision tree

Appraised to be of acceptable quality	
3 E-B clinical practice guidelines	✓
3 Systematic reviews	✓
1 Original study reports	✓

Figure 18-1 Poster

nurse specialist for your unit. A 15-minute search on CINAHL—using the terms *delirium*, *hip fracture*, and *interventions*, with the *research only* and *evidence-based practice* filters on—turns up two EbCPGs, an SR, and several research articles about preventing and managing delirium in patients with hip fracture; they indicate that pain relief is clearly important.

To talk to the clinical nurse specialist or nurse leader, it is best to make an appointment. Catch-as-catch-can in the hallway usually does not work; interruptions are bound to occur, or you may catch him when he has something else on his mind. Here are some suggestions for preparing for your appointment:

- Be able to give some recent examples of why you think delirium prevention and management is a problem on your unit. Specific patient examples would support your claim that delirium care is not as good as it could be.

- Briefly describe the research evidence you found on your quick search. It might be good to give him a copy of several of the research abstracts or URLs you found.
- If your unit already has a protocol about this topic, look at it before your appointment. If the protocol is evidence based and well written, maybe the appropriate action would be to bring it anew to the staff's attention along with any new research. If the protocol is not helpful, up to date, or consistent with newer research, point out its shortcomings.
- Ask his opinion about how to get things moving to make a change, but have an idea or two in mind beforehand.

There is no guarantee you will get a positive response and good follow-through, but the chances are good and the cause is a good one.

Contribute to a Patient Care Conference

Care design is not done just by organizational teams for populations of patients. It is also done in multidisciplinary patient care conferences. When a patient's care presents difficult problems or requires complex discharge arrangements, a patient care planning conference will often be called. The goal of such a conference is to bring together all the information about the patient's situation (from the chart, from the family, or from the various disciplines working with the patient) and develop a specific plan of care.

These planning sessions design more effective strategies when someone is assigned to spend an hour looking for research evidence relative to a key issue or issues in the management of the patient's problems. Perhaps there is an evidence-based guideline that is relevant to the patient's sleeping problem. Maybe a systematic review that addresses the issue of whether a teenager can take a shower even though he has external skeletal pins in place can be identified. Increasingly, evidence-based information is being brought to the table at patient care planning conferences.

If a conference is called and you will be involved, you should give some thought to the problems or issues that may be, or should be, discussed. There may be one or two issues for which it would be helpful for all participants to understand effective approaches that are supported by research evidence. If the person who leads the conference does not assign anyone to look at the research evidence about the problem, you might lead the way by doing so.

At the conference, you could bring what you found in your brief search to the table—not in a lecturing way, but in a contributing way. In that regard, I warn against the overused and vague phrase, "research shows." Instead, say something like, "I found one systematic review that looked at five studies about sleeping problems in hospitalized adolescents. The reviewers reached the conclusion that . . ." Have the article with you so anyone who chooses to can look at it. The inclusion of research-based information into the discussion will most likely be valued and will serve to take the exchange beyond opinions to more objective knowledge as the basis for care planning.

Build Your EBP Knowledge and Skills

If the transfer of scientific knowledge into practice really interests you, you should consider developing your EBP skills beyond what you have learned in the course you are now taking. You could take a graduate course or continuing education course about EBP. Some clinical congresses offer EBP presessions or multiday EBP workshops. Alternatively, you might ask your nurse manager to give you paid time to attend an in-depth EBP workshop such as the following:

- The Hirsh Institute of the Bolton School of Case Western Reserve University offers 2-day basic and intermediate EBP certificate programs. http://fpb.case.edu/Centers/Hirsh/basic_quikpay.shtm and http://fpb.case.edu/Centers/Hirsh/intermediate.shtm
- University of Iowa Hospitals and Clinics has basic EBP internships. http://www.uihealthcare.org/otherservices.aspx?id=22792, a 3-day, advanced EBP institute: http://www.uihealthcare.org/otherservices.aspx?id=225169 and a Web-based CEU course: http://www.uihealthcare.org/otherservices.aspx?id=225170
- The Joanna Briggs Institute and collaborating centers around the world offer intensive training residencies. http://www.joannabriggs.edu.au/Joanna%20Briggs%20Collaboration and http://www.ebnp.org/fellows/fellowsresources.html
- Two organizations offer online EBP courses: Institute for Johns Hopkins Nursing: www.ijhn.jhmi.edu/programDetail_class.asp?id=1278 and University of Oklahoma College of Nursing: www.nursing.ouhsc.edu/CE/evidence_based_practice.cfm

The active learning that occurs in these kinds of programs will prepare you to fully participate in—even lead—EBP projects in your clinical unit or agency. Another option would be that when seeking employment at a large medical center, you ask about in-house EBP training. Quite a few medical centers have them. For instance, the Hospital of the University of Pennsylvania in Philadelphia offers 1-year fellowships in which staff participates in an EBP project (Barnsteiner, Cheeks Reeder, Palma, Preston, & Walton, 2010).

So, there are numerous ways to be involved in evidence-based practice and thereby contribute to good patient care.

http://go.jblearning.com/brown3e

References

Barnsteiner, J. H., Cheeks Reeder, V., Palma, W. H., Preston, A. M., & Walton, M. K. (2010). Promoting evidence-based practice and translational research. *Nursing Administration Quarterly, 34*(3), 217–225.

Vanderwee, K., Grypdonck, M., & Defloor, T. (2008). Alternating pressure air mattresses as prevention for pressure ulcers: A literature review. *International Journal of Nursing Studies, 45*(5), 784–801.

CHAPTER NINETEEN

Research-Informed Practice

Point-of-care design occurs when an individual nurse adapts an evidence-based clinical protocol to a patient's preferences; this tailoring or individualizing of care was described earlier in Chapter 17. In addition, point-of-care design occurs when a nurse encounters a situation in caring for a patient that is not addressed or not addressed in detail by an existing agency. In fact, a great deal of care is designed at the point of care by direct-care providers. Generally speaking, this happens in one of two ways: (1) in the case of a patient who has perplexing or unusual nursing care needs or (2) in the nurse's approach to care of all patients with a particular problem or need.

Many aspects of care are not spelled out in detail in clinical protocols, and this provides an opportunity to use research evidence in individual practice. For instance, many asthma protocols in hospitals, rehabilitation facilities, and home care agencies require that patients with asthma be taught how to take their aerosol medications using an inhaler. However, the type of inhaler device used and the method of teaching the patient are may be left to the discretion of the clinicians working with the particular patient—and there is research evidence relative to these issues (Brocklebank et al., 2001; Dolovich et al., 2005; Brocklebank et al., 2001; Vincken, Dekhuijzen, Barnes, & ADMIT Group, 2010). Let's say a nurse is working with a 10-year-old with newly diagnosed asthma and he is having difficulty using a press-and-breathe inhaler. The nurse could go to the TRIP database (http://www.tripdatabase.com/) from her PDA. Entering *"asthma inhaler child"* into the search box, she could view an easy-to-read technological guide produced by the

National Institute for Clinical Excellence (NICE), *Inhaler Devices for Routine Treatment of Chronic Asthma in Older Children (aged 5–15 years).* NICE is a respected producer of e-b guidance. This would give her some ideas about techniques to assure that the child is getting the correct dose of medication. The nurse who seeks out this research evidence or becomes aware of it at a specialty congress or workshop can enhance the effectiveness of the care she delivers by incorporating that research evidence into her individual patient teaching.

Generally, use of research evidence by the individual nurse is not as rigorous as the way evidence-based quality management (EBQM) EBP project teams use several forms sources of evidence to develop care protocols (Eddy, 2005). It just cannot be because the individual does not have the time, access to data, or appraisal skills that the team has. Usually, the individual nurse uses a care design process that is less comprehensive and systematic. The search for research evidence is not as sweeping, the appraisal is quicker, and the integration across a body of evidence is less systematic (see **Table 19–1**). The individual nurse also relies more on evidence that has been preappraised by others. Thus, an individual nurse's use of research evidence to design care is often informed by the research evidence available but not really truly based on it—hence the term **research-informed practice** (RIP). The rigor of the process used to incorporate research into individual practice can be enhanced considerably by relying mainly on evidence-based

TABLE 19–1 EBP Vis-à-Vis RIP

Characteristic	Evidence-Based Practice	Research-Informed Practice
Who does it?	Project group with skills and resources	Individual clinician
Question/issue	Well framed, often guided by organizational data	Arises in an individual's practice
Search	Extensive, librarian-assisted	Quick, broad, or limited
Appraisal and summary	Systematic, criteria-based	Varies widely, preappraised, short format is best
Translation	Methodical, strategically planned	Informal, often just one clinician
Evaluation	Planned and analytical	Often not planned, anecdotal

clinical practice guidelines (EbCPGs) and systematic reviews (SRs) rather than individual study findings. This is even more important for RIP than it was for protocol development.

RIP Opportunities

Opportunities for research-informed practice occur when during the course of actually giving care, a nurse recognizes she needs additional knowledge regarding management of a patient problem—and needs it immediately. Searching and retrieval of research-based information from the point-of-care can often help the nurse make a research-informed decision about care for a patient she is taking care of at the time. In some clinical settings, she also could search healthcare databases and evidence-based practice Internet sites for relevant sources from a wireless computer terminal, smartphone, or other personal digital assistant (PDA). If there is any doubt about using the research-informed approach found during that search, it would be best to discuss it with the most experienced nurse available at the time.

- Know what you do not know.
- Seek the information you need.
- Check it out with a clinical leader.

Another RIP opportunity presents when a nurse reads an integrative research review article in his specialty journal that provides solid research evidence in support of a particular approach to care or method of care, but the method is not used in his setting. Either there is no protocol addressing that issue or the protocol does not specify the actions that the review addresses. In either case, this nurse should discuss using the research-based method with the unit's clinical leader to be certain it would not confuse or create a problem for other care providers. It may be a method he can use in care of patients without any official approval, or it may be something that an authoritative clinical leader should endorse. This action may also lead to a unit-wide consideration of the method.

When a nurse uses research evidence in the ways just described, she or he is engaging in research-informed practice. It is a different process from the use of research findings by a team developing an evidence-based clinical protocol, which spells out important and critical actions for a patient population. Because the protocol addresses the most important aspects of care and will affect so many patients, it is important that the team use a rigorous process to produce it. Locating and summarizing all the relevant evidence on an issue and then using it to design a clinical guideline or protocol is a very demanding undertaking in terms of the knowledge, skills, discipline, and time required—and is beyond what an individual nurse can do on her or his own. Still, research evidence can be incorporated into an individual's practice.

Specific RIP Activities

Consider further how an individual might engage in RIP:

- Reflect on the effectiveness of the clinical actions you perform
- When care dilemmas, new issues, or poor outcomes occur in your practice, make the effort to search the healthcare databases and professional Internet sites for a relevant evidence-based guideline or research summary
- Participate in a journal club where research articles are discussed
- Regularly read research summaries and report articles that are published in clinical journals
- Conduct a basic level appraisal to determine if a summary, study, or guideline that comes to your attention was soundly produced
- Conduct a basic level appraisal of whether the conclusions, findings, or recommendations would be applicable to the patients you care for and to the setting in which you practice
- Adjust or fine-tune your own practice based on credible findings—within the context of what is possible or changeable in your setting
- Regularly check websites that post evidence-based information related to your area of clinical practice

The Information Intersection

In a very real sense, the point-of-care is an information intersection (Porter O'Grady, 2010). It is the point at which scientific knowledge, patient-specific information, e-b clinical protocols, available clinical services, and personal expertise converge as the basis for care design (see **Figure 19–1**). At present, electronic patient records, clinical decision support systems, bibliographic databases, electronic scheduling systems, and email help clinicians access various sources of information. In the future, Porter-O'Grady (2010) sees healthcare information systems as providing clinicians with a

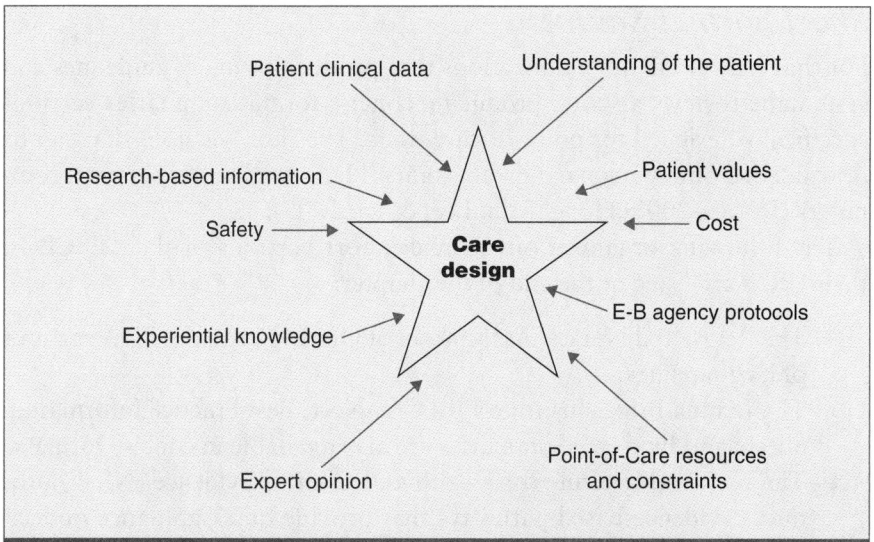

Figure 19-1 Information Intersection

"seamless intersection of data" on which to decide and act (p. 22). Such an information system would make patient data, agency standards, research evidence, assessment guides, and decision support tools available at the point of care in easily searched and quick-to-read formats. Wireless hand-held and mobile devices will increase access to information and provide decision- making support. However, only the human decider can synthesize all the information to make a decision about what care should be given to a particular patient.

Point-of-Care Formats Resources

As you have seen in this part of the book, evidence-based clinical practice guidelines, systematic reviews, and individual study reports can be quite lengthy. At the point of care, nurses need shorter versions of these documents—sometimes called synopses. There is also a need for summaries of the evidence about managing specific conditions and interventions—what we know with certainty, what we know tentatively, and what we have no research evidence about. Increasingly, electronic sources meeting these needs are becoming available.

Short Format Sources

For that reason, many organizations that produce or index guidelines and systematic reviews also are producing concise format summaries versions specifically designed for point-of-care users. The short versions that can be downloaded onto personal data assistants (PDAs) and tablet personal computers (Doran, 2009; Hong, Kim, Lee, & Ki, 2009).

The following organizations provide short versions of their EbCPGs; their URLs are listed at the end of the chapter:

- The Registered Nurses' Association of Ontario provides PDA versions of its guidelines.
- The Joanna Briggs Institute's JBI COnNect, Best Practice Information Sheets and Evidence Summaries are also available in concise formats.
- The National Institute for Health and Clinical Evidence (NICE) produces evidence-based pathways that provide quick guidance in decision tree format on a variety of clinical topics.
- The Oncology Nursing Society makes available *Putting Evidence Into Practice (PEP)* quick views of recommendations for more than 15 topics about oncology nursing on its website and via iPhone apps; links to the evidence base are provided.

In similar fashion, there are several sources for synopses of SRs. These synopses are one- to two-page summaries of SR conclusions, often with short commentaries regarding the soundness of the methodology. These sources include:

- *Evidence-Based Nursing* provides synopses of SRs and study reports accompanied by commentaries that provide methodological assessment and highlight key findings. This is a subscription resource.
- Centre for Reviews and Dissemination, University of York DARE database contains 15,000 abstracts of systematic reviews, including more than 6,000 quality-assessed reviews and details of all Cochrane reviews and protocols. A methodological commentary accompanies the abstracts.
- Summaries and abstracts of the Cochrane Collaboration's SRs are available at no charge from their website.
- The TRIP database indexes and provides links to guidelines, SRs, and other high-quality, international resources. The database is searched

by entering key terms, and the retrieved list can be ordered by date or relevance.

- The abstracts available at the PubMed website especially for handheld devices also serve as a condensed summaries of research evidence; the site has several different approaches to searching, including PICO questions

Some of the sources just listed include a brief commentary about the methodological quality of the EbCPG or SR; others do not. Obviously, the nurse at the bedside would like to know that the EbCPG or SR has been preappraised by a respected organization.

Information Services

Another emerging type of resource from the point of care is web-based information services for healthcare providers (Health Lib Wiki Canada, n.d.). Hospitals and healthcare agencies purchase these information services from vendors, sometimes at considerable cost, to support the decision making of the clinical staff. Some of these services just provide background or factual information; that is, the type of information that is found in textbooks. This would include sign and symptoms of medical conditions and *basic* information about pathophysiology, treatment, or drug information.

Other services go beyond general information and make available e-b summaries of what is known about a particular clinical topic and update the summaries when new evidence becomes available. They are designed especially as point-of-care references. By purchasing these e-b summary services, agencies are in essence outsourcing the early steps in the evidence-based practice process (i.e., search, appraisal, and evidence summarization)

Two Levels of Preappraisal

1st Level :	SR or EbCPG that used a quality filter to determine which individual studies were used as the basis for conclusions or recommendations
2nd level :	SR or EbCPG that has passed a quality filter or been appraised as evidenced in a methodological commentary

Two Levels of Preappraisal

that were formerly performed in-house. The judgment about the application of the evidence still is the responsibility of the agency and/or the individual care provider.

A list of the more widely information services that are widely subscribed to by hospitals, clinics, and healthcare libraries is provided later in Appendix I. Ones specifically for nurses include:

- JBI COnNECT+ Joanna Briggs Institute
- Nursing Reference Center—EBSCO
- ProQuest Nursing & Allied Health Source

You should know that an evaluation of clinical information services designed mainly for physicians found that the quality of these services varied quite widely—in terms of the degree to which the information they provide is: comprehensive, truly evidence based, and frequently updated (Banzi, Liberati, Moschetti, Tagliabue, & Moja, 2010). When considering purchasing one of the electronic summary services, the agency should first evaluate it using the following criteria suggested by Banzi and colleagues:

1. Is a systematic literature search or surveillance the basis of content development?
2. Is the critical appraisal method fully described?
3. Are systematic reviews preferred over other types of publication?
4. Is there a system for grading the quality of evidence?
5. When expert opinion is included is it clear when it was the basis of a recommendation?

Banzi and colleagues appraised 18 online evidence-based practice point-of-care information summary providers; those appraisals are detailed in the article.

Ideally,
Research evidence accessed at the point-of-care should be:
preappraised and concisely summarized.

At this time, these online e-b summary services should be viewed as reference resources as opposed to authoritative sources. But ask an expert nurse in the agency whether she thinks the information provided by the summary service to which they subscribe is trustworthy. These services are evolving quickly, so the quality is likely to continue to improve, and we are likely to see more of them and EBP apps designed specifically for nurses in the near future.

Even now there is a wealth of evidence-based information for point-of-care information seekers. Just using a mobile device app for medication reference information, signs and symptoms of diseases, dosage calculations, normal lab values, and for communication is playing at the edges of what information technology can contribute to patient care.

SHORT-FORMAT EVIDENCE* FOR POINT-OF-CARE USERS

- **EbCPGs short versions**
- **Synopses of SRs**
- **Synopses of individual studies**
- **E-B summaries from commercial information services**

*All best if accompanied by a brief commentary about or indication of methodological quality. If accessed directly from the organization that produced it, the production method used by that organization should be available in another document.

Clinical Decision Support

The new generation of clinical information systems (CIS), in addition to managing patient information, also supports the clinical decision making of care providers. When patient data is entered, the CIS links the patient information to relevant agency protocols and external research evidence. Thus, the provider does not have to know or look to see if there is a relevant agency protocol; it will be brought forward by the CIS. Similarly, she doesn't have to go in search of evidence-based information in the form of an EbCPG, systematic review, study report, or other summarized evidence-based information. Rather, based on the inputted patient data, the CIS will make relevant information sources available via an information button (DiCenso, Bayley, & Haynes, 2009; Lobach et al., 2012). This high degree of integration of patient data and relevant information sources should enhance the degree to which care provided to individual patients incorporates evidence-based practice and is consistent with agency regulatory and accrediting standards (Lobach et al., 2012). CISs with this capability are increasingly being put in place in healthcare agencies and practices.

My Ending—Your Beginning

Having come to the end of this book, I would like to bring together in one place the specific EBP and RIP professional behaviors that have been recommended. In **Box 19–1**, notice the value placed on individual nurses being observant, reflective, and curious about their daily delivery of care. Other behaviors pertain to participating in the quality management activities of your unit, clinical service, or agency. Still others relate to continuing to develop EBP and RIP skills.

BOX 19–1 Professional Evidence-Based Practice Behaviors of the BSN Nurse

1. **Deliver care in accord with your unit's or agency's evidence-based protocols.**
2. **Constantly monitor the effectiveness of the care you are providing.**
3. **When you identify a patient situation where an e-b protocol does not seem to be effective or safe, consult with a nurse leader before deviating from the protocol.**
4. **Actively support implementation of evidence-based protocols in your unit, service, or agency.**
5. **Participate in the development of evidence-based protocols involving your clinical unit.**
6. **Be aware of quality improvement activities in your agency; actively participate.**
7. **Create an EBP folder in your company's Bookmarks or Favorites menu; add links to EBP resources that you find useful and to the EBP page of your specialty professional association.**
8. **Read research articles published in the clinical journals for your area of practice.**
9. **Bring credible e-b clinical methods to the attention of your peers and unit leaders.**
10. **Develop and maintain your knowledge and skills in evidence appraisal by appraising one research guideline/review/study report per month.**

Hopefully you have gotten my not-too-subtle message that *evidence-based practice is not a spectator sport.* It's an intellectually challenging, rewarding, and ethically required professional activity. I hope you will take up the challenge as a way of contributing to the health and well-being of patients and their families.

http://go.jblearning.com/brown3e

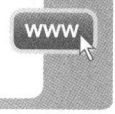

References

Banzi, R., Liberati, A., Moschetti, I., Tagliabue, L., & Moja, L. (2010). A review of online evidence-based practice point-of-care information summary providers. *Journal of Medical Internet Research, 12* (3). doi: 10.2196/jmir.1288. Retrieved May 25, 2012 from http://www.ncbi.nlm.nih.gov/pmc/articles/PMC2956323/?tool=pubmed.

Brocklebank, D., Ram, F., Wright, J., Barry, P., Cates, C., Davies, L., et al. (2001). Comparison of the effectiveness of inhaler devices in asthma and chronic obstructive airway diseases: A systematic review of the literature. *Health Technology Assessment, 5*(26), 1–149.

DiCenso, A., Bayley, L., & Haynes, R. B. (2009). Accessing pre-appraised evidence: Fine-tuning the 5S model into a 6S model. *Evidence Based Nursing, 12*, 99–101.

Dolovich, M. B., Ahrens, R. C., Hess, D. R., Anderson, P., Dhand, R., Rau, J. L., Guyatt, G. et al. (2005). Device selection and outcomes of aerosol therapy: Evidence-based guidelines: American College of Chest Physicians/American College of Asthma, Allergy, and Immunology. *Chest, 127*(1), 335–371.

Doran, D. (2009). The emerging role of PDAs in information use and clinical decision making. *Evidence Based Nursing, 12*, 35–38.

Eddy, D. (2005). Evidence-based medicine: A unified approach: Two approaches to using evidence to solve clinical problems, and how to unify them. *Health Affairs, 24*(1), 9–17.

Health Lib Wiki Canada. (n.d.). *Point of care decision-making tools—Overview.* Retrieved May 25, 2012 from http://hlwiki.slais.ubc.ca/index.php/Point_of_care_decision-making_tools_-_Overview

Hong, H. S., Kim, I. K., Lee, S. H., & Ki, H. S. (2009). Adoption of a PDA-based home hospice care system for cancer patients. *Computers, Informatics, and Nursing, 27*(6), 365–371.

Lobach, D., Sanders, G. D., Bright, T. J., Wong, A., Dhurjati, R., Bristow, E., et al. (2012). *Enabling health care decisionmaking through clinical decision support and knowledge management*. Rockville, MD: Agency for Healthcare Research and Quality.

Porter-O'Grady, T. (2010). A new age for practice: Creating the framework for evidence. In K. Malloch & T. Porter-O'Grady (Eds.), *Introduction to evidence-based practice in nursing and health care* (2nd ed., pp. 1–30). Sudbury, MA: Jones and Bartlett.

Vincken, W., Dekhuijzen, P. R., Barnes, P., & ADMIT Group. (2010). The ADMIT series—Issues in inhalation therapy. (4) How to choose inhaler devices for the treatment of COPD. *Primary Care Respiratory Journal, 19*(1), 10–20.

Resources

Centre for Reviews and Dissemination, University of York DARE database:
http://www.york.ac.uk/inst/crd/

Cochrane Collaboration:
http://www.cochrane.org/cochrane-reviews

Evidence-Based Nursing:
http://ebn.bmj.com

The Joanna Briggs Institute's JBI COnNect:
http://www.jbiconnect.org/agedcare/ebhc/summarise/search-form.php

The National Institute for Health and Clinical Evidence (NICE):
http://guidance.nice.org.uk/CG

Oncology Nursing Society Putting Evidence into Practice resources:
http://www.ons.org/Research/PEP

PubMed for Handhelds:
http://pubmedhh.nlm.nih.gov/

The Registered Nurses' Association of Ontario:
http://www.rnao.org/

TRIP Database:
http://www.tripdatabase.com/

APPENDIX A

Appraisal Guide:

Recommendations of a Clinical Practice Guideline

Citation:

_____

_____

_____

Synopsis

What does the guideline address? Clinical questions, issues, subissues.

What population of patients is the guideline intended to address?

Did the panel use existing SRs or did they conduct their own?

What clinical outcomes was the guideline designed to achieve?

What group or groups produced the guideline?

What is the date on it and how recent are the cited evidence sources?

What are the main recommendations?

Credibility

Was the panel made up of people with the necessary expertise?	❑ Yes	❑ No	❑ Not clear
Was the organization and/or the panel free of conflict of interest?	❑ Yes	❑ No	❑ Not clear
*Were the SRs used of high quality?	❑ Yes	❑ No	❑ Not clear
*Does the production process meet recognized standards?	❑ Yes	❑ No	❑ Not clear
*Is the evidence supporting each recommendation graded, indicated, summarized, or discussed?	❑ Yes	❑ No	❑ Not clear
Was the guideline reviewed by outside experts and a member of the public *or* field tested?	❑ Yes	❑ No	❑ Not clear
Is the guideline current?	❑ Yes	❑ No	❑ Not clear
ARE THE RECOMMENDATIONS CREDIBLE?	❑ All	❑ Some	❑ No

Clinical Significance

Were patient concerns, values, and risks addressed?	❑ Yes	❑ No	❑ Not clear
Are the projected benefits of the guideline indicated?	❑ Yes	❑ No	❑ Not clear
*Is the degree of confidence that each recommendation will result in the intended effect indicated (by a grade or otherwise)?	❑ Yes	❑ No	❑ Not clear
Were all important decisions and actions the nurse would have to make addressed?	❑ Yes	❑ No	❑ Not clear
ARE THE RECOMMENDATIONS CLINICALLY SIGNIFICANT?	❑ All	❑ Some	❑ No

Applicability

Does the guideline address a problem, weakness, or decision we are examining in our setting? ❑ Yes ❑ No

Did the research evidence involve patients similar to ours and was the setting similar to ours? ❑ Yes ❑ No ❑ Some

What changes, additions, training, or purchases would be needed to implement and sustain a clinical protocol based on these conclusions? Specify

_____

_____

*Is what we will have to do to implement the new protocol realistically achievable by us (resources, capability, commitment)? ❑ Yes ❑ No ❑ Not clear

Which departments and/or providers will be affected by a change? Specify

_____

_____

*How will we know if our patients are benefiting from our new protocol? Specify

_____

_____

SHOULD WE IMPLEMENT THE GUIDELINE IN ITS ENTIRETY OR MODIFY IT? ❑ Yes ❑ Modify ❑ No

* = Important criteria

Comments

_____

_____

APPENDIX B

Completed Appraisal:

Recommendations of a Clinical Practice Guideline

Citation:

Scottish Intercollegiate Guidelines Network. (2010). *Non-pharmaceutical management of depression in adults: A national guideline*. Retrieved from http://www.sign.ac.uk/pdf/sign114.pdf

The appraisal considers only exercise and lifestyle modification—not psychological therapies, self-help, herbal and nutritional remedies, or alternative therapies.

Synopsis

What does the guideline address? Clinical questions, issues, subissues.
Nonpharmaceutic treatments of depression in adults, including psychological therapies, self-help, exercise and lifestyle changes, meditation, herbal remedies and nutritional supplements, and complementary and alternative therapies as alternatives to/instead of prescription medications.

What population of patients is the guideline intended to address?
Adults with mild to moderate depression.

Did the panel use existing SRs or did they conduct their own?
They conducted some SRs and meta-analyses using SIGN methodology and used existing SRs and meta-analyses that met quality standards.

What clinical outcomes was the guideline designed to achieve?
Reduction in depressive symptoms as measured by a recognized depression scale, illness duration, quality of life, or patient satisfaction.

What group or groups produced the guideline?
A 22-member panel of clinical and academic mental health experts from various disciplines and Scottish agencies.

What is the date on it and how recent are the cited evidence sources?
Issued in January 2010; 90 references with dates up to 2008.

What are the main recommendations?
The only recommendation that was made (in the treatments under consideration in this appraisal) related to exercise and lifestyle modification was: Structured exercise may be considered as a treatment option. No recommendation regarding lifestyle modification, but a Best Practice Point was offered.

Credibility

Was the panel made up of people with the necessary expertise? ☑ Yes ❑ No ❑ Not clear

Could have benefitted from a home care nurse.

Was the organization and/or the panel free of conflict of interest? ☑ Yes ❑ No ❑ Not clear

All members of the guideline development group made declarations of interest. Section 11.2 of the guideline online.

Were the SRs used of high quality? ☑ Yes ❑ No ❑ Not clear

SIGN has explicit standards about this at http://www.sign.ac.uk/guidelines/fulltext/50/section6.html

*Does the production process meet recognized standards? ☑ Yes ❑ No ❑ Not clear

The widely respected SIGN standards for CPG production are explicitly set forth in the Developer's Handbook on the website.

*Is the evidence supporting each recommendation graded, indicated, summarized, or discussed? ☑ Yes ❑ No ❑ Not clear

Levels of evidence are rated 1++ through 4 and are defined in terms of evidence type and quality. For exercise, the evidence ranged from 1++ to 1+. The body of evidence about exercise, was graded as B, and narrative judgments were offered regarding several aspects of exercise.

Was the guideline reviewed by outside experts and a member of the public *or* field tested? ☑ Yes ❑ No ❑ Not clear

Yes to peer review and patient involvement. (from sections 11.3 and 11.2.1 of the guideline online).

Is the guideline current? ☑ Yes ❑ No ❑ Not clear

Issued 2010.

ARE THE RECOMMENDATIONS CREDIBLE? ☑ All ❑ Some ❑ No

Clinical Significance

Were patient concerns, values, and risks addressed? ☑ Yes ❑ No ❑ Not clear

The comprehensive nature of issues considered impressed us. Risk was taken into consideration in the discussion of evidence related to exercise.

Are the projected benefits of the guideline indicated? ☑ Yes ❑ No ❑ Not clear

Reduction in symptoms as described in sections 1.2 and 1.5.

*Is the degree of confidence that each recommendation will result in the intended effect indicated? (by grade or otherwise) ☑ Yes ❑ No ❑ Not clear

Implicitly in the recommendation grades; A, B, C, and D are defined. We found the inclusion of best practice points helpful. The benefits of each recommendation are addressed in the discussion of evidence regarding each. However, the discussion of the evidence in section 5.1 does not specify the outcomes it affects; presumably the main outcome studies are level of depression. In the absence of research about the effects of healthy lifestyle, the best practice point is helpful and resonates with our experience. However, we have never formalized an approach to it or offered it as a discrete service.

Were all important decisions and actions the nurse would have to make addressed? ☑ Yes ❑ No ❑ Not clear

All possible nonpharmaceutic modalities we might use were considered, although recommendations about many of them were not made due to lack of evidence.

ARE THE RECOMMENDATIONS CLINICALLY SIGNIFICANT? ☑ All ❑ Some ❑ No

Applicability

Assume a community mental health center that is considering what nonpharmaceutical treatments to offer as alternatives to medication therapies. Effectiveness in reducing depressive symptoms will be the main consideration, but community preference will also be considered.

*Does the guideline address a problem, weakness, or decision we are examining in our setting? ☑ Yes ❑ No

Eighteen percent of our patients express a wish to avoid prescription medication if at all possible. The low number of nonprescription modalities supported by research evidence is disappointing.

Did the research evidence involve patients similar to ours, and was the setting similar to ours? ☑ Yes ❑ No ❑ Some

We think many of our patients who decline medication therapy would be open to structured exercise and/or healthy lifestyle support. We would have liked to learn if older patients are receptive to structured exercise and how committed they are to it once underway.

What changes, additions, training, or purchases would be needed to implement and sustain implementation of a clinical protocol basis on this guideline? Specify

We need to decide if we should offer structured exercise under our auspices or refer patients to community programs. Under our auspices, we would

have to find and rent a space and hire an instructor; we need a cost analysis; there are clear benefits to going this route. Alternatively, we could just compile a list of community programs offering structured exercise programs; the counselors should have this list readily available. We could also put up posters about these programs around the agency. A healthy lifestyle support group would definitely be best offered under our auspices. We have some expertise on staff, but an expert consultation should be contracted to help develop some of the content. We will submit a report to the Board of Directors about the options for making structured exercise and healthy lifestyle counseling available as primary treatment modalities to our patients.

*Is what we will have to do to implement the guideline or parts of it realistically achievable by us (resources, capability, commitment)?	☑ Yes ❑ No ❑ Not clear

Options for delivering exercise-as-a-primary-treatment options will undergo cost analysis. Healthy lifestyle support group require little additional cost beyond the initial consultation; investigate whether such an offering is reimbursable by insurance.

Which departments and/or providers will be affected by a change?	Specify

Counselors need education about the value of these therapies and the mechanisms for getting patients enrolled in them.

*How will we know if patients benefit from our incorporating the guideline recommendations or some of them into the care we give?	Specify

We could: (1) set up a system to identify patients who prefer nonmedication approaches, (2) determine what percent are offered structured exercise and/or membership in a healthy lifestyle support group, (3) find out how many of those actually enroll in an exercise activity (ours or in the community) or lifestyle support group and (4) after 4 months evaluate their level of depression and their impressions regarding the effects of their nonmedication therapy.

SHOULD WE IMPLEMENT THE GUIDELINE IN ITS ENTIRETY OR MODIFY IT? ☑ Yes ❑ Modify ❑ No

If the cost analysis is favorable or even equivocal, we will recommend to the Board of Directors that we move ahead with both the exercise recommendation and the healthy lifestyle best practice point.

* = Important criteria

Comments

_____

_____

APPENDIX C

Appraisal Guide:

Conclusions of an Integrative Research Review

Citation:

_____

_____

_____

Synopsis

How many persons were involved in conducting the review?

What topic or question did the integrative research review address?

How were potential research reports identified?

What determined if a study was included in the analysis?

How many studies were included in the review?

What research designs were used in the studies?

What were the consistent and important across-studies conclusions?

Credibility

Was the topic clearly defined?	❑ Yes	❑ No	❑ Not clear
Was the search for studies and other evidence comprehensive and unbiased?	❑ Yes	❑ No	❑ Not clear
Was the screening of citations for inclusion based on explicit criteria?	❑ Yes	❑ No	❑ Not clear
*Were the included studies assessed for quality?	❑ Yes	❑ No	❑ Not clear
Were the design characteristics and findings of the included studies displayed or discussed in sufficient detail?	❑ Yes	❑ No	❑ Not clear
*Was there a true integration (i.e., synthesis) of the findings—not merely reporting of findings from each study individually?	❑ Yes	❑ No	❑ Not clear
*Did the reviewers explore why differences in findings might have occurred?	❑ Yes	❑ No	❑ Not clear
Did the reviewers distinguish between conclusions based on consistent findings from several good studies and those based on inferior evidence (number or quality)?	❑ Yes	❑ No	❑ Not clear
Which conclusions were supported by consistent findings from two or more good or high-quality studies?	List		

_____

_____

_____

ARE THE CONCLUSIONS CREDIBLE? ❑ All ❑ Some ❑ No

Clinical Significance

*Across studies, is the size of the treatment or the strength of the association found or the meaningfulness of qualitative findings strong enough to make a difference in patient outcomes or experiences of care? ❑ Yes ❑ No ❑ Not clear

Are the conclusions relevant to the care the nurse gives? ❑ Yes ❑ No ❑ Not clear

ARE THE CONCLUSIONS CLINICALLY SIGNIFICANT? ❑ All ❑ Some ❑ No

Applicability

Does the IRR address a problem, situation, or decision we are addressing in our setting? ❑ Yes ❑ No ❑ Not clear

Are the patients in the studies similar to those we see, either overall or in a subgroup of patients? ❑ Yes ❑ No ❑ Not clear

What changes, additions, training, or purchases would be needed to implement and sustain a clinical protocol based on these conclusions? Specify

_____

_____

_____

Is what we will have to do to implement the new protocol realistically achievable by us (resources, capability, commitment)? ❑ Yes ❑ No ❑ Not clear

How will we know if our patients are benefiting from our new protocol? Specify

SHOULD WE PROCEED TO DESIGN A PROTOCOL INCORPORATING THESE CONCLUSIONS? ❑ All ❑ Some ❑ No

* Important criteria

Comments

APPENDIX D

Completed Appraisal:

Conclusions of an Integrative Research Review

Citation:

Crowe, M., Wilson, L., & Inder, M. (2011). Patients' reports of the factors influencing medication adherence in bipolar disorder—An integrative review of the literature. *International Journal of Nursing Studies, 48*, 894–903.

Synopsis

How many persons were involved in conducting the review?
3

What topic or question did the integrative research review address?
The perceptions of patients with bipolar disorder about medication adherence.

How were potential individual research reports identified?
Databases were searched and hand searches were done. Search strategy is reported.

What determined if a study was included in the analysis?
There were explicit inclusion and exclusion criteria.

How many studies were included in the review?
13

What research designs were used in the studies?
Mostly descriptive quantitative studies, one mixed methods study, and one qualitative study.

What were the consistent and important across-studies conclusions?
The factors that influence medication adherence are numerous; they can be categorized as illness related, personal attitudes and beliefs, medication related, and environmental/contextual. There is some confirmation from one study to another regarding the influence of patients' beliefs about the illness itself, their view of self, and what taking medication means to them. The importance of the relationship with the prescribing provider was also found in several studies.

Credibility

Was the topic clearly defined? ☑ Yes ❑ No ❑ Not clear

The inclusion of the phrase "from the patients' perspective" is important.

Was the search for studies and other evidence comprehensive and unbiased? ☑ Yes ❑ No ❑ Not clear

They searched several databases.

Was the screening of citations to select studies for inclusion based on explicit criteria? ☑ Yes ❑ No ❑ Not clear

We do however question why several studies of which we are aware did not meet the inclusion criteria, e.g., Fleck, D. E., Keck, P. E., Corey, K. B., & Strakowski, S. M. (2005). Factors associated with medication adherence in African American and white patients with bipolar disorder. Journal of Clinical Psychiatry, 66, 646–652.

Were the included studies assessed for quality? ☑ Yes ❑ No ❑ Not clear

The criteria used were listed, and it was stated that they all met minimum criteria, but the variability of the quality of the studies was not described.

Were the design characteristics and findings of the included studies displayed or discussed in sufficient detail? ☑ Yes ❑ No ❑ Not clear

However, we found the information about design types a bit confusing; we would have preferred to have this included on Table 3. We also wished we knew the country in which each study was conducted and a brief profile of the patients who participated in each as there may be some unique cultural influences regarding the disorder and about taking medications. That only one qualitative study and one mixed methods study were located surprised us.

Was there a true integration (i.e., synthesis) of the findings—not merely reporting of findings from each study individually? ☑ Yes ❑ No ❑ Not clear

It is not clear if the reviewers created the four categories of factors influencing adherence or if they came from elsewhere. Either way, presenting the findings of the review in this framework is quite helpful. While the review confirmed that patients have complex views of their illness and that these views influence adherence, the relationship between mood state and medication adherence was not illuminated.

Did the reviewers explore why differences in findings might have occurred? ☑ Yes ❑ No ❑ Not clear

They noted the variety of measures of adherence used and that adherence status was not linked to specific medications in most studies. Only one study followed patients over the long term.

Did the reviewers distinguish between conclusions based on consistent findings from several good studies and those based on inferior evidence (number or quality)? ☑ Yes ❑ No ❑ Not clear

We found this aspect to be a bit weak but this could be due to the varied nature of the studies and the limited amount of evidence available about diverse issues. The reviewers did interface the findings of this review with evidence from other studies that studied the issue from a different perspective.

Which conclusions were supported by consistent findings from two or more good or high-quality studies? List

The many factors involving the interplay of beliefs about the disease, view of self, and the meaning of taking medications that control mood were confirmed by several studies. Also, the influence of patients' perceptions of their relationship with the prescribing provider was noted in several studies, including one large one.

ARE THE RECOMMENDATIONS CREDIBLE? ☑ Yes ❑ No ❑ Not clear

But our confidence in the conclusions is constrained by the diverse nature of the studies.

Clinical Significance

Across studies, is the size of the treatment or the strength of the association found or the meaningfulness of qualitative findings strong enough to make a difference in patient outcomes or experiences of care? ☑ Yes ❑ No ❑ Not clear

The complex web of patients' beliefs about the illness, their sense of self, and what the medications actually do for them was confirmed, but the dynamics of the web remain elusive—and therefore difficult to build on in practice. Certainly, the importance of the relationship with the provider and the information given about the medication stand out as influencing adherence. The extent to which the provider being sensitive to the factors identified actually will affect patient outcomes is assumed but was not addressed because it was beyond the objectives of this IRR.

Are the conclusions relevant to the care nurses give? ☑ Yes ❑ No ❑ Not clear

We find the problem of adherence in this population to occur frequently and to be an important issue for their quality of life. However, we are disappointed that the issues of whether patients view the medications as helpful

and how their view of effectiveness affects adherence were not directly addressed by any study. Also, the extent to which front-end discussions with patients about taking the medication vis-à-vis ongoing discussions promote adherence remains unexamined.

ARE THE CONCLUSIONS CLINICALLY SIGNIFICANT? ❑ Yes ❑ No ☑ Not clear

Importantly, incorporating the factors identified into clinical care carries no risk of harm.

Applicability

Assume an outpatient mental health clinic.

Does the IRR address the problems, situation, or decision we are addressing in our setting? ☑ Yes ❑ No ❑ Not clear

We have the sense that it is a problem but have no data.

Are the patients in the studies similar to those we see, either overall or in a subgroup of patients? ❑ Yes ❑ No ☑ Not clear

Cannot tell because the patients in the studies are not described.

What changes, additions, training, or purchases would be needed to implement and sustain a clinical protocol based on these conclusions? Specify

We will use this review and the findings of a few other studies to develop a protocol for clinicians who treat patients with bipolar disorder. The protocol will (1) remind providers to assess how patients view their illness and taking medications at the time of considering medication, (2) remind them to discuss expected benefits as well as side effects, (3) set forth issues that should be discussed on follow-up, and (4) recommend issues that should be explored should medication nonadherence become a problem.

The time involved in developing the protocol needs to be set aside. Also, the protocol (with reminders) will need to be incorporated into the clinical information system.

Is what we will have to do to implement the new protocol realistically achievable by us (resources, capability, commitment)?	☑ Yes ❑ No ❑ Not clear

This problem has come up in many patient planning meetings, and there is consensus that we need to include it in our standards of care.

How will we know if our patients are benefiting from our new protocol?	Specify

We need to get some hard data regarding medication nonadherence in our patients; at this point we only believe it to be a problem because of anecdotal reporting. With a protocol that is well introduced, we would hope to see a 20% reduction in patients reporting nonadherence at the time of follow-up visits.

SHOULD WE PROCEED TO DESIGN A PROTOCOL INCORPORATING SOME OR ALL OF THESE CONCLUSIONS?	❑ All ☑ **Some** ❑ No

Comments

These authors have a more recent study about the effectiveness of interventions to improve medication adherence in bipolar disorder (http://anp.sagepub.com/content/46/4/317.full).

Also, there is an SR about medication adherence in older persons with bipolar disorder (http://www.ncbi.nlm.nih.gov/pmc/articles/PMC2921250/). And there is a clinical trial under way about enhancing medication adherence in patients with bipolar disorder (http://clinicaltrials.gov/ct2/show/NCT00830310). So there are other sources to check out as well.

APPENDIX E

Appraisal Guide:

Findings of a Qualitative Study

Citation:

_____

_____

_____

Synopsis

What experience, situation, or subculture does the researcher seek to understand?

Does the researcher want to produce a description of an experience, a social process, or an event, or is the goal to generate a theory?

How was data collected?

How did the researcher control his or her biases and preconceptions?

Are specific pieces of data (e.g., direct quotes) and more generalized statements (themes, theories) included in the report?

What are the main findings of the study?

Credibility

Is the study published in a source that required peer review?	❑ Yes	❑ No	❑ Not clear
Were the methods used appropriate to the study purpose?	❑ Yes	❑ No	❑ Not clear
Was the sampling of observations or interviews appropriate and varied enough to serve the purpose of the study?	❑ Yes	❑ No	❑ Not clear
*Were data collection methods effective in obtaining in-depth data?	❑ Yes	❑ No	❑ Not clear
Did the data collection methods avoid the possibility of oversight, underrepresentation, or overrepresentation from certain types of sources?	❑ Yes	❑ No	❑ Not clear
Were data collection and analysis intermingled in a dynamic way?	❑ Yes	❑ No	❑ Not clear
*Is the data presented in ways that provide a vivid portrayal of what was experience or happened and its context?	❑ Yes	❑ No	❑ Not clear
*Does the data provided justify generalized statements, themes, or theory?	❑ Yes	❑ No	❑ Not clear
ARE THE FINDINGS CREDIBLE?	❑ All	❑ Some	❑ No

Clinical Significance

*Are the findings rich and informative? ❑ Yes ❑ No ❑ Not clear

*Is the perspective provided potentially useful in providing insight, support, or guidance for assessing patient status or progress? ❑ Yes ❑ No ❑ Not clear

❑ All ❑ Some ❑ No

* = Important criteria

Comments

_____

_____

APPENDIX F

Appraisal Guide:

Findings of a Quantitative Study

Citation:

_____

_____

_____

Synopsis

What was the purpose of the study (research questions, purposes, and hypotheses)?

How was the sample obtained?

What inclusion or exclusion criteria were used?

Who from the sample actually participated or contributed data (demographic or clinical profile and dropout rate)?

What methods were used to collect data (e.g., sequence, timing, types of data, and measures)?

Was an intervention tested? ❑ Yes ❑ No

1. How was the sample size determined?
2. Were patients randomly assigned to treatment groups?

What are the main findings?

Credibility

Is the study published in a source that required peer review?	❑ Yes	❑ No	❑ Not clear
Was the design used appropriate to the research question?	❑ Yes	❑ No	❑ Not clear
*Did the data obtained and the analysis conducted answer the research question?	❑ Yes	❑ No	❑ Not clear
Were the measuring instruments reliable and valid?	❑ Yes	❑ No	❑ Not clear
*Were important extraneous variables and bias controlled?	❑ Yes	❑ No	❑ Not clear
*Was the study free of extraneous variables introduced by how, when, and where the study was done?	❑ Yes	❑ No	❑ Not clear
*If an intervention was tested, answer the following five questions:	❑ Yes	❑ No	❑ Not clear
1. Were participants randomly assigned to groups and were the two groups similar at the start (before the intervention)?	❑ Yes	❑ No	❑ Not clear
2. Were the interventions well defined and consistently delivered?	❑ Yes	❑ No	❑ Not clear
3. Were the groups treated equally other than the difference in interventions?	❑ Yes	❑ No	❑ Not clear
4. If no difference was found, was the sample size large enough to detect a difference if one existed?	❑ Yes	❑ No	❑ Not clear
5. If a difference was found, are you confident it was due to the intervention?	❑ Yes	❑ No	❑ Not clear
Are the findings consistent with findings from other studies?	❑ Yes	❑ No	❑ Not clear
ARE THE FINDINGS CREDIBLE?	❑ All	❑ Some	❑ No

Clinical Significance

Note any difference in means, r^2s, or measures of clinical effects (ABI, NNT, RR, OR)

*Is the target population clearly described? ❑ Yes ❑ No ❑ Not clear

*Is the frequency, association, or treatment effect impressive enough for you to be confident that the finding would make a clinical difference if used as the basis for care? ❑ Yes ❑ No ❑ Not clear

ARE THE FINDINGS CLINICALLY SIGNIFICANT? ❑ All ❑ Some ❑ No

* = Important criteria

Comments

_____

_____

_____

APPENDIX G

Completed Appraisal:

Findings of a Quantitative Study

Citation:

Evangelista, L. S., Moser, D. K., Westlake, C., Pike, N., Ter-Galstanyan, A., & Dracup, K. (2008). Correlates of fatigue in patients with heart failure. *Progress in Cardiovascular Nursing, 23*(1), 12–17.

Synopsis

What was the purpose of the study (research questions, purposes, and hypotheses)?
"To examine the prevalence of fatigue and identify its demographic, clinical, and psychological correlates in patients with systolic heart failure (HF)." They were also interested in predictors of fatigue.

How was the sample obtained?
A convenience sample was recruited at an outpatient HF clinic of a tertiary care, university –affiliated medical center on the US West Coast. That is all the detail provided about recruitment and setting.

What inclusion or exclusion criteria were used?
Over age 18; able to read, write, and speak English; left ventricular ejection fraction < 40%; symptoms of HF for 6 months or longer.

Who from the sample actually participated or contributed data (demographic or clinical profile, and dropout rate)?
The sample included 150 patients with HF awaiting transplant and being seen at the outpatient clinic of a tertiary referral center. Average age = 55; 73% men; average ejection fraction = 26.7%; 66% had some college or completed college.

What methods were used to collect data (e.g., sequence, timing, types of data, and measures)?
Questionnaires that took 10 to 15 minutes to complete measured fatigue (POM-F); quality of life (Minnesota Heart Failure subscales: total, physical health, and emotional health); and depression (Beck Depression Inventory). The participants were recruited during routine clinic visits.

Was an intervention tested? ❑ Yes ☑ No

1. How was the sample size determined?
2. Were patients randomly assigned to treatment groups?

What are the main findings?

a. *About 51% of the sample reported a high level of fatigue, and 28% scored in the depression range.*
b. *Ejection fraction had a low level of correlation with fatigue.*
c. *Maximal workload, quality of life total, physical health, emotional health, and depression had high correlations with fatigue.*
d. *About 51% of the variance in fatigue was predicted by a model consisting of maximal workload, physical health, emotional health, and depression.*

Credibility

Is the study published in a source that required peer review? ☑ Yes ❑ No ❑ Not clear

Was the design used appropriate to the research question? ☑ Yes ❑ No ❑ Not clear

They were interested in exploring the relationship between clinical and psychological states and fatigue, so correlational design was appropriate.

*Did the data obtained and the analysis conducted answer the research question? ☑ Yes ❑ No ❑ Not clear

They obtained data on physiological and psychological variables that could be related to and predict fatigue. Pearson rs *and multiple regression are the appropriate statistics for this data and their question.*

Were the measuring instruments reliable and valid? ☑ Yes ❑ No ❑ Not clear

The instruments are widely used and have reliability and validity histories. The fatigue and depression instruments have normative cut points; however, no validity information was provided about their validity with HF patients.

*Were important extraneous variables and bias controlled? ☑ Yes ❑ No ❑ Not clear

Controls were not highly important in this observational study, other than defining inclusions: age, diagnosis, and capability to complete written questionnaires.

*Was the study free of extraneous variables introduced by how, when, and where the study was done? ☑ Yes ❑ No ❑ Not clear

It is possible that asking the patients to complete the questionnaires would make them think about their psychological state more than patients who were not asked extensively about these issues. This could lead to scores that reflect more problems than patients who are not asked extensively about their quality of life, fatigue, depression, emotional health, and physical health. There is no way to get around this, but it could represent a Hawthorne effect.

Also, the lack of control for type 1 conclusion error, which was a possibility because of the high number of tests of significance that were run, is of some concern. However, when Bonferroni correction was applied to these results, the conclusions of the study did not change in important ways.

*If an intervention was tested, answer the following five questions: ❑ Yes ❑ No ❑ Not clear

1. Were participants randomly assigned to groups and were the two groups similar at the start (before the intervention)? ❑ Yes ❑ No ❑ Not clear
2. Were the interventions well defined and consistently delivered? ❑ Yes ❑ No ❑ Not clear
3. Were the groups treated equally other than the difference in interventions? ❑ Yes ❑ No ❑ Not clear
4. If no difference was found, was the sample size large enough to detect a difference if one existed? ❑ Yes ❑ No ❑ Not clear
5. If a difference was found, are you confident it was due to the intervention? ❑ Yes ❑ No ❑ Not clear

Are the findings consistent with findings from other studies? ☑ Yes ❑ No ❑ Not clear

Yes, as indicated in the discussion section, the findings are generally consistent with what studies of other HF populations have found.

ARE THE FINDINGS CREDIBLE? ☑ All ❑ Some ❑ No

Clinical Significance

Note any difference in means, r^2s, or measures of clinical effects (ABI, NNT, RR, OR)

*Is the target population clearly described? ❑ Yes ❑ No ☑ Not clear

The lack of detail about the recruitment process and the nature of the clinic in which they were recruited leave us unclear regarding the target population.

*Is the frequency, association, or treatment effect impressive enough for you to be confident that the finding would make a clinical difference if it were used as the basis for care? ☑ Yes ❑ No ❑ Not clear

The R^2 for the multivariate predictive model is 51%, which is quite substantial. As the authors point out, three of the four independent predictors of fatigue (i.e., emotional health, physical health, and depression) are potential targets for intervention to combat fatigue. This finding could lead to future studies that try to alter the levels of these variables to reduce fatigue. Interventions directed at them could be studied one at a time or as a group of interventions.

We think these findings establish that fatigue is related to overall physical health and emotional health as well as to heart function. Fatigue is undoubtedly a physical experience, but there is also a response to the experience that affects mental outlook and functional level; this response may be a target for intervention.

ARE THE FINDINGS CLINICALLY SIGNIFICANT? ☑ All ❑ Some ❑ No

Yes, we find all the main findings clinically significant, but are surprised at the low correlation between ejection fraction and fatigue. The lack of clarity regarding the population to whom the findings apply does constrain our confidence in the clinical significance of these findings for our patient population.

* = Important criteria

Comments

_____

_____

_____

APPENDIX H

Completed Findings Table

Topic: Fatigue in Patients With Congestive Heart Failure **Date: July 2010**

Author(s) and date	Questions, variables, objectives, hypotheses	Design, sample, setting	Findings	Notes
Evangelista et al., 2008	Fatigue-inertia, psychosocial and cardiac variables, QOL, depression, emotional health, physical health	Correlational 150 persons with HF awaiting transplant at tertiary center; mean age = 55; men = 73%; mean ef = 27% USA	1. 51% had high level of F 2. Maximal workload, physical health, emotional health, and depression explain 51% of F 3. Depression in > 28%	POMS-F; Minnesota Living with HF QOL overall; MN QOL physical; MN QOL emotional; Beck
Hägglund et al., 2008	Living with HF Experience of F	Qualitative Interviews and content analysis 10 women from outpatient clinic; mean age = 83 Sweden	1. Loss of physical energy 2. Experience of feebleness and unfamiliar body sensations 3. Experience unpredictable variations in physical ability 4. Need help from others 5. Strive for independence 6. Acknowledge remaining abilities 7. Being forced to adjust	

Topic: Fatigue in Patients With Congestive Heart Failure *(continued)* **Date: July 2010**

Author(s) and date	Questions, variables, objectives, hypotheses	Design, sample, setting	Findings	Notes
Stephen, 2008	F intensity, global fatigue, symptom severity, trait negativity, functional status, exercise routine, QOL, satisfaction with life	Correlational 53 elders with stable HF, average age = 77; mean = 68%; average ef = 31% USA	1. F prevalence = 96% 2. F associated with QOL, perceived health, satisfaction with life 3. No relationship between F intensity and functional status 4. Being married predicted F 5. Regular exercisers reported less F	POMS-F; Visual analogue F; HF functional status inventory; MN overall; MN Satisfaction with Life Scale
Falk et al., 2009	General F, physical F, mental F, activity, motivation, anxiety, depression, symptom distress	Correlational 112 community-dwelling persons with worsening HF who sought care; average age = 77; men = 60% Sweden	1. F associated with emotional distress 2. Most intense symptoms: F, difficulty breathing, insomnia 3. Depression associated with activity	Multidimensional Fatigue Inventory; Symptom Distress Scale; Hospital Anxiety and Distress Scale

(continues)

Topic: Fatigue in Patients With Congestive Heart Failure *(continued)* **Date: July 2010**

QOL = quality of life

HF = heart failure

F = fatigue

POMS-F = Profile of Mood States Scale, fatigue subscale

MN = Minnesota Living with Heart Failure Questionnaire

ef = ejection fraction

References

Evangelista, L. S., Moser, D. K., Westlake, C., Pike, N., Ter-Galstanyan, A., & Dracup, K. (2008). Correlates of fatigue in patients with heart failure. *Progress in Cardiovascular Nursing, 23*(1), 12–17.

Falk, K., Patel, H., Swedberg, K., & Ekman, I. (2009). Fatigue in patients with chronic heart failure—A burden associated with emotional and symptom distress. *European Journal of Cardiovascular Nursing, 8*, 91–96.

Hägglund, L., Boman, K., & Lundman, B. (2008). The experience of fatigue among elderly women with chronic heart failure. *European Journal of Cardiovascular Nursing, 7*, 290–295.

Stephen, S. A. (2008). Fatigue in older adults with stable heart failure. *Heart & Lung, 37*, 122–131.

APPENDIX I

List of Evidence-Based, Point-of-Care, Summary Resources

STAT!Ref
http://www.statref.com/content/solutions.html

BestBETs
http://www.bestbets.org/

BMJ Clinical Evidence
http://clinicalevidence.bmj.com/x/index.html

BMJ Point-of-Care
http://group.bmj.com/products/evidence-centre/bmj-point-of-care-1/

Mobile Clin-eguide
http://www.unboundmedicine.com/news/unbound_wkhealth_clineguide

DynaMed—EBSCO
http://dynamed.ebscohost.com/

Essential Evidence Plus—formerly InfoPOEMs/InfoRetriever
http://www.essentialevidenceplus.com/

Evidence-Based Medicine Guidelines (EBMG)—Wiley
http://www.wiley.com/WileyCDA/WileyTitle/productCd-047001184X.html

Evidence Matters
http://evidencematters.com/

JBI COnNECT+—Joanna Briggs Institute
http://connect.jbiconnectplus.org/

NHS Clinical Knowledge Summaries
www.cks.nhs.uk/

Nursing Reference Center—EBSCO
http://www.ebscohost.com/pointOfCare/nrc-about

OvidMD
http://www.ovid.com/site/resources/prodinfo_ovidmd.jsp

ProQuest Nursing & Allied Health Source
http://www.proquest.com/en-US/catalogs/databases/detail/pq_nursingahs.shtml

Rehabilitation Reference Centre—EBSCO
http://www.ebscohost.com/pointOfCare/rrc_about

Thomson Clinical Xpert
http://www.micromedex.com/products/clinicalxpert/

UpToDate—WoltersKluwer
http://www.uptodate.com/index

ZynxEvidence
http://www.zynxhealth.com/Solutions/ZynxEvidence.aspx

Glossary

Absolute benefit increase (ABI) The difference between the percentage of persons in one treatment group who attained a clinical milestone and the percentage of persons in another treatment group who attained it.

Across-studies analysis Comparison, contrast, and pattern searching in findings from two or more studies; the analysis examines the studies as a body of evidence.

Algorithm A step-by-step instruction for solving a clinical problem; often consists of a series of yes/no questions leading to one of several possible decisions or actions.

Applicability The relevance of research evidence to a particular setting considering the similarity of the setting's patients to those in the studies, as well as the safety, feasibility, and expected benefit of implementing the findings.

Appraisal Making objective, systematic judgments regarding the credibility, clinical significance, and applicability of research evidence to determine if changes in practice should be made based on the evidence.

Bias A study influence or action (such as preconceptions or research methods) that produces distorted results, i.e. results that deviate from actuality. The most common sources of research methods bias are design bias, selection bias, measurement bias, and procedural bias.

Blinding Steps taken in experimental studies to keep study staff and participants from knowing which treatment group a person is in; the function of blinding is to prevent personal predilections from influencing responses to the treatment or rating of responses.

Bonferroni correction A change in the level at which a *p*-value is considered significant; it is used to prevent a type 1 conclusion error resulting from multiple tests on the same data.

Care bundle A group of e-b interventions related to a health condition that, when executed together, result in better outcomes than when implemented individually.

Care design The process of using knowledge, information, and data to develop a plan of care for a patient population or for an individual patient.

Case-control study A study in which patients who have an outcome of interest and similar patients who do not have the outcome are identified; then, the researcher looks back to determine exposures and experiences that could have contributed to the outcome occurring or not occurring.

Chance variation The variability in sample averages that is expected whenever one measures a trait, behavior, physiological state, or outcome in two or more samples from the same population.

Clinical decision support The function of a computerized clinical information system that uses inputted patient data to provide agency protocols, information, and more general knowledge relevant to the care of the patient.

Clinical practice guideline A generic set of recommendations regarding the management of a clinical condition, problem, or situation. Ideally, the guideline is produced by a panel of experts and is based on rigorous analysis of research evidence.

Clinical protocol An agency standard of care that sets forth care that should be given to patients with a specified health condition, treatment, or circumstances. Protocols take a variety of forms including care maps, decision algorithms, standard order sets, clinical procedures, care bundles, and standardized plans of care; they guide care in combination with clinical judgment and patient preference.

Clinical significance In quantitative studies, an appraiser's judgment that a research finding indicates a large enough intervention effect or association between variables to have clinical meaning in terms of patients' health or well-being. In qualitative studies, an appraiser's judgment that the findings are informative and useful. The term can be applied in a more general sense to recommendations of clinical practice guidelines and conclusions of systematic reviews.

Coefficient of determination (r^2) The proportion (or percentage) of a variable that is associated with, or explained by, another variable.

Cohen's kappa In a test of an observational instrument, a statistic used to establish the degree of interrater reliability (agreement among raters) when classifying observations into categories is required. If all raters assign the same category to all observations, the kappa is +1.00. Generally, Cohen's kappa values should be above 0.70.

Cohort study A study in which two groups of people are identified, one with an exposure of interest and another without the exposure. The two groups are followed forward to determine if the outcome of interest occurs.

Comparison group In an experimental study, the group that was not given the experimental treatment.

Conclusion error A wrong statistical conclusion reached because of a chance statistical result, a sample size that is too small, large variations in scores, or extraneous variables.

Confidence interval (CI) An extraneous interval that estimates the result that would be found if the whole target population were included in the study; it is an interval around the sample result.

Confounding variable An influence on the outcome that is present at different levels in the groups being compared. The influence either was not recognized before the study but could not be controlled by study design. Its effect can be statistically controlled or analyzed.

Consecutive series sampling A method of obtaining a sample in which starting at a certain point, every person who meets the inclusion criteria is asked to participate in the study, and enrollment continues until the predetermined sample size is reached. It is essentially a convenience sample, although it is less prone to bias than the researcher inviting persons to participate based on his own schedule and inclinations.

Control Study methods that (1) decrease, isolate, or eliminate the influence of extraneous variables; (2) prevent bias from influencing the results; and (3) limit the amount of chance variation.

Control group See *Comparison group*.

Convenience sample A sample that is drawn from an accessible group of people who the researcher thinks are part a larger target population.

Correlation A relationship between two interval or rank-order variables in which their values move in accordance with one another to a lesser, moderate, or greater degree.

Correlational research Research in which the relationship between two or more variables is studied without active intervention by the researcher.

Credibility A characteristic conferred on a finding. The judgment that a finding is trustworthy and not determined by bias, error, extraneous variables, or inaccurate interpretation of the data.

Database A structured, updated collection of informational records about articles, books, and other resources; access to the records is managed with computer software. Some examples are CINAHL, MEDLINE, and PsycINFO.

Data saturation In qualitative research, the point in enrollment of study participants at which the researcher is obtaining only redundant information and not learning anything new from the most recently recruited study participants.

Delivery system The context in which direct clinical care is given; it is made up of a network of logistics including patient flow, scheduling, communications, supplies and equipment availability, role responsibilities, work patterns, accountability structures, and other work dynamics that support direct patient care.

Dependent variable Also called the outcome variable. In experimental research, the response or outcome that is expected to depend on or be caused by the independent variable. It occurs later in time than the independent variable.

Descriptive study A quantitative study that aims to portray a naturally occurring situation, event, or response to illness; data consists of counts of how often something occurs and breakdowns of various aspects of the situation into categories or levels.

Dichotomous variable A variable that has only two possible values, for example, readmitted/not readmitted.

Effect size A statistical representation of the strength of a relationship between two variables; commonly, the size of an intervention's impact on an outcome variable relative to the impact of the comparison intervention.

Error Distortion of data or results caused by mistakes in sampling or measuring or failure to follow study procedures.

Ethnographic research A qualitative research tradition that examines cultures and subcultures to understand how they work and the meaning of members' behaviors.

Evidence Objective knowledge or information used as the basis for a clinical protocol, clinical decision, or clinical action. Evidence sources include research, agency data regarding system performance and patient outcomes, large healthcare databases, and expert opinion.

Evidence-based clinical practice guideline A set of recommended clinical actions for a clinical problem or population that are based to some degree on research evidence.

Evidence-based practice (EBP) The use of care methods that have been endorsed by an agency because available evidence indicates they are effective.

Experimental group In an experimental study, the group that received the treatment of interest, which may be new or not yet definitively tested.

Experimental study A study aimed at comparing the effects of two or more interventions on clinical outcomes. It is characterized by random assignment of participants to treatment groups, careful measurement of outcomes, and control of as many extraneous variables as is feasible to achieve maximum confidence in causal conclusions.

External validity The extent to which study results can be generalized beyond the study sample to a specified population

Extraneous variable A variable that is outside the interests of the study but that may influence the data being collected and lead to wrong conclusions. Researchers try to identify them in advance so as to eliminate or control their influence.

Findings The interpretation of study results into statements that are slightly more general than the statistical results.

Generalizability A judgment about the extent to which the findings of a study will be similar outside the sample in which they were found, i.e., in other practice populations.

Grounded theory method A qualitative tradition of inquiry that is conducted to capture social processes that play out in situations of interest; the goal is to incrementally generate a theory that accounts for behavior or decisions.

Guideline See *Clinical practice guideline.*

Hawthorne effect A change in participants' responses or behaviors because they are aware they are in a study.

Hypothesis A formal statement of the expected results of a study. Hypotheses are tested by data collection and analysis.

Impact As used with the evidence-based practice impact model, it is the effect evidence-based practice has on patients' outcomes and experiences of health, illness, and health care.

Independent variable Also called the intervention/treatment variable. In an experimental study, the variable that is manipulated or varied by the researcher to create an effect on the dependent variable. It occurs first in time relative to the dependent variable.

Institutional review board (IRB) An agency or university committee that reviews the design and procedures of studies prior to their being conducted in the care setting. The purpose of the review is to ensure that the research is ethical and that the rights of study participants will not be violated. IRBs are federally regulated.

Instrument Also referred to as a measurement tool. A way of measuring something. The instrument can be a laboratory test, a questionnaire, a rating guide for observations, or a scored assessment form, to name a few.

Instrument validity The degree to which a measuring instrument captures the concept it is intended to measure instead of another similar concept.

Integrative research review (IRR) A type of systematic review in which the findings from various studies are integrated using logical reasoning augmented by findings tables and lists. The goal of an IRR is to summarize the research knowledge regarding a topic.

Internal consistency An evaluation of the extent to which the items/questions that comprise a measurement instrument capture the underlying concept. A commonly used measure of internal consistency is Cronbach's α.

Interrater reliability The degree to which two or more raters who independently assign a code or score to something assign the same or very similar codes/scores.

Intervention See *Treatment.*

Measurement error The difference in a value obtained by a measurement activity and the actual/true value

Level of significance probability *p*-level See *p*-level.

Meta-analysis A systematic research review involving a statistical pooling of the results from several (or many) quantitative studies examining an issue to produce a statistical result with the larger sample size.

Metasynthesis A systematic research review in which findings from several (or many) qualitative studies examining an issue are merged to produce generalizations and theories.

Number needed to treat (NNT) A representation of treatment effect indicating the number of persons who would need to be treated with the more effective treatment to achieve one additional good outcome (over what would be achieved by using the less effective treatment).

Outcome measure The instrument or tool used to quantify a dependent variable.

Outlier Data contributed by a single study participant that is extreme and considerably outside the range of the other scores in the data set.

Phenomenological research A qualitative research tradition used to examine human experiences. The methods seek to understand how the context of the persons' lives affect the meaning they assign to their experiences; the methods rely on inductively building understanding of the experience across several, a few, or a small number of persons.

PICOTS An acronym standing for the elements that should be considered when conducting an evidence-based project and when searching a database for studies. P= population; I = intervention or issue; C = comparison intervention; O= outcome(s); T=timing; S=setting.

***p*-level** The prespecified decision point for the level of significance; data-based *p*-values above this level are considered statistically not significant.

Point-of-care design Care planning for a particular patient that takes place at the bedside or in the patient–nurse encounter; it includes either modification of a protocol or new courses of action not specified by an existing protocol.

Point-of-care evidence Research evidence presented in short formats that summarize the research evidence or present part of a larger evidence document.

Population A group of persons or entities with an important characteristic or characteristics in common.

Power analysis A way of determining sample size that factors in the size of the difference or association expected, the *p*-value cut point, and the probability of finding a difference or relationship that exists.

Prespecification design Care design for a population of patients that incorporates the best evidence available into a care protocol; it is done away from the demands of moment-to-moment care responsibilities.

Projected population Based on the profile of a sample, the population to which the results of a study are believed to apply.

Protocol See *Clinical protocol.*

***p*-value** The data-based probability that the obtained result is attributable to chance variation. This probability is compared to a previously chosen level of significance *p*-level to reach a conclusion about whether the relationship or difference found is statistically significant, i.e., likely to exist in the target population.

Qualitative content analysis A group of data analysis techniques used by qualitative researchers to derive meaning from the content of textual data. It typically involves developing a series of codes from the data.

Qualitative description A qualitative research method that produces straightforward descriptions of participants' experiences in language as similar to the participants' native language as possible.

Qualitative filter An assessment of the methodological quality of studies using explicit criteria; it is used in conducting systematic reviews to separate studies of different methodological soundness or to eliminate poorly conducted studies.

Qualitative research Inquiry regarding human phenomena that refrains from imposing assumptions on study participants and situations. Its purposes include exploration, description, and theory generation.

Quality improvement An agency's programs aimed at improving the safety, timeliness, patient-centeredness, and efficiency of care delivery systems.

Quantitative research Inquiry that (1) examines preidentified issues; (2) uses designs that control extraneous variables; (3) uses numeric measures to determine levels of various variables; and (4) analyzes data using statistical or graphing methods.

Quasi-experimental research A type of intervention research in which either random assignment to control groups or control over the intervention and setting is not possible.

Random assignment A chance-based procedure used to assign study participants to a treatment or comparison group. Each participant has an equal chance of being assigned to either treatment group. It serves to distribute participant characteristics evenly in both groups.

Randomized clinical trial (RCT) An experimental study that involves advanced testing of an intervention using defined study protocols typically with a large, diverse sample.

Random sample A sample created by one of several methods by which every person in the population has a greater than zero chance of being included in the sample.

Relationship In research, a connection between two variables in which one influences the other, both influence each other, or both are influenced by a third variable.

Reliability The degree to which a measuring instrument consistently obtains the same or similar measurement values.

Research design A framework or general guide regarding how to structure studies conducted to answer a certain type of research question.

Research evidence Findings of individual studies, conclusions of systematic reviews of research, and research-based recommendations of soundly produced clinical practice guidelines.

Research-informed practice (RIP) The use of research evidence by an individual nurse in the care of an individual patient or in her/his practice.

Results The outcomes of the numerical and statistical analysis of raw data.

Rigor A quality of a research study that reflects its adherence to recognized standards for its type of study.

Sample Persons chosen from a target population to participate in a study. The ideal sample is representative of the target population.

Scientific knowledge production The series of inquiry activities that start with a knowledge question and end with clinical recommendations based on conclusions reached by thorough review of all studies about the question. Scientific knowledge production typically plays out over many years and is always considered open to revision.

Scope The range or breadth of a question, project, review, or guideline including a description of what is included.

Search In the context of EBP, a pursuit to identify all research conducted relevant to a topic. More particularly, the use of a computer search engine to comb through bibliographic databases and other indexes to identify relevant research articles.

Simple random sample A sample that is randomly selected from a list of population members.

Statistical significance A statistical conclusion that a difference or association would likely be found in the population. It is based on a low probability of the result being just due to chance variation.

Study plan A term used in quantitative research to describe how the study will be conducted, including how the sample will be obtained; how the data will be measured, collected, and analyzed; and any control that will be used.

Systematic review (SR) A comprehensive and systematic identification, analysis, and summary of research evidence related to a specified issue. An SR can use statistics, tabulation, compare-and-contrast methods, or pattern-identification to reach conclusions based on the body of studies in the review.

Target population The entire group of individuals or organizations to which the sample results are considered applicable. It may be the entire population from which the sample was randomly drawn or a projected population based on a convenience sample's profile.

Test-retest reliability A way of evaluating the consistency with which persons score themselves similarly on the questionnaire at two completions of the questionnaire separated by an appropriate period of time.

Theory Assumptions, concepts, definitions, and/or propositions that provide a cohesive (although tentative) explanation of how a phenomenon is thought to work.

Translational research Also called implementation research. The field of study that investigates how research evidence can effectively be integrated into agency and individual practice.

Treatment In the research context, clinical interventions, therapies, action, or courses of action that are evaluated in the study. The treatment is the independent variable, and its effect on the dependent variables (outcomes) is what is being tested by the study.

Treatment effect measures Various numerical representations of the clinical effectiveness of treatments, therapies, and interventions, including absolute benefit increase (ABI), number needed to treat (NNT), relative risk (RR), and odds ratio (OR).

Type 1 conclusion error The conclusion that there is a significant relationship between variables or a significant difference in groups' outcomes when in fact there is not a significant relationship or difference.

Type 2 conclusion error The conclusion that there is not a significant relationship between variables or a significant difference in groups' outcomes when in fact there is a significant relationship or difference.

Valid finding A finding of a study or conclusion of an SR that is credible, that is trustworthy, because it was produced by sound methods that controlled extraneous variables and bias.

Validity See *Instrument validity.*

Variable An attribute of a person, social group, thing, or situation that when measured has two or more categories or possible values.

Index

A

absolute benefit increase (ABI)
  clinical significance, 331
  defined, 435
  experimental research, 177, 191
  intervention comparisons, 342
abstracts
  cohort research exemplar, 198
  defined, 27
  descriptive research exemplar, 84–85
  experimental research exemplar, 159–160
  integrative research review exemplar, 225–226
  qualitative research exemplar, 44
  research reports, 27–28
  systemic review, 21
accrediting agencies, 286, 287
across-studies analysis, 343–346, 435
active reading, 25
Agency for Healthcare Research and Quality (AHRQ), 357
AGREE system, 322–323
AHRQ. *See* Agency for Healthcare Research and Quality
algorithms, 7, 353, 435
allied health journals, 298–299
Allied Health Source, 390
alternative explanations for findings, 34
American Journal of Nursing, 11
American Nurses Association database links, 297–298
analysis of data. *See* data analysis
annotating articles, 25
appendices, descriptive research exemplar, 101–102
applicability
  of clinical practice guidelines, 326
  defined, 435
  of evidence, 316–318
  of integrative research reviews, 332
  research-practice connection, 13
appraisal, 311–333
  overview, 311–312
  AGREE and GRADE systems, 322–323
  applicability, 326
  clinical guide to. *See* appraisal guide
  clinical significance, 315–316, 325–326
  of conclusions, 224, 329
  credibility, 323–325
  defined, 435
  evaluation instruments, 322
  of evidence, 311–319
  of integrative research review, 219, 329–333
  of integrative research review conclusions, 325, 405–408
  of preappraised evidence, 384, 389, 390
  of recommendations, 321–327
  research-practice connection, 13
  of study findings. *See* appraisal, of original study findings
  synopsis, 323
  of systematic review, 329

appraisal, of original study findings, 335–346
across-studies analysis, 343–346
design appropriateness, 336–337
peer review, 337
qualitative research
clinical significance, 338–339
credibility, 336–338
sample guide, 415–417
quantitative research
applicability, 342–343
clinical significance, 342
completed guide, 423–427
conclusion errors, 339–341
credibility, 336–337, 338, 339–342
sample guide, 419–421
appraisal guide
applicability, 397, 402–404, 407–408, 413–414
citation, 395, 399, 405, 409, 415, 419, 423
clinical significance, 396, 401–402, 407, 412–413, 417, 421, 426–427
Conclusions of an Integrative Research Review, 405–408
credibility, 396, 400–401, 406, 410–412, 416, 420, 424–426
Findings of a Qualitative Study, 415–417
Findings of a Quantitative Study, 419–421, 423–427
Recommendations of a Clinical Practice Guideline, 395–397, 399–404
synopsis, 395, 399–400, 405, 409–410, 415, 419, 423–424
for use by nurse with a BSN, 322–327
appraise, 435
article availability, 299
asking clinical questions. *See* clinical questions, asking
assumptions
assumed population, in descriptive research, 104
in qualitative research, 37
in research report, 28
authors
experimental research exemplar, 172
qualitative research exemplar, 59
averages, pitfalls of, 157

B

background
cohort research exemplar, 198
descriptive research exemplar, 85
integrative research review exemplar, 227–228
Beck Depression Inventory (BDI), 127
benefit expectations, 316–317
Best Practice Sheets (JBI), 260
bias
controlling, 147, 152–153, 156, 341
defined, 435
in integrative research reviews, 216, 223, 330
from missing data, 154–156
in systematic review, 217
biomedical journals, 298–299
bipolar disorder medication IRR exemplar, 224–250
profile and commentary, 248–250
bivariate correlational analysis, 122
blinding, defined, 436
blinding data collectors, 153
bone healing delay and cigarette smoking exemplar, 198–212
profile and commentary, 206–212
Bonferroni correction, 141, 436
Boolean operators, 301, 302
borderline results, 188
bridge metaphor, EBP care design, 350–351
browse box, 302

C

care
design and delivery, 7–9, 383–384
individualized, 383–384
protocols, 352–353. *See also specific types of protocols*
care bundle, 7, 352–353, 436
care conferences, patient, 375, 379–380
care delivery. *See* delivery system
care design, 350–351, 436
case studies, evidence-based practice, 11
case-control studies, 195–197, 436
causation, and correlations, 119
cause-and-effect relationships, 119, 193
Centers for Disease Control and Prevention (CDC), 293
Centers for Medicare and Medicaid Services (CMS), 287, 357
Centre for Evidence Based Physiotherapy (CEPD), 297
Centre for Reviews and Dissemination (CRD), 296, 388
chance variation
defined, 436
descriptive research, 108
experimental research, 179
as extraneous, 340

CI. *See* confidence intervals
cigarette smoking and bone healing delays exemplar, 198–212
  profile and commentary, 206–212
"Cigarette Smoking Delays Bone Healing: A Prospective Study of 200 Patients Operated On by the Hemicallotasis Technique" (Dahl and Toksvig-Larsen), 198–206
CINAHL database, 21, 297–308, 378
CIS. *See* clinical information systems
citation features, 307
citations, in research reports, 34
clinical decision support, 391, 436
Clinical Guidelines (NICE), 296
clinical information systems (CIS), 391
clinical perspective on experimental research, 176–178
clinical practice, 252
clinical practice guidelines. *See also* evidence-based clinical practice guidelines (EbCPG)
  appraisal of, 321–327. *See also* appraisal guide
  comorbidity, 261
  defined, 436
  evidence strength, 254–257
  forerunner to clinical protocols, 251–253
  formats, 259–261
  knowledge building for, 15–16
  non-pharmaceutical management of depression exemplar, 261–275
  production of, 253–258
  recommendations in, 16, 20–24
  research-practice connection, 12
  searching for, 293–294
  sources of, 294–298
clinical protocols
  building, 16
  defined, 252, 436
  EbCPGs integration benefits, 252
  evidence for, 6–7
  evidence-based practice project implementation plan, 362–365
  forerunner to, 251–253
  formats of, 7
  nursing development role, 9–10
  qualitative research, 343
  reevaluating, 286
  for specific populations, 352
clinical questions, asking, 285–292
  clinical practice, 286
  forming a useful project question, 288–292
  professional standards, 287
  quality data, 286–287
  questions not answered by evidence, 287–288
  triggers, 285–287
clinical significance
  overview, 315
  appraising, 315–316
  defined, 436–437
  evidence, appraisal of, 315–316
  integrative research reviews, 331–332
  qualitative research, 338–339
  quantitative research, 342
  of recommendations, 325–326
  of treatment differences, 185–187
cluster sampling, 78, 79
CMS. *See* Centers for Medicare and Medicaid Services
Cochrane Collaboration, Oxford University, 11, 213, 295, 388
Cochrane Nursing Care Network (CNCN), 295
coding data, 41–42
coefficient of determination, 121, 437
Cohen's kappa, 437
cohort research, 193–212
  overview, 193, 197
  vs. case-control studies, 195–197
  cigarette smoking and bone healing delays exemplar, 198–212
  confounding variables, 194–195
  design, 193–194, 206–207
  discussion, 212
  limitations, 198
  outcomes, 207
  purposes of studies, 206
  results, 207–212
  risk factors, 206–207
  sampling, 207
cohort study, 437
comparison groups, 147, 150, 437
"Comparison of Inhalation of Isopropyl Alcohol *vs.* Promethazine in the Treatment of Postoperative Nausea and Vomiting (PONV) in Patients Identified as at High Risk for Developing PONV" (Pellegrini *et al*), 159–172
comparisons
  interventions, 289–290, 342
  statistics, 151
  treatment effectiveness, 178, 179, 189–190
computer systems. *See* databases
concepts, searching by, 302

concern presentations, 375, 377–379
conclusion errors, 339–341, 437
conclusions
  from across-studies analysis, 344–345
  appraising conclusions of integrative research reviews, 325, 405–408
  appraising IRR, 329–333
  in correlational research exemplar, 134
  in descriptive research exemplar, 85, 98–99
  as essential study element, 26–27
  integrative research review exemplar, 226, 243
  as interpretations, 224
  research reports, 33–34
  significance of, 180–181
confidence intervals (CI), 76, 210, 437
confirmation of findings, 15–16
confounding variables
  in case-control studies, 196
  in cohort research, 194–195, 210–212
  defined, 437
consecutive series, sampling, 158, 206, 437
consistency of data/evidence, 70
content analysis, qualitative, 41
control
  of bias, 74, 152–153
  defined, 437
  of extraneous influence, 147, 152–153, 156
control group. *See* comparison groups
controlled vocabulary, 302
convenience samples, 80, 104, 438
"Correlates of Fatigue in Patients with Heart Failure" (Evangelista *et al*), 123–136
correlation, 438
correlation coefficients, 122
correlation quantitative research design, 20
correlation statistics, 112
correlational research, 111–144
  data analysis, 139
  defined, 111, 438
  design, 122–123, 136
  discussion, 142–143
  fatigue in patients with heart failure exemplar, 123–143, 492–493
  measurement, 137–139
  purposes of studies, 136
  relationships in, 18, 111–121
  results, 139–142
  sampling, 136–137
CRD. *See* Centre for Reviews and Dissemination
credibility
  of clinical practice guidelines, 323–325
  defined, 438
  evidence, appraisal of, 312, 313–315
  of evidence, 312, 313
  integrative research reviews (IRRs), 330–331
  linked to evidence, 324
  original studies, 336–337
  peer review, 337
  qualitative, 336–338
  quantitative research, 336–337, 338, 339–342
  reading research articles, 35
  validity *vs.*, 341–342
cross-sectional design, 136

D

DARE. *See* Database of Abstracts of Reviews of Effects
data
  in correlational research, 139
  descriptive research exemplar, 89–90
  missing, 154–156
  in qualitative research, 38–41
  quality of, 70, 157, 286
  reliability of, 70–71, 73
  from surveys, 82
data analysis
  correlational research exemplar, 128, 139
  descriptive research exemplar, 90
  as essential study element, 26–27
  from integrative research reviews, 219–223
  in qualitative research, 38–41
  qualitative research exemplar, 49, 63
  statistical, 176
data collection
  as essential study element, 26
  missing data, experimental research, 147, 154–156
  qualitative research exemplar, 63
  quality improvement, 356–357
  in research reports, 32
data saturation, 63, 438
Database of Abstracts of Reviews of Effects (DARE), 296–297
databases
  in cohort research, 194
  defined, 438
  search for evidence, 295–308
  searching, 218–219

sources of, 295–297
switching between databases, 308–309
systematic *vs.* literature reviews, 215
datasets, hypothetical, 114–118
decision algorithms, 353
decision points for significance, 180–181
decision trees of clinical protocols, 7
delivery systems
defined, 438
quality improvement, 355, 358–360
dependent variables, 438
depression, non-pharmaceutical management of, exemplar, 261–275
profile and commentary, 274–275
descriptive quantitative research design, 20
descriptive research, 67–110
classification, 68
design, 103
discussion, 109
endotracheal suctioning practices exemplar, 84–109
ethics review, 105
extraneous variables, 74–75
measurement, 104–105
natural conditions, 67–68
purposes of studies, 103
results, 83–84, 105–109
sampling, 75–82, 104
surveys, 82
target populations, 75–82
variables, 68–75
descriptive studies, 68, 438
design
of care, 7–9, 383–384
point-of-care design, 351, 383, 387–391
question-design match, 313–314
of research. *See* research design
dichotomous outcomes
cohort research, 208–210
experimental research, 176–178, 190–191
dichotomous variable, 438
discipline, nursing as, 11
disclaimer, experimental research exemplar, 172
discourse analysis, 38
discretionary acts, 8
discriminate analysis, 123
discussion
cohort research exemplar, 203–205, 212
correlational research exemplar, 131–134, 142–143
descriptive research exemplar, 96–98, 109
experimental research exemplar, 168–171, 191–192
integrative research review exemplar, 239–243, 249
purpose of, 28
qualitative research exemplar, 57–59, 64
research reports, 33–34
dispersion of data, 83
dropouts, 155–156

E

EbCPG. *See* evidence-based clinical practice guidelines
EBP. *See* evidence-based practice
EBQM. *See* evidence-based quality management
EBSCO Nursing Resource Center, 390
EBSCOhost (database vendor), 308
effect size, 439
end-of-life wishes, 288
endotracheal suctioning practices exemplar, 84–109
profile and commentary, 103–109
errors
conclusion errors, 339–341, 437
controlling, 147, 152–153
defined, 439
integrative research reviews, 216, 223
and reliability, 70
ethics
descriptive research exemplar, 90, 105
qualitative research exemplar, 61–62
review/questions, 287–288
ethnographic research, 38, 39, 439
evaluation. *See also* appraisal
of EBP project impact, 366
evidence, 257–258
instruments for, 322
evidence
applicability of, 316–318
appraisal of, 311–319
building knowledge for clinical practice, 15–16
for clinical protocols, 6–7
clinical questions not answered by, 287–288
credibility linked to, 324
defined, 439
EB clinical *vs.* care team investigation, 24
eliminate poor quality, EBP projects, 362
evaluating, 257–258. *See also* evidence, appraisal of

in evidence-based practice, 11–12
fit, 316
grading hierarchies, 256
grading recommendations, 257–259
preappraised, 384, 389, 390
questions not answered by, 287–288
from research, 5
safety and expected benefits, 316–317
scientific, for protocols, 11
search for, 293–309
strength of, clinical practice guidelines, 254–257
types of, 15–24
evidence, appraisal of, 311–319
applicability, 316–318
appraisal systems, 312
clinical significance, 315–316
credibility, 312, 313–315
feasibility of implementation, 317–318
goals of, 312–313
practical considerations, 318–319
preappraised, 384, 389, 390
production methods, 314
question-design match, 313–314
similarity to findings from other studies, 314–315
synopsis, 313
evidence, search for, 293–309
clinical practice guidelines, 24
databases, 295–308
EBP projects, 362
evidence-based practice projects, 362
for reports/protocols/guidelines, 293–294
research sources, 294–298
techniques
advanced, 303–307
basic, 300–301
intermediate, 301–303
evidence, types of, 15–24
grading, 256
overview, 23
qualitative research, 17
quantitative research, 17–18
recommendations of an EbCPG, 16, 22–24
single original study, 15, 16–20
systematic reviews, 16, 20–21
evidence-based care, 7–9
evidence-based clinical practice guidelines (EbCPG), 251–277
appraising recommendations, 321
clinical protocol forerunners, 251–253
clinical protocols, 9
comorbidity, 261
defined, 439
in E-B protocols, 22, 23–24
EBP, 385, 388, 389, 391
exemplar, 271–272
formats, 259–261
methods, 274–275
non-pharmaceutical management of depression exemplar, 261–275
nursing practice, 11
production process, 253–258
recommendations, 275–276
sources of, 293–298
topic, 274
evidence-based practice (EBP)
overview, 11–14
care design, 350–351
defined, 439
impact model, 281–283
individualized care, 353–354
list of resources, 433–434
as a movement, 11–12
organizational integration, 366–367
participation scenarios, 375–381
professional action, 349–350
projects, 360–366
protocols, 352–354
quality improvement, 354–360
research-informed practice, 384–385, 392
research-practice lag, 368–369
short format sources, 388–389
evidence-based practice (EBP) participation scenarios, 375–381
build your EBP knowledge and skills, 375, 380–381
contribute to a patient care conference, 375, 379–380
join a project team, 375–376
present an idea or concern, 375, 377–379
submit a poster, 375, 376–377, 378
evidence-based practice (EBP) projects, 360–366
action steps, 360–361
design a clinical protocol, 362
eliminate poor quality evidence, 362
extract information, 362
impact evaluation, 366
plan protocol implementation, 362–365
project work-group formation, 361–362
respond to identified need, 361
revisit and revise, 366
search for evidence, 362

targeted adopters, 364–365
work-setting dynamics, 365
evidence-based practice (EBP) protocols
care protocols, 352–353
individualized protocols/care, 353–354
evidence-based (E-B) protocols
asking clinical questions, 285–292
development of, 22, 23–24
evidence-based quality management (EBQM), 384
experimental groups, 150, 439
experimental intervention. *See* interventions
experimental quantitative research design, 20
experimental research, 145–192
overview, 145–146, 156
characteristics of sound, 156
defined, 439
design, 147, 173–175
evidence grading, 256
features, 147–156
bias and extraneous influence control, 147, 152–153, 156
intervention delivery, 147, 153–154, 156
missing data, 147, 154–156
random assignment, 147, 150–152, 156
sample size, 147, 149–150, 156
target population, 147, 148–149, 156
interventions, 174–175
methods, 147–159
features, 147–156
limitations of randomized experiments, 157
measurement of outcome variables, 156
PONV treatments exemplar, 159–175
quasi-experimental design, 157–159
outcomes, 175
postoperative nausea and vomiting (PONV) treatment exemplar, 159–175
purposes of studies, 173
results, 176–192
clinical perspective, 176–178, 185–187
outcomes reporting, 187
PONV treatments exemplar, 188–192
statistical perspective, 179–187
sampling, 173–174
systematic review, 217
experimental treatment. *See* interventions
expert opinions, 256
expertise, clinical practice guidelines panel, 253–254
Explode feature, 303–305
external validity, 439
extraction, from integrative research reviews, 219–223
extraneous influence, experimental research, 74–75, 147, 152–153, 156
extraneous variables
conclusion errors, 340–341
defined, 439
descriptive research, 74–75
experimental research, 152–153
quasi-experimental designs, 158

F

facilitation strategies for EBP projects, 363–364
facts stated, qualitative research exemplar, 46
false hits, 300
fatigue in patients with heart failure correlational exemplar, 123–143, 492–493
feasibility of implementation, 317–318, 326
figures, in research report, 33
findings
from across-studies analysis, 344–345
alternative explanations for, 34
appraisal. *See* appraisal, of original study findings
biased, 155
combining, 16
defined, 5, 32, 439
differences in, 315
erroneous, 82
as essential study element, 26–27
evidence. *See* evidence
influences on, 33–34, 75, 121–122
integration of, 20–21
in integrative research reviews, 219–223
from original study, 16–20
from other studies, appraisal of evidence, 314–315
pitfalls of, 157
in research reports, 32–33, 34
research-practice connections, 5–6
results. *See* results
review of. *See* integrative research reviews (IRR); systematic review (SR)
significance of, 180–181
focus, forming a useful project question, 289–292
formats. *See also specific types of research*
of clinical practice guidelines, 259–261
of clinical protocols, 7
of research reports, 27–34
full text availability, 299

G

generalizability, 109, 157, 440
Google, 298, 299–300
government-funded research implementation, 11–12
GRADE system, 322–323
grading evidence, recommendations, 257–259
grounded theory methods, 4, 38, 40, 42, 440
guidelines. *See also* clinical practice guidelines; evidence-based clinical practice guidelines (EbCPG)
  definition, 10
  evidence-based, 11, 22–24
  protocols as, 8–9

H

Hawthorne effect, 75, 109, 440
Headings tab, 301
healthcare information systems, research-informed practice, 385, 386–387
healthcare variables of interest, 70
heart failure, fatigue in patients with, correlational exemplar, 123–143, 492–493
Hirsh Institute, Case Western Reserve University, 380
historical analysis, 38
human experiences, 38
hypothesis
  defined, 440
  as essential study element, 26, 27
  purpose, in research report, 30
  in qualitative studies, 42–43
  study method, 19
  study purpose, 30
  testing, descriptive research exemplar, 106–107
hypothetical correlational studies, 113
hypothetical datasets, 114–118

I

idea presentations, 375, 377–379
identified need, EBP project response, 361
impact, 440
impact model, EBP, 281–283
implementation feasibility, 317–318, 326
implemented research, 12
incidence of PONV, 188–189
inclusion, systematic *vs.* literature reviews, 215
independence *vs.* relationships, 112
independent variables, 147, 440. *See also* interventions
index headings, 299, 301–302
individualized protocols/care, 353–354, 383–384
inductive methods, 38
inference, population, 76
inferential statistics, 179
influences
  controlling, 152–153
  controlling extraneous, 74–75, 147, 152–153, 156
  in integrative research reviews, 223
  in IRR production process, 216
  outliers as, 121–122
information, extracting, 362
information intersection, 385, 386–387
information services, 389–391
innovation in EBP projects, 363–364
Institute for Johns Hopkins Nursing, 380
Institute for Medicine, 216
Institutional Review Board (IRB), 31, 61–62, 440
instructions for reaching a decision, 353
instrument validity, 440. *See also* validity
instruments
  correlational research exemplar, 126–127
  defined, 69, 440
  for evaluating, 322
  qualitative research exemplar, 48–49
  used, in research reports, 32
integrative research reviews (IRRs)
  applicability, 332, 342, 346
  appraisal of, 329–333
  appraising conclusions of, 325, 405–408
  bipolar disorder medication IRR exemplar, 224–250
  clinical significance, 331–332
  conclusions, 405–408
  defined, 214, 440
  discussion, 249
  EBP impact evaluation, 366
  findings, 219–223
  methods, 248
  production process, 216–224
  purposes of studies, 248
  relevance screening, 218–219
  reports, 223–224
  results, 249–250
  scope, 216–217
  search for studies, 218–219
  SR production steps, 216
  synopsis, 330

topic formulation, 216–218
types of studies, 217–218
using, 224
internal consistency, 138, 440
Internet, 385–391
interquartile range (IQR), 83–84
interrater reliability, 105, 138, 441
interval level scale, 112, 178, 179, 210
interventions. *See also* treatments
overview, 147
comparison of, 289–290, 342
consistent delivery of, 153–154
delivery, in experimental research, 147, 153–154, 156
EbCPG exemplar, 272–273
effectiveness, 176, 178
experimental research exemplar, 174–175
meta-analysis improvements, 214
quantitative comparison of, 18
interviews, 38, 41
introduction
cohort research exemplar, 199
correlational research exemplar, 124–125
descriptive research exemplar, 85–86
EbCPG exemplar, 265–268
experimental research exemplar, 160–161
integrative research review exemplar, 226–227
purpose of, 28
qualitative research exemplar, 45
research reports, 28–31
IQR. *See* interquartile range
IRB. *See* Institutional Review Board
IRRs. *See* integrative research reviews
isopropyl alcohol. *See* postoperative nausea and vomiting (PONV) treatment exemplar

J

JBI. *See* Joanna Briggs Institute
Joanna Briggs Institute (JBI), 213, 216, 294–295, 380, 388, 390
Best Practice Sheets, 260
The Joint Commission, 287
journals, in databases, 298–299

K

key questions, EbCPG exemplar, 273–274
key words
descriptive research exemplar, 85
experimental research exemplar, 160
integrative research review exemplar, 225
qualitative research exemplar, 45
knees, total knee replacement (TKR) exemplar report, 43–64
knowledge building
for clinical practice, 15–16
evidence-based practice, 375, 380–381
transformations in clinical practice guidelines, 252

L

levels of evidence, EbCPG exemplar, 274
licensing agencies, 286, 287
limitations
in cohort research, 198
in descriptive research, 109
descriptive research exemplar, 98
qualitative research exemplar, 58–59
in research report, 34
limited generalizability, 109
limiting searches, 301, 303, 305–306
literature reviews. *See also* research articles, reading
descriptive research exemplar, 86–88
systematic reviews *vs.,* 215
low statistical power, 150

M

manipulation of interventions, 147
McMaster Medical School, 11
mean outcome scores, 178, 179
means, 83
measurement
correlational research, 137–139
descriptive research, 104–105
descriptive research exemplar, 104–105
relationships, 112–121
variables, 69–74, 157
measurement error, 71, 441
median, 83
medical terminology challenges, 300
medication adherence in bipolar disorder IRR exemplar, 224–250
profile and commentary, 248–250
Medline, 298–308
Medline database, 297
meta-analysis, 214, 254, 256, 441
metasynthesis, 214, 441
methods
cohort research exemplar, 198–201
descriptive research exemplar, 85, 88–91

EbCPG exemplar, 274–275
experimental research exemplar, 162–164
integrative research review exemplar, 226, 228–231, 248
to obtain evidence, 17–20
in qualitative research exemplar, 44, 47–50, 61–63
in research reports, 31–32
rigor of, 338
missing data, experimental research, 154–156
mixed design/methods, 335–336
moderate relationships, 112
multiple regression analysis, 123, 141

N

NAON. *See* National Association of Orthopaedic Nurses
narrative reviews. *See* integrative research reviews
narrowing searches, 301, 303, 305–306
National Association of Orthopaedic Nurses (NAON), 376–377
National Database of Quality Indicators, 358
National Guideline Clearinghouse (NGC), 295–296
National Health Service, 296
National Institute for Clinical Excellence (NICE), 296, 384, 388
National Institute of Nursing Research, 11
National Library of Medicine, 308
natural conditions in descriptive research, 67–68
negative relationships, 111, 112
NGC. *See* National Guideline Clearinghouse
NICE. *See* National Institute for Clinical Excellence
NNT. *See* number needed to treat
nonexperimental designs, descriptive research, 68
non-participant structured observation, 103
non-pharmaceutical management of depression exemplar, 261–275
profile and commentary, 274–275
number needed to treat (NNT)
clinical significance, 331
defined, 441
experimental research, 177–178, 190–191
intervention comparisons, 342
nurses' associations databases, 297–298
nursing art, 8
Nursing Best Practice Guidelines (RNAO), 294
nursing journals, 298–299, 303
Nursing Reference Center, EBSCO, 296, 390

O

observation, structured, 103
observational designs, 68, 217–218, 256
"An Observational Study on the Open-System Endotracheal Suctioning Practices of Critical Care Nurses" (Kelleher and Andrews), 84–102
odds ratio (OR), 211–212
Oncology Nursing Society, 258, 388
opportunities for research-informed practice, 385–386
OR. *See* odds ratio
original studies
overview, 335–336
across-studies analysis, 343–346
applicability, 342–343
appraisal of findings. *See* appraisal, of original study findings
credibility, 336–337
essential elements, 26–27
findings from, 16–20
qualitative research, 338–339
quantitative research, 339–342
single, as evidence, 15, 16–20
outcome measure, 153, 175, 441
outcomes
attainment of, 176–178
bias. *See* bias
in cohort research, 201, 207
dichotomous. *See* dichotomous outcomes
differences in, 150, 179
interval level scale, 210
mean outcome scores, 178, 179
predicting, 123, 141
quantitative comparison of, 18
reporting, 187
variables in, 157
outliers, 120–121

P

panel, clinical practice guidelines development, 253–254
patients. *See also specific topics*
advocacy for, 8
care conferences, 375, 379–380
provider dialogue, 38
"Patients' Perspectives on Total Knee Replacements" (Jacobson et al), 44–61
"Patients' Reports of the Factors Influencing Medication Adherence in Bipolar Disorder - an Integrative Review of the Literature" (Crowe *et al*), 225–248
PDA-formats, 260, 385, 388

Pearson *r* coefficient, 112–113, 119–121, 140–141
PEDro database, 297
peer review, 327
percentages, to report results, 83
phenomena, 18
phenomenological research, 38, 39, 441
physiological measure, as psychological state indicator, 73
Physiotherapy Evidence Database (PEDro), 297
PICOT format, 289–290, 376, 441
placebo interventions, 153–154
p-level, 441
point-of-care design, 351, 383, 387–391
point-of-care evidence
  defined, 441–442
  EBP, 353–354
  list of resources, 433–434
  research-informed practice, 383, 387–391
POMS-F. *See* Profile of Mood States-Fatigue
PONV. *See* postoperative nausea and vomiting (PONV) treatment exemplar
population
  clinical protocols for, 352–353
  convenience samples, 80
  defined, 6, 442
  in descriptive research, 104
  estimates of, clinical practice guidelines, 255
  random sampling, 44, 77–79, 107, 151, 443
  representativeness, erosion of, 81
  sampling, 75–82, 104, 316
  validity in, 157
positive relationships, 111, 112
posters, making, 375, 376–377, 378
postoperative nausea and vomiting (PONV) treatment exemplar, 159–175
  profile and commentary, 173–175, 188–192
power analysis, 149–150, 442
preappraised evidence, 384, 389, 390
predictor variables, 123, 139–140, 141
prespecification design, 351, 442
prevention-of-ventilator-associated-pneumonia bundle, 352–353
production process
  credibility, 323–324
  methods, appraisal of, 314
  systematic *vs.* literature reviews, 215
professional action, 349–350
professional standards, 287
Profile of Mood States-Fatigue (POMS-F), 126–127, 138, 139
projected population, 80, 104, 442
promethazine. *See* postoperative nausea and vomiting (PONV) treatment exemplar
propositions, in research report, 28
ProQuest Nursing, 390
prospective studies, 206. *See also specific types of studies*
protocols, 10. *See also specific types of protocols*
PsycArticles, 308
psychology journals, 298–299
psychosocial variables, 73–74
PsycINFO, 298–299, 308
publication types, 303
PubMed database, 21, 297–299, 308, 389
purpose of research
  overview, 19–20
  cohort research exemplar, 206
  correlational research exemplar, 136
  descriptive research exemplar, 84, 88, 103
  in descriptive research reports, 103
  experimental research exemplar, 172
  integrative research review exemplar, 248
  qualitative research exemplar, 61
  research reports, 27, 30–31
  systematic *vs.* literature reviews, 215
  words and phrases, in research reports, 30
Putting Evidence Into Practice (PEP) (Oncology Nursing Society), 388
p-values, 107–108, 179–185, 442

Q

QQL. *See* quality of life (QQL) measure
qualitative content analysis, 442
qualitative description, 442
qualitative filter, 442
qualitative research, 37–65
  overview, 17
  applicability of, 343
  clinical significance, 338–339
  credibility of, 336–338
  data collection and analysis, 38–41
  defined, 38, 442
  essential elements in, 27
  evidence from, 17
  features of, 335–336
  original studies, 338–339
  phenomena in, 18
  purpose of, 19, 30, 37
  qualitative description, 41–42
  with quantitative research, 41–42
  results/findings, 33
  systematic review, 217–218

total knee replacement (TKR) exemplar report, 43–64
uniqueness of, 42–43
qualitative systematic reviews. *See* integrative research reviews (IRR)
quality data, asking clinical questions, 286–287
quality filter, in systematic reviews, 215
quality improvement (QI), 354–360
defined, 443
delivery system improvement, 358–360
delivery systems, 355
and EBP relationship, 360
EBP *vs.*, 354–356
organizational integration of EBP, 366–367
programs, 356–360
research-practice connection, 13
standards of care, 357–358
quality of life (QQL) measure, 127, 139–141
quantitative research
overview, 17–18
clinical significance, 342
consistency of data/evidence, 70
credibility, 336–337, 338, 339–342
defined, 443
essential elements in, 27
evidence from, 17–18
features of, 335–336
purpose of, 19, 31
with qualitative research, 41–42
research design, 20
results/findings, 32–33
systematic review, 217
quasi-experimental design, 157–159
defined, 443
evidence grading, 256
quantitative, 20
question-design match, 313–314
questions, asking clinical. *See* clinical questions, asking
quick reference guides for guidelines, 260
quota sampling, 104

R

R^2 statistic, 123
random assignment
cohort research, 193
defined, 443
experimental research, 147, 150–152, 156
random missing data, 154–155
random sampling, 44.107, 77–79, 151, 443
randomization, 151
randomized clinical trials (RCT), 146, 256, 443
randomized controlled experiments, 157
randomized experiments, 157
range of scores, 83
rapid response teams (RRT), 213
rating, strength of evidence, 254
RCT. *See* randomized clinical trials
reading research articles. *See* research articles, reading
recommendations
appraisal guide: Recommendations of a Clinical Practice Guideline, 395–397, 399–404
appraising, 321–327
in clinical practice guidelines, 16, 22–24
in descriptive research, 109
descriptive research exemplar, 97
of EbCPG, evidence from, 16, 22–24
EbCPG exemplar, 262–263, 269–271, 272, 275–276
grading evidence, 257–259
references
cohort research exemplar, 205–206
correlational research exemplar, 134–135
descriptive research exemplar, 99–100
experimental research exemplar, 171–172
integrative research review exemplar, 244–247
qualitative research exemplar, 46, 49–50, 60–61
research reports, 34
refining searches, 301
Registered Nurses Association of Ontario (RNAO), 22, 260, 294, 388
relationships
in correlational research, 111–121
defined, 443
in quantitative research, 18
relative risk (RR), 208–210, 342
reliability
of data, 70–71, 157
defined, 443
descriptive research exemplar, 90
interrater, 105, 138
test-retest, 138
reliable data, 70
representativeness, erosion of, 81
research articles, reading, 25–36
overview, 25–26
approach to, 34–36
format of reports, 27–34
goals in reading, 26, 35

literature reviews, 86–88, 215
starting point, 26–27
research design
appropriateness of, 336–337
clinical protocol, evidence-based practice, 362
cohort research, 193–195, 206–207
cohort research exemplar, 206–207
correlational research, 122–123
correlational research exemplar, 126–127, 136
defined, 19–20, 443
descriptive research exemplar, 85, 88, 103
descriptive research reports, 103
experimental research exemplar, 147, 172–175
observational designs, 68, 217–218, 256
qualitative research exemplar, 47, 61
research evidence, 5, 443. *See also* evidence
research reports, 27–34. *See also specific types of research*
abstract, 27–28
discussion or conclusion, 33–34
format of, 27–34
integrative research reviews, 223–224
introduction, 28–31
methods, 31–32
references, 34
results/findings, 32–33
study purpose, 30–31
systematic *vs.* literature reviews, 215
theoretical frameworks, 28–30
title, 27–28
research-informed practice (RIP), 383–394
overview, 383–384
clinical decision support, 391
clinical information systems, 391
defined, 384, 443
evidence-based practice, 384–385, 392
information intersection, 385, 386–387
information services, 389–391
opportunities, 385–386
point-of-care design, 351, 383, 387–391
short format sources, 388–389
research-practice connection, 5–14
clinical protocols, 6–7
evidence-based practice, 11–14
findings, 5–6
results
borderline, 188
cohort research exemplar, 198, 201–203, 207–212
correlational research exemplar, 128–134, 139–142
defined, 443
in descriptive research, 83–84, 105–109
descriptive research exemplar, 85, 91–95, 105–109
erroneous, 82
as essential study element, 26–27
experimental research exemplar, 165–168, 188–192
influences on, 33–34, 74–75, 121–122
integrative research review exemplar, 226, 231–239, 249–250
interpreted. *See* findings
percentages to report, 83
qualitative research exemplar, 44, 50–57, 64
in research reports, 32–33
scores, 83–94
retrospective studies, 359. *See also* descriptive research
revisit and revise EBP projects, 366
rigor, 444
rigor of methods, 42, 338
RIP. *See* research-informed practice
risk factors
cohort research, 193
in cohort research, 206–207
RNAO. *See* Registered Nurses Association of Ontario
RR. *See* relative risk
RRT. *See* rapid response teams

S

safety, 316–317
sample
cohort research exemplar, 198, 207
defined, 444
descriptive research, 104
descriptive research exemplar, 88–89, 104
experimental research exemplar, 172–173
qualitative research exemplar, 63
sample size
adequacy of, 147, 149–150, 156
descriptive research, 81
qualitative research, 43
qualitative research exemplar, 47–48
range of, 27
reading research articles, 25
research report, 32
sampling
cohort research, 207
convenience sampling, 80
correlational research exemplar, 136–137

descriptive research, 75–82, 104
populations, 75–82, 316
random, 44, 77–79, 107, 151, 443
scatter diagrams, 113
scatter plots, 119
scientific knowledge production, 444
scope
defined, 444
in integrative research reviews, 216–217
score continuum, 83
scores, 176
scoring directions, 138
Scottish Intercollegiate Guidelines Network (SIGN), 253, 261, 263, 275
seamless intersection of data, 385, 386–387
search
defined, 444
for evidence, 24, 293–309, 362
systematic *vs.* literature reviews, 215
selection, systematic *vs.* literature reviews, 215
setting, descriptive research exemplar, 88–89
SIGN. *See* Scottish Intercollegiate Guidelines Network
significance
clinical. *See* clinical significance
decision points for, 180–181
p-values, experimental research, 180–185
statistical, 180–185
simple random sample, 44, 77
single original study, evidence from, 15, 16–20
skewed distribution of scores, 83
skills building, EBP, 375, 380–381
social processes, 38
specialty nurses' associations databases, 297–298
SR. *See* systematic review
stakeholders, clinical practice guidelines development, 253–254
standards of care, 7, 357–358
state-of-the-science summaries. *See* integrative research reviews (IRR)
statistical significance, 444
statistically significant results, 140
statistics
analysis of, 176
in cohort research, 201
experimental research, 179–187
inferential, 179
meta-analysis of findings, 214
odds ratio, 211–212
statistical significance, 180–185, 444
stratified random sampling, 78, 79
strength-of-evidence recommendation grading, 256, 257–258
stroke descriptive study, 68
strong relationships, 112
structured observation, 103
studies. *See also* specific types of research
hypothetical, 113
methods overview, 17–20
original. *See* original studies
searching for, 218–219
study plan, 20, 444
Subheadings feature, 305–306
subject heading searches, 299, 302
subjectivity of psychosocial variables, 73
SurveyMonkey, 82
surveys in descriptive research, 82
switching between databases, 308–309
synopsis
appraising guide, 323, 395, 399–400, 405, 409–410, 415, 419, 423–424
clinical practice guidelines, appraising, 323
evidence, appraisal of, 313
integrative research reviews (IRRs), 330
synthesis from integrative research reviews, 219–223
systematic review (SR), 213–250. *See also* integrative research reviews (IRR)
abstract of, 21
appraising conclusions, 329
bipolar disorder medication IRR exemplar, 224–250
conclusions of, 21
credibility linked to evidence, 324
defined, 20, 444
in E-B protocols, 23
evidence from, 16, 20–21
evidence grading, 256
join an EBP project team, 376
literature reviews *vs.*, 215
process of, 21
production steps, 216
rapid response teams, 213
searching for, 293–294
short format sources, 388–389
sources of, 293–298
strength of evidence, clinical practice guidelines, 254
types of, 214–215

T

table of contents, EbCPG exemplar, 263–265
tables, in research report, 33
tag-flag-nag approach, 364

tangibility of psychosocial variables, 73
target populations
  defined, 444
  descriptive research, 75–82
  in descriptive research, 104
  experimental research, 147, 148–149, 156
  in research reports, 32
targeted adopters, evidence-based practice projects, 364–365
team, evidence-based practice projects, 375–376
test intervention. *See* interventions
test-retest reliability, 138, 445
text word searching, 300
themes in data coding, 42
theoretical frameworks in research report, 28–30
theory, 28, 445
theory of community empowerment, as example, 28–29
third-party payers as research driver, 293
titles
  cohort research exemplar, 198
  correlational research exemplar, 124
  descriptive research exemplar, 84
  experimental research exemplar, 159
  integrative research review exemplar, 225
  qualitative research exemplar, 44
  research reports, 27–28
topic, EbCPG exemplar, 274
total knee replacement (TKR) exemplar, 43–64
  profile and commentary, 61–64
translational research, 12, 445
treatment effect measures, 445
treatments. *See also* interventions
  clinical protocols, 6
  comparative effectiveness, 178, 179, 189–190
  defined, 445
  descriptive research exemplar, 90–91
triggers for questions, 285–287
TRIP database, 383–384, 388–389
t-tests, 108–109, 179–180
type 1 conclusion error, 339–341, 445
type 2 conclusion error, 339–341, 445

U

U.K. National Health Service, 296
underpowered studies, 150
understanding, as qualitative research goal, 17
University of Iowa Hospitals and Clinics, 380
University of Oklahoma College of Nursing, 380
University of Pennsylvania, 381
U.S. Copyright Law, 299

V

valid, as term, 342
valid finding, 445
valid measures, 70
validity
  in case-control studies, 195–197
  correlational research, 122
  credibility *vs.*, 341–342
  of data, 71–73, 157
  descriptive research exemplar, 90
  instrument validity, 440
  of variables, 71–72, 73
variables
  cause-and-effect relationship, 119
  comparison statistics on, 151
  correlational research, 139–140
  data quality, 70
  defined, 18, 445
  in descriptive research, 68–75
  extraneous. *See* extraneous variables
  independent. *See* interventions
  measurement of, 69–74, 157
  psychosocial, 73–74
  reliability, 70–71, 73
  validity, 71–72, 73

W

weak relationships, 112
work flow in care delivery systems, 358–360
work-group formation, EBP projects, 361–362
work-setting dynamics, EBP projects, 365